Perinatal Growth
and Nutrition

Perinatal Growth and Nutrition

Edited by **Ian J. Griffin**

University of California-Davis Children's Hospital
Sacramento, California, USA

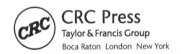

CRC Press
Taylor & Francis Group
Boca Raton London New York

CRC Press is an imprint of the
Taylor & Francis Group, an **informa** business

CRC Press
Taylor & Francis Group
6000 Broken Sound Parkway NW, Suite 300
Boca Raton, FL 33487-2742

First issued in paperback 2017

© 2014 by Taylor & Francis Group, LLC
CRC Press is an imprint of Taylor & Francis Group, an Informa business

No claim to original U.S. Government works

ISBN-13: 978-1-4665-5853-3 (hbk)
ISBN-13: 978-1-138-03368-9 (pbk)

Library of Congress Cataloging-in-Publication Data

Perinatal growth and nutrition / editor, Ian J. Griffin.
   p. ; cm.
   Includes bibliographical references and index.
   ISBN 978-1-4665-5853-3 (hardback : alk. paper)
   I. Griffin, Ian J., editor of compilation.
   [DNLM: 1. Infant Nutritional Physiological Phenomena. 2. Infant,
Premature--growth & development. 3. Fetal Development. 4. Infant, Newborn--growth
& development. 5. Metabolic Diseases--etiology. 6. Nutritional Requirements. WS 120]

RJ216
618.92'01--dc23

2014001362

Visit the Taylor & Francis Web site at
http://www.taylorandfrancis.com

and the CRC Press Web site at
http://www.crcpress.com

To my Mum and Dad for their love and encouragement;
to Deborah for her love and support; and
to my teachers for their patience.

Contents

SECTION I Causes and Assessment of Ex Utero Growth Restriction in Preterm Infants

SECTION II The Effects of In Utero and Ex Utero Growth in Term and Preterm Infants

SECTION III Can We Be Better? Reducing Ex Utero Growth Restriction in Preterm Infants

Preface

Humans, like all mammals, have an inborn desire to nurture and suckle their young and the act of feeding is important for the bonding between mother and child. The birth of a critically ill preterm infant disrupts this, but for a mother, the use of her milk to feed her infant may be the most tangible role she has in the medical care of her critically sick child. Parents and caregivers see growth and feeding as important milestones first demonstrating increasing stability, then signaling the start of recovery, and finally showing readiness for discharge home.

Despite our intuitive and emotional connection with growth, preterm infants grow poorly after birth and very commonly develop *ex utero* growth restriction (EUGR) or postnatal growth failure. There are many reasons for this including the associated medical conditions of prematurity, but inadequate nutrient intake plays a large part. This results both from technical difficulties in providing adequate nutrition, and from fears about the complications associated with doing so, including metabolic derangements such as hyperglycemia and hyperlipidemia, and diseases such as necrotizing enterocolitis.

At the time of hospital discharge, many preterm infants are profoundly growth retarded, and their average weight is as little as 70% of that expected for their peers who were not born prematurely. Preterm infants show variable amounts of catch-up growth after discharge, but typically remain smaller than the term-born peers throughout childhood and adolescence.

This pattern of early growth restriction followed by variable amounts of catch-up growth has drawn parallels with the *in utero* growth-restricted (IUGR), small-for-gestational-age, infant. The IUGR infant is at increased risk of long-term metabolic complications, such as insulin resistance, type 2 diabetes, and hypertension, and the risks are worsened by rapid postnatal catch-up growth. This has led to the belief that catch-up growth in the *preterm* infant is undesirable, and even that slower early (in-hospital) growth may be beneficial. This idea is seductive. It means that the goal that is so difficult to achieve (reducing EUGR or ensuring catch-up growth) is not actually in the newborn infant's best interest. The alternative, tolerating poor postnatal growth, is not only easier but is to be preferred. It is not surprising that such an idea is popular, but what is sometimes overlooked is the real evidence addressing the risks and benefits of different growth rates in preterm infants.

In this volume, we will discuss three main areas. We will begin by discussing the advances in growth standards for preterm infants, the diagnosis of EUGR, the causes of EUGR in preterm infants, and whether other assessments may assist in the evaluation of the nutritional adequacy of the diet we are feeding preterm infants.

We will next consider the extensive human literature examining the effect of IUGR, EUGR, and catch-up growth on long-term metabolic outcomes (including obesity, insulin resistance, type 2 diabetes, dyslipidemia, hypertension, and cardiac disease) and long-term neurodevelopmental outcomes (including cognition). We will assess the evidence for the effect of growth on these outcomes in term infants (either appropriate-, small-, or large-for-gestational-age) and in preterm infants. From this review, the risk–benefit balance between relatively slower and relatively more rapid growth in preterm infants is clear.

Finally, given the benefits of avoiding EUGR, we will consider how we might reduce the incidence of EUGR in preterm infants, and optimize catch-up growth if it does occur. To achieve this, we have two main choices to make: to concentrate on inputs (e.g., optimizing nutrient intakes) or concentrate on outputs (e.g., growth or other proxy markers); and to customize targets (and adjust them based on individual needs) or to generalize targets (and aim for similar nutrient intakes or similar growth rates in a broad group of infants). These are not mutually exclusive. For example, one may modify energy intake to reach a general goal for growth, or customize protein intake to achieve a general goal for blood urea nitrogen concentration. Optimizing nutrient intakes is especially difficult for the human-milk-fed intake due to the wide variability in the composition of human milk. We will review approaches to improving the nutritional management of preterm infants, both from enteral and parenteral sources, customizing human-milk fortification to account for differences in baseline composition, and assessing growth to more quickly identify growth faltering when it develops.

EUGR is common in preterm infants and has serious long-term adverse consequences. However, we must continue to try to prevent EUGR, and new tools and techniques may provide methods that can help us do better.

Additional Files

Additional files that allow the calculation of age- and gender-specific Z-scores for term and preterm infants, display the results graphically, and identify periods of growth faltering are available online at www.iangriffin.net.

About the Editor

Ian Griffin studied medicine at Leeds University, U.K., before training in pediatrics in Glasgow. He has been involved in research on the growth and nutrition of preterm infants since the 1990s, and was involved in a large study of post-discharge nutrition in Newcastle-upon-Tyne in the United Kingdom before moving to the United States. He was a member of the neonatal faculty at Baylor College of Medicine in Houston, Texas, before moving to the University of California–Davis in Sacramento, California, in 2008. His research interests include the growth and nutrition of newborn infants, and mineral requirements of preterm infants. He has spoken at meetings across the world, and is the author of over 80 peer-reviewed publications.

Contributors

Enrico Bertino
Neonatal Unit
University of Turin
AO Città della Salute e della Scienza
Turin, Italy

Richard J. Cooke
Department of Pediatrics
University of St. Louis
St. Louis, Missouri

Elizabeth A. Davis
School of Paediatrics and Child Health
University of Western Australia
Crawley, Western Australia, Australia

Paula Di Nicola
Neonatal Unit
University of Turin
AO Città della Salute e della Scienza
Turin, Italy

Magnus Domellöf
Department of Clinical Sciences
   (Pediatrics)
Umeå University
Umeå, Sweden

Nicholas D. Embleton
Newcastle Neonatal Service
Royal Victoria Infirmary
Newcastle-upon-Tyne, United Kingdom

Tanis Fenton
Alberta Children's Hospital Research
   Institute
University of Calgary
Calgary, Alberta, Canada

Giorgio Gilli
Neonatal Unit
University of Turin
AO Città della Salute e della Scienza
Turin, Italy

Frank R. Greer
Department of Pediatrics
University of Wisconsin School of
   Medicine and Public Health
Madison, Wisconsin

Ian J. Griffin
UC Davis Medical Center
University of California–Davis
Sacramento, California

Sharon Groh-Wargo
Department of Pediatrics
MetroHealth Medical Center
Case Western Reserve University
   School of Medicine
Cleveland, Ohio

Rae-Chi Huang
School of Paediatrics and Child Health
University of Western Australia
Crawley, Western Australia, Australia

Matthew J. Hyde
Institute of Health & Society
Newcastle University
Newcastle-upon-Tyne, United Kingdom

Jae H. Kim
Department of Pediatrics
Rady Children's Hospital
University of California–San Diego
San Diego, California

Luciana Occhi
Neonatal Unit
University of Turin
AO Città della Salute e della Scienza
Turin, Italy

Giovanna Prandi
Neonatal Unit
University of Turin
AO Città della Salute e della Scienza
Turin, Italy

Jennifer Scoble
UC Davis Medical Center
University of California–Davis
Sacramento, California

Dirk Wackernagel
Department of Clinical Sciences
  (Pediatrics)
Umeå University
Umeå, Sweden

Claire Wood
Section of Neonatal Medicine
Faculty of Medicine
Imperial College London
London, United Kingdom

Ekhard E. Ziegler
Department of Pediatrics
University of Iowa
Iowa City, Iowa

Section I

Causes and Assessment of Ex Utero Growth Restriction in Preterm Infants

INTRODUCTION

Preterm birth represents a profound and sudden divergence from the expected trajectory for growth and development. It is therefore difficult to consider what "normal" postnatal growth should be in such an abnormal condition. Aiming to match the growth of other infants in similar conditions lets us define normal growth in a statistical sense, but has no real physiological meaning.

Our current goals for growth are typically to match the *in utero* growth that might have occurred had the baby not been born prematurely. In recent years, there have been significant advances in the amount of data available to construct such growth references, and in the mathematical techniques used to do so (Chapter 1). These growth references allow us to examine how closely we meet these targets, and which babies are most at risk of poor growth (Chapter 3).

Growth is, however, a crude and imprecise assessment. Slow growth may result from a variety of causes including an inadequate protein intake, inadequate energy intake, electrolyte imbalances, etc. Conversely, just because body size and weight gain are within the normal range, does not mean that the composition of weight gain is either normal or appropriate. Nor should it reassure us that the intake of all individual nutrients is adequate. For this reason, biochemical assessments are often used in addition to growth measures to assess nutritional adequacy in preterm infants (Chapter 2). There is now increasing interest in the use of metabolomic profiling to identify novel markers for nutritional adequacy in preterm infants (Chapter 2), although none are ready for clinical use at present.

1 Growth Charts for Preterm Infants and Related Tools for Growth Monitoring

Tanis R. Fenton

INTRODUCTION

Growth charts help health professionals provide size-appropriate care to preterm infants. Preterm infants are not mature enough to adequately communicate their nutritional needs as do older infants, so health professionals must determine each baby's individual needs. Without awareness of an infant's growth pattern, nutrition decisions are based on average estimated needs, which is not likely appropriate for all individuals.

For example, enteral energy requirements likely vary from 110 to 135 kcal/kg/day, in healthy preterm infants.[1] If an infant requires the upper end of the range, but is being fed at the lower end, the infant will not likely grow at a desirable rate, which would show its growth curve as flatter than desired.

Health professionals need to know three things about the growth chart they are using:

1. What type of growth reference it represents (fetal estimates, previous preterm infants, or term infants)
2. The strengths of that methodology
3. The limitations of the methodology

This chapter will review the history of growth chart development for preterm infants, outline the strengths and weakness of each type, discuss the use of additional tools (percentiles and z-scores), as well as provide some perspectives on the growth goals of preterm infants.

Growth charts also can provide a quick assessment of whether an infant's head and length are growing appropriately relative to the infant's weight gain. A check of head size against a growth reference could identify pathological head growth such as hydrocephalus. Evaluation of length assists assessment of whether the infant might be gaining too much weight for its length growth. Growth of very low birth weight infants has been observed to be a predictor of neurodevelopmental outcomes.[2–7] Low weight,[2–4,7] head,[5] and length[6] growth have all been associated with poorer development. Recognizing instances of faltering growth enables the health care team to institute changes that not only may improve growth outcomes but also may improve neurodevelopmental outcomes.

HISTORY OF GROWTH CHARTS FOR PRETERM INFANTS

GROWTH STANDARDS AND GROWTH REFERENCES

With the production of the World Health Organization's (WHO) recent growth charts based on their Multicentre Growth Reference Study, a growth standard now exists for term infants.[8] This new growth standard has been designed to represent "healthy children living under conditions likely to favor the achievement of their full genetic growth potential."[9]

These charts are growth *standards* that would describe "what growth should be." However, there is no growth standard for preterm infants. Thus, the growth charts available for use are all growth *references*. Growth references provide a comparison of growth with others who may have been representative of a population. Without the designation as a growth standard, growth references just provide a comparison, or reference, to another population. Thus, preterm growth charts, being growth references, describe "what growth is"[10] without a claim about health status.

Historically, three types of growth references have been used for preterm infants, and these have usually been referred to in the literature as postnatal, intrauterine, and fetal-infant growth charts. It is helpful to understand the development, advantages, and limitations of these growth charts to use them to their best advantage.

POSTNATAL GROWTH CHARTS

The first growth chart developed specifically to monitor the growth of low birth weight and preterm infants was published in 1948 by Dancis et al.[11] This chart was a postnatal or peer growth chart that extended to 50 days, and it demonstrated the actual growth pattern of low birth weight infants after birth. Postnatal growth charts display the initial weight loss experienced by the infants after birth, regain of birth weight, as well as the subsequent growth pattern.

The smallest babies represented in the Dancis chart had birth weights of approximately 750 g, although none of these small infants survived.[11] Despite still being used until recently,[12] this growth chart had limitations especially because the population represented likely differed from the infants in the NICU decades later.[13] For example, at the time this growth chart was developed, low birth weight infants who were likely to survive were likely near term but small for gestational age, since neonatal care in the 1940s could not support very preterm infants.

More recent postnatal growth charts for preterm infants have been developed including the large multicenter growth survey by the National Institute of Child Health and Human Development of infants born in 1994–1996[14] and the widely distributed survey by the Infant Health and Development Program of infants born in 1985.[15] These surveys were conducted prior to widespread use of early parenteral protein on the birth or first day of life. Postnatal growth charts are limited by the fact that the growth patterns displayed in these charts are influenced by the medical and nutritional care for the time and may not represent ideal growth of preterm infants at a future date. Recent reports suggest that present day very low birth weight infants do not lose as much weight after birth, and also regain their birth weight faster than they did in the past.[16, 17] Improved recent weight status may be due at least in part to earlier and better protein nutrition in the early weeks of life.[18–20]

An additional limitation to postnatal charts, beyond the fact that these charts reflect the care the infants received, is the limitation that these charts only illustrate the mean curves for each infant weight category. Postnatal charts do not show the distributions, the variation above and below the averages, so it is not possible to evaluate how well or poorly an infant is growing relative to the chart, or to calculate infant percentiles or z-scores.

INTRAUTERINE GROWTH CHARTS

Intrauterine growth charts, which are sometimes referred to as fetal or birth-size growth charts, are based on the size at birth of infants born at various gestational ages. These charts are considered to provide estimates of the size of the fetus at each week of gestation.

Perhaps the most well known of the intrauterine charts are those published by Lubchenco et al. in 1966,[21] sometimes referred to as the Denver charts. These charts are still used as a growth reference[22–24] and were recommended for the classification of size for gestational age as recently as 2010.[25] This may be in part because this chart was endorsed by the American Academy of Pediatrics for the assessment of intrauterine growth restriction in 1967.[26] A limitation of this chart is that the infants' gestational ages were classified prior to the routine assessment of gestational age, so their sample likely included infants with misclassified gestational ages.

Intrauterine growth charts have been criticized as not representative of fetal size because some growth-restricted infants may be preferentially delivered before term. The birth of growth-restricted infants might create a difference in the size from those who remain *in utero*. No solution to this problem has been found to date. Some have considered ultrasound measurements of healthy fetuses; however, this method may not be ideal because ultrasound estimates of weight and head circumference are determined from two-dimensional measurements.

Inaccuracies in assessments of gestational age in the earlier intrauterine studies of size at birth created bimodal or exaggerated S-shape curves due to misclassification of gestational age. For example, the 90th centile at 33 weeks of a large intrauterine study was 3536 g,[27] likely due to some term infants being considered preterm based on inaccurate maternal dates.[28] In contrast, others have estimated the 90th percentile at 33 weeks to be 2400[21] and 2600 g.[12] This bimodal shape is not representative of the growth patterns of infants. Additionally, the Lubchenco et al.[21] data were collected at a time when maternal weight gain restriction was encouraged for various obstetric goals[29, 30]. Restricted maternal weight gains have been associated with lower birth weights.[30, 31] For these reasons, older intrauterine growth charts are likely not representative of the growth pattern of more recent infants.

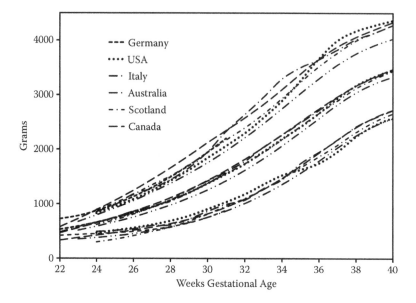

FIGURE 1.1 Girls' birth weight percentiles (3rd, 50th, and 97th) from six countries: Germany, Italy, United States, Scotland, Australia, and Canada.

More recent intrauterine-type growth charts for preterm infants are based on larger sample sizes—for example, the British charts based on 9443 infants[32] and several large (45,000 to 2,300,000 infants) intrauterine studies of birth weight from Germany,[33] Italy,[34] United States,[22] Scotland,[35] Australia,[36] and Canada[28] (Figure 1.1), and of birth length and head circumference from the United States[22] and Italy.[34] The birth weights of these six large studies[22, 32–36] show similar patterns and close agreement for the 50th and 3rd centiles. The 97th percentiles of these studies show some differences, with the lowest values for the Italian infants and the highest values for the Canadian (before 32 weeks gestation), Australian (between 32 and 35 weeks), and American (after 35 weeks) datasets.

FETAL INFANT GROWTH CHARTS

Fetal infant growth charts for preterm infants are based on two types of merged sets of reference data: data on the size of the fetus (estimates from intrauterine data) and the term infant (usually postnatal surveillance data of term infants). Typically, fetal infant growth charts include weight, head, and length parameters on one chart.

Currently, the growth goal for preterm infants is to approximate the growth patterns of the normal fetus and of the term-born infant. Fetal infant growth charts incorporate both of these growth references, with some degree of smoothing between the datasets. Therefore, fetal infant growth charts reflect the recommended growth goals for preterm infants: the fetus and the term infant. These charts demonstrate a distribution of sizes at the various ages, usually illustrated as major percentiles.

Gairdner and Pearson[37] and Babson and Benda[38] developed the first fetal infant growth charts in the 1970s. Babson and Benda referred to their chart as a "fetal infant growth chart." These early charts extended from 28 weeks gestational age to 2 years[37] or 26 weeks preterm to 1 year post-term.[38] With *x*-axes of these early charts beginning at 26 to 28 weeks of gestational age, younger gestational age preterm infants (i.e., 23 to 25 weeks gestational age) could not be plotted during their first weeks of life, a time of some of the greatest growth and assessment challenges for the neonatal health care team.

A more recent fetal infant growth chart was developed in 2003,[12] and recently revised in 2013.[39] This growth chart extended from 22 weeks to 50 weeks (10 weeks post-term) of post-menstrual age, to support growth monitoring through the transition to term growth charts.

The 2013 revision of the 2003 Fenton preterm growth chart was set equal to the WHO Growth Standard at 10 weeks post-term age (longitudinally measured). We defined the curves for younger than 40 weeks based on a systematic review and meta-analysis with strict inclusion criteria.[39] The 2013 version used the large recent intrauterine studies from Germany,[33] Italy,[34] United States,[22] Scotland,[35] and Canada[28] for the fetal estimates, which had a combined sample size of almost 4 million babies (Figure 1.2). This fetal infant growth chart is consistent with the fetal estimate data to 36–38 weeks, and thus can be used to assign newborn size for gestational age up to and including 36 weeks.

An advantage of fetal infant growth charts is that they provide an assessment of whether a preterm infant is achieving catch-up growth or if growth velocity may be

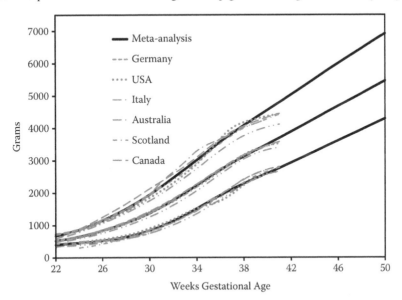

FIGURE 1.2 Comparison of the Fenton/Kim 2013 boys' meta-analysis percentiles (3rd, 50th, and 97th) (black solid) along with the six recent population-based birth-size studies' percentiles from developed countries: Germany, Italy, United States, Scotland, Australia, and Canada (grey dashed).

TABLE 1.1

Table of Strengths and Weaknesses of the Various Types of Preterm Growth Charts

Type	Strengths	Weaknesses
Postnatal/peer	Illustrates the growth pattern of preterm infants after birth, including weight loss after birth Longitudinal data	Growth patterns reflect the neonatal care received Inability to calculate percentiles and z-scores
Intrauterine/fetal, or birth-size	Usually based on large numbers Based on the size of infants at birth, estimated to reflect the size of the fetus Ability to calculate percentiles and z-scores	Cross-sectional data Gestational age errors lead to misclassification, which appears as an exaggerated S-shape Infants who are born may not be the same size as those who remain *in utero*
Fetal-infant	Combines intrauterine data on the size of infants at birth, estimates of the size of the fetus with a term growth chart to permit growth comparisons with the recommended growth reference: the fetus and the term infant Ability to calculate percentiles and z-scores The World Health Organization Growth Standard can be used for the infant estimates.	Cross-sectional data (for the fetal estimates) Gestational age errors lead to misclassification, which appears as an exaggerated S-shape Infants who are born may not be the same size as those who remain *in utero*

inadequate or excessive relative to the recommended growth references for preterm infants: the fetus[1, 40, 41] and then the term infant.[40, 41]

ACCURACY OF MEASUREMENTS

Growth assessments are only as accurate as the precision of the infant measurements. If inaccurate, the measurements will not provide a correct growth assessment, regardless of the choice of growth chart (Table 1.1). Typically, weight measurements are fairly accurate when calibrated electronic scales are used, and any equipment attached to the infant (ventilator tubes, arm or leg boards) are correctly accounted for.

Length is more difficult to measure accurately than is weight or head circumference.[42] Several infant length measurement techniques have been compared (including laying the infant on top of a tape measure, marking a paper laying under the infant, or using a head/foot board to ensure vertical barriers for the measurement) and all were found to have standard deviation errors of 0.6 to 1 cm,[43] while smaller errors were obtained by others using a limited number of trained measurers implementing a head and foot board.[44] To obtain the most accurate length measurements, experts recommend that whichever techniques are used, they be used consistently and that the length measurements should be interpreted with some caution.[45]

PERCENTILES AND Z-SCORES

Health practitioners find it useful to be able to define a child's size as a percentile or z-score. With size defined by these numerical values, one can determine whether the child is catching up or losing status relative to a growth reference. For example, an infant may have a percentile value of 40 (z-score = −0.25) at birth, decrease to the 11th percentile (z-score = −1.2) at one week of age, have a percentile value of 20 (z-score = −0.8) at discharge, and then gradually regain percentiles to be close to the birth percentile (35th percentile (z-score = −0.4)) by two months of corrected age.

Percentiles and z-scores are related but different measurement tools, and each has its uses. Z-scores define how far a measurement is above or below the median, expressed in standard deviation units. Percentiles define a child's position within a reference population, in numbers that range from 0 to 100.[10] Percentiles are most useful when the measurements fall between the 2nd and the 98th percentiles, and they become almost meaningless outside of this range (Table 1.2, Figure 1.3). In contrast, z-scores are still very useful when measurements are outside of this range. For example, a small-for-gestational-age infant who has a percentile value of 0.1 (z-score = −3) at birth, may have a percentile value of 2 (z-score = −2) at discharge. The z-score change from −3 to −2 shows a meaningful change while the percentile values at the extreme changed only from 0.1 to 2, which may be harder to interpret.

Z-scores and percentiles are derived from the distribution of the infants at each age from a growth reference. LMS parameters are used in the background to

TABLE 1.2

Comparison of Percentiles and the Equivalent Z-Scores

z-score	4	3	2	1	0	−1	−2	−3	−4
Percentile	99.99	99.9	97.7	84	50	16	2.3	0.1	0.01

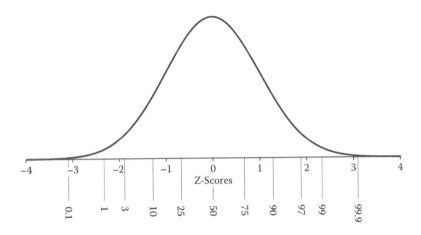

FIGURE 1.3 Percentiles (lower numbers) and z-scores (upper numbers) in relation to the normal distribution.

calculate percentiles or z-scores. The LMS parameters summarize the distribution at each age: L refers to any skew in the distribution, M refers to the mid-point or the median, and S summarizes the width of the distribution.[46] To date, only intrauterine and fetal-infant growth charts have LMS parameters summarized.

GROWTH VELOCITY ESTIMATES

Clinically it can be useful to add a calculation of growth velocity to a growth assessment. Although various calculations have been used, perhaps the most valid calculation uses the average weight from the time interval as the denominator.[19]

$$\frac{(\text{end weight} - \text{start weight}) / \text{average weight}}{\text{time interval}}$$

If an early weight is used as the denominator, for example,

$$\frac{(\text{end weight} - \text{start weight}) / \text{start weight}}{\text{time interval}}$$

as has been done in some studies,[47] growth rates are overestimated.[19] For example, if the early weight is used as the denominator, growth estimates can be as high as 22 to 24 g/kg/day, while when the average weight is used, the growth estimates were 15 to 16 g/kg/day.[19] This overestimate of 7 to 8 g/kg/day was due to the choice of denominator in the calculation. If growth over a longer time interval were estimated, the error would be magnified. It is important that any comparisons made between studies or infants use the same calculation method.

A recent study of growth velocity, based on a systematic review of size at birth studies, with strict inclusion criteria,[39] found that the estimated growth velocity (g/kg/day) of the fetus is not constant between 22 and 40 weeks.[17] The estimates of fetal growth velocity ranged from a high of approximately 18 g/kg/day between 24 and 30 weeks, to a low of about 5 g/kg/day at 38 to 39 weeks. Overall, a growth velocity rate of 15 g/kg/day, which is often quoted,[48–50] was found to be a reasonable growth rate for infants up to about 36 weeks.[17]

The historic target for weight gain of 15 g/kg/day should be considered a minimum goal and not a maximum. There is no firm evidence to support recommendations for a maximum desirable gain; the desirable growth rate for a given infant at a specific point in time will depend on his or her size for gestational age, weight loss after birth, time to regain birth weight, and current percentile or z-score. If an infant was small for his or her genetic potential at birth, had a larger than expected weight loss after birth (e.g., 15 to 20%), took an extended time to regain his or her birth weight, and had periods of suboptimal feeding for a variety of reasons, one might expect that this infant may achieve a higher growth velocity once receiving adequate nutrition than the infant born with an appropriate birth percentile size, had less weight loss (e.g., 5 to 10%),[20] and took to feedings well.

A few weeks after birth preterm infants have been noted to place low in weight percentiles relative to fetal estimates,[13, 14, 51, 52] due to postbirth weight loss. If the time to regain their birth weight is lengthy, their weight percentiles are further reduced relative to the reference fetus. However, if this weight loss and the time to regain birth weight can be minimized[16, 17] due to earlier and better nutrition in the first days and weeks of life,[18–20] the need for catch-up growth will be dramatically reduced.

Some cautions should be taken with the use of growth velocity calculations. These calculations of growth in g/kg/day should not be conducted on too short an interval, as daily weight fluctuations can obscure the longer-term growth trends and lead to micromanagement of the nutrition care. Ideally, calculations of growth velocity are part of a growth assessment that includes consideration of the infant's genetic potential, of which parental height is an imperfect but helpful guide,[53, 54] nutrition history, as well as the infant's placement and trajectory on a growth chart.

Over the years in an attempt to estimate the range of fetus growth rates, clinicians have calculated the growth velocity of intrauterine charts along the 3rd, 50th, and 97th percentiles. This method is problematic for several reasons, primarily because the data was cross-sectional, and thus it is not known whether infants actually grew following along the various percentiles. Ideally, growth velocity is calculated using longitudinally collected data, as was done by the WHO in preparation of their Growth Standard data for the first 2 years of life.[55] Second, it has been established that term infants often cross percentiles as they grow,[56, 57] presumably as they find their genetically determined growth trajectory, and preterm infants may do the same. Given these limitations, perhaps the most valid calculation of growth velocity is to estimate along the median (50th percentile), while noting that some variation is always present in biological systems.

GROWTH-RESTRICTED INFANTS

Beginning in the first days of life, growth-restricted infants tend to follow a slightly different growth pattern compared to appropriately grown infants. Since growth restriction is defined as size smaller than the 10th percentile, this category includes normally small infants as well as infants with a pathological reason for their small size. The etiology of their small size will determine subsequent growth potential. Small size at birth can be due to genetically small size, maternal origins (such as preeclampsia, malnutrition, and exposure to drugs, tobacco, or alcohol), placental and cord origins, and infant origins (congenital conditions). If an infant's small size does not originate with the infant, growth-restricted infants have a potential to lose less weight relative to their larger cohorts, and then their subsequent growth is often faster.[13, 14, 20] Some small-for-gestational-age infants grow rapidly and achieve weights much higher than their birth percentiles.[58] Adult-onset diseases have been associated with small infants growing faster;[13] however, a superior or ideal pattern of growth has not been defined for these infants.[59–61]

BALANCING THE RISKS—NEURODEVELOPMENT AND CARDIOVASCULAR RISKS

Slow growth of preterm infants has been associated with poorer neurodevelopmental status[2-7] (see Chapter 8), and rapid growth of infants born small for gestational age has been associated with higher risk of metabolic syndrome[62] (see Chapters 3 and 8). It is biologically plausible that for optimal brain growth, infant growth should not be interrupted in the phase of very rapid brain growth. Of importance, not all studies have supported that the association between rapid infant growth and higher risk of metabolic syndrome is of importance as the development of adult obesity may have a greater impact.[63] Further, for infants born small for their genetic potential, perhaps the most important part of the insult may be the growth restriction, which in the case of intrauterine growth restriction has already taken place prior to admission to the neonatal unit.

What should health practitioners do to balance the risks between neurodevelopment and metabolic syndrome in later life? Perhaps the optimum balance between these risks is to find the middle ground, to minimize postnatal weight loss through nutrition support on the infant's birthday, followed by optimal nutrition to support growth throughout the neonatal period. Ziegler advocates for aggressive nutrition support,[64] designed to meet the estimated nutritional needs of the infants. While Ziegler refers to these guidelines as aggressive, they are actually *adequate* nutrition support. Adequate nutrition support has been shown to reduce or prevent extra uterine growth restriction.[18, 19] Of importance, more involvement of dietitians in neonatal units is associated with superior nutrition support.[65]

APPROPRIATE GROWTH GOALS

Parents have difficulties understanding growth charts and some parents wish their children to have high percentiles.[66, 67] Perhaps this desire for high percentiles is a wish for high "marks" for their child or perhaps it is a reassurance that they are doing well at nourishing their child, a primary parental responsibility.[68] In spite of wishes for large children, it is normal for sizes in a population to range between the first and ninety-ninth percentiles.

Experts on child feeding recommend that a child's eating be guided by their hunger and satiety, and not by artificial guides of finishing a portion of food.[69] For the first months of life, preterm infants are unable to adequately express their hunger and satiety, and are schedule fed. Prior to discharge, parents need to be instructed to focus on hunger and satiety cues, so they can learn the division of feeding responsibilities. Satter recommends a division of feeding responsibilities: the role of parents is to supply nutritious food, while a child's responsibility is to decide how much to eat or whether to eat at all.[69]

Appropriate growth goals need to be set for preterm infants, to help the transition from the high focus on the need to aggressively nourish newborn preterm infants in the first weeks of life to prepare for discharge under the parents care, keeping in mind parents' desires for high percentiles. Nutrition post-discharge should be provided as cue-based feeding; that is, the amount taken should be decided by the infant. Growth goals should generally aim for size within the growth chart distribution range, perhaps in some cases to return to an infant's birth percentiles, with appropriate weight-for-height, while considering whether the infant is genetically small or growth restricted. Although nutrition and medical care has changed and what is achievable may have changed over time, in the past not all small-for-gestational-age infants were able to fully "catch up" in height.[70, 71] Thus, if full catch-up is not achievable, catch-up should not be set as the goal because pushing calories may only increase weight and body fat.

IMPORTANCE OF EARLY NUTRITION TO SUPPORT GROWTH

Adequate early protein and energy nutrition are required to support infant growth.[18–20] There is also observational evidence of an association between linear growth and adequate bone mineralization,[72, 73] thus suggesting that adequate calcium and phosphorus are also important to enable preterm infants to achieve their growth genetic potential.

In conclusion, growth charts are useful tools for nutrition and growth assessments of preterm infants. Health practitioners have several preterm growth charts to choose from, and each has strengths and weaknesses. Knowing the strengths and weakness of the growth charts can help health practitioners make the most accurate assessments of infant size and growth, and then set appropriate growth goals and appropriate provision of nutrition for the individual infant. Size and growth assessments can be by a visual analysis of the growth trajectories, or by using a detailed comparison of percentiles, z-scores, and possibly an assessment of growth velocity.

REFERENCES

1. Agostoni C, Buonocore G, Carnielli VP, De CM, Darmaun D, Decsi T, et al.: Enteral nutrient supply for preterm infants. A comment of the ESPGHAN Committee on Nutrition.
2. Franz AR, Pohlandt F, Bode H, Mihatsch WA, Sander S, Kron M, Steinmacher J: Intrauterine, early neonatal, and postdischarge growth and neurodevelopmental outcome at 5.4 years in extremely preterm infants after intensive neonatal nutritional support. *Pediatrics* 2009, 123: e101–e109.
3. Belfort MB, Rifas-Shiman SL, Sullivan T, Collins CT, McPhee AJ, Ryan P, Kleinman KP, Gillman MW, Gibson RA, Makrides M: Infant growth before and after term: effects on neurodevelopment in preterm infants. *Pediatrics* 2011, 128: e899–e906.
4. Ehrenkranz RA, Dusick AM, Vohr BR, Wright LL, Wrage LA, Poole WK: Growth in the neonatal intensive care unit influences neurodevelopmental and growth outcomes of extremely low birth weight infants. *Pediatrics* 2006, 117: 1253–1261.
5. Georgieff MK, Hoffman JS, Pereira GR, Bernbaum J, Hoffman-Williamson M: Effect of neonatal caloric deprivation on head growth and 1-year developmental status in preterm infants. *J Pediatr* 1985, 107: 581–587.
6. Ramel SE, Demerath EW, Gray HL, Younge N, Boys C, Georgieff MK: The relationship of poor linear growth velocity with neonatal illness and two-year neurodevelopment in preterm infants. *Neonatology* 2012, 102: 19–24.
7. Powers GC, Ramamurthy R, Schoolfield J, Matula K: Postdischarge growth and development in a predominantly Hispanic, very low birth weight population. *Pediatrics* 2008, 122: 1258–1265.

8. de Onis M., Onyango AW, Borghi E, Garza C, Yang H: Comparison of the World Health Organization (WHO) Child Growth Standards and the National Center for Health Statistics/WHO international growth reference: implications for child health programmes. *Public Health Nutr* 2006, 9: 942–947.

9. World Health Organization: WHO Child Growth Standards: Head Circumference-for-age, Arm Circumference-for-age, Triceps Skinfold-for-age and Subscapular Skinfold-for-age. Methods and development. 2007.

10. Dietitians of Canada, Canadian Pediatric Society, College of Family Physicians of Canada, Community Health Nurses of Canada: Promoting optimal monitoring of child growth in Canada: using the new WHO growth charts. *Can J Diet Pract Res* 2010, 71: 1–22.

11. Dancis J, O'Connell JR, Holt LE, Jr.: A grid for recording the weight of premature infants. *J Pediatr* 1948, 33: 570–572.

12. Fenton TR: A new growth chart for preterm babies: Babson and Benda's chart updated with recent data and a new format. *BMC Pediatr* 2003, 3: 13.

13. Fenton TR, McMillan DD, Sauve RS: Nutrition and growth analysis of very low birth weight infants. *Pediatrics* 1990, 86: 378–383.

14. Ehrenkranz RA, Younes N, Lemons JA, Fanaroff AA, Donovan EF, Wright LL, Katsikiotis V, Tyson JE, Oh W, Shankaran S, Bauer CR, Korones SB, Stoll BJ, Stevenson DK, Papile LA: Longitudinal growth of hospitalized very low birth weight infants. *Pediatrics* 1999, 104: 280–289.

15. Guo SS, Roche AF, Chumlea WC, Casey PH, Moore WM: Growth in weight, recumbent length, and head circumference for preterm low-birthweight infants during the first three years of life using gestation-adjusted ages. *Early Hum Dev* 1997, 47: 305–325.

16. Christensen RD, Henry E, Kiehn TI, Street JL: Pattern of daily weights among low birth weight neonates in the neonatal intensive care unit: data from a multihospital health-care system. *J Perinatol* 2006, 26: 37–43.

17. Fenton TR, Nasser R, Eliasziw M, Kim JH, Bilan D, Sauve R: Validating the weight gain of preterm infants between the reference growth curve of the fetus and the term infant. *BMC Pediatr.* 2013;13(1):92. http://www.biomedcentral.com/1471-2431/13/92

18. Valentine CJ, Fernandez S, Rogers LK, Gulati P, Hayes J, Lore P, Puthoff T, Dumm M, Jones A, Collins K, Curtiss J, Hutson K, Clark K, Welty SE: Early amino-acid administration improves preterm infant weight. *J Perinatol* 2009.

19. Senterre T, Rigo J: Reduction in postnatal cumulative nutritional deficit and improvement of growth in extremely preterm infants. *Acta Paediatr* 2012, 101: e64–e70.

20. Senterre T, Rigo J: Optimizing early nutritional support based on recent recommendations in VLBW infants and postnatal growth restriction. *J Pediatr Gastroenterol Nutr* 2011, 53: 536–542.

21. Lubchenco LO, Hansman C, Boyd E: Intrauterine growth in length and head circumference as estimated from live births at gestational ages from 26 to 42 weeks. *Pediatrics* 1966, 37: 403–408.

22. Olsen IE, Groveman SA, Lawson ML, Clark RH, Zemel BS: New intrauterine growth curves based on United States data. *Pediatrics* 2010, 125: e214–e224.

23. Giancotti A, Spagnuolo A, D'ambrosio V, Pasquali G, Muto B, De GF: Pregnancy in lupus patients: our experience. *Minerva Ginecol* 2010, 62: 551–558.

24. Fidanci K, Meral C, Suleymanoglu S, Pirgon O, Karademir F, Aydinoz S, Ozkaya H, Gultepe M, Gocmen I: Ghrelin levels and postnatal growth in healthy infants 0–3 months of age. *J Clin Res Pediatr Endocrinol* 2010, 2: 34–38.

25. Carney LN, Blair J: Assessment of nutrition status by age and determining nutrient needs. In *The A.S.P.E.N. Pediatric Nutrition Support Core Curriculum.* Corkins MR, Ed. Silver Springs, MD: The American Society of Parenteral and Enteral Nutrition; 2010: 409–432.

26. American Academy of Pediatrics. Committee on fetus and newborn. Nomenclature for duration of gestation, birth weight and intra-uterine growth. *Pediatrics* 1967, 39: 935–939.

27. Alexander GR, Himes JH, Kaufman RB, Mor J, Kogan M: A United States national reference for fetal growth. *Obstet Gynecol* 1996, 87: 163–168.

28. Kramer MS, Platt RW, Wen SW, Joseph KS, Allen A, Abrahamowicz M, Blondel B, Breart G: A new and improved population-based Canadian reference for birth weight for gestational age. *Pediatrics* 2001, 108: E35.

29. Pomerance J, Johnson R, Kagal S, Brooks P, Margolin M, Allen A: Attitudes toward weight gain in pregnancy. *West J Med* 1980, 133: 289–291.

30. Simpson JW, Lawless RW, Mitchell AC: Responsibility of the obstetrician to the fetus. II. Influence of prepregnancy weight and pregnancy weight gain on birthweight. *Obstet Gynecol* 1975, 45: 481–487.

31. Miller HC, Hassanein K, Chin TD, Hensleigh P: Socioeconomic factors in relation to fetal growth in white infants. *J Pediatr* 1976, 89: 638–643.

32. Cole TJ, Williams AF, Wright CM: Revised birth centiles for weight, length and head circumference in the UK-WHO growth charts. *Ann Hum Biol* 2011, 38: 7–11.

33. Voigt M, Zels K, Guthmann F, Hesse V, Gorlich Y, Straube S: Somatic classification of neonates based on birth weight, length, and head circumference: quantification of the effects of maternal BMI and smoking. *J Perinat Med* 2011, 39: 291–297.

34. Bertino E, Spada E, Occhi L, Coscia A, Giuliani F, Gagliardi L, Gilli G, Bona G, Fabris C, De CM, Milani S: Neonatal anthropometric charts: the Italian neonatal study compared with other European studies. *J Pediatr Gastroenterol Nutr* 2010, 51: 353–361.

35. Bonellie S, Chalmers J, Gray R, Greer I, Jarvis S, Williams C: Centile charts for birth-weight for gestational age for Scottish singleton births. *BMC Pregnancy Childbirth* 2008, 8: 5.

36. Roberts CL, Lancaster PA: National birthweight percentiles by gestational age for twins born in Australia. *J Paediatr Child Health* 1999, 35: 278–282.

37. Gairdner D, Pearson J: A growth chart for premature and other infants. *Arch Dis Child* 1971, 46: 783–787.

38. Babson SG, Benda GI: Growth graphs for the clinical assessment of infants of varying gestational age. *J Pediatr* 1976, 89: 814–820.

39. Fenton TR, Kim JH: A systematic review and meta-analysis to revise the Fenton growth chart for preterm infants. *BMC Pediatr.* 2013;13:59. http://www.biomedcentral.com/1471-2431/13/59

40. Committee on Nutrition American Academy Pediatrics: Nutritional needs of preterm infants. In *Pediatric Nutrition Handbook*, 6th ed. Elk Grove Village, IL: 2009.

41. Nutrition Committee Canadian Paediatric Society: Nutrient needs and feeding of premature infants. *CMAJ* 1995, 152: 1765–1785.

42. Johnson TS, Engstrom JL, Gelhar DK: Intra- and interexaminer reliability of anthropometric measurements of term infants. *J Pediatr Gastroenterol Nutr* 1997, 24: 497–505.

43. Johnson TS, Engstrom JL, Warda JA, Kabat M, Peters B: Reliability of length measurements in full-term neonates. *J Obstet Gynecol Neonatal Nurs* 1998, 27: 270–276.

44. Doull IJ, McCaughey ES, Bailey BJ, Betts PR: Reliability of infant length measurement. *Arch Dis Child* 1995, 72: 520–521.

45. Johnson TS, Engstrom JL, Haney SL, Mulcrone SL: Reliability of three length measurement techniques in term infants. *Pediatr Nurs* 1999, 25: 13–17.

46. Cole TJ: Using the LMS method to measure skewness in the NCHS and Dutch national height standards. *Ann Hum Biol* 1989, 16: 407–419.

47. Martin CR, Brown YF, Ehrenkranz RA, O'Shea TM, Allred EN, Belfort MB, McCormick MC, Leviton A: Nutritional practices and growth velocity in the first month of life in extremely premature infants. *Pediatrics* 2009, 124: 649–657.

48. Anderson DM: Nutritional assessment and therapeutic interventions for the preterm infant. *Clin Perinatol* 2002, 29: 313–326.

49. Griffin IJ: Nutritional assessment in preterm infants. *Nestle Nutr Workshop Ser Pediatr Program* 2007, 59: 177–188.

50. Klein CJ: Nutrient requirements for preterm infant formulas. *J Nutr* 2002, 132: 1395S–1577S.

51. Lubchenco LO, Hansman C, Dressler M, Boyd E: Intrauterine growth as estimated from liveborn birth-weight data at 24 to 42 weeks of gestation. *Pediatrics* 1963, 32: 793–800.

52. Bertino E, Coscia A, Mombro M, Boni L, Rossetti G, Fabris C, Spada E, Milani S: Postnatal weight increase and growth velocity of very low birthweight infants. *Arch Dis Child Fetal Neonatal Ed* 2006, 91: F349–F356.

53. Cole TJ, Wright CM: A chart to predict adult height from a child's current height. *Ann Hum Biol* 2011, 38: 662–668.

54. Galobardes B, McCormack VA, McCarron P, Howe LD, Lynch J, Lawlor DA, Smith GD: Social inequalities in height: persisting differences today depend upon height of the parents. *PLoS One* 2012, 7: e29118.

55. World Health Organization: The WHO Child Growth Standards, http://www.who.int/childgrowth/standards/en/.

56. Mei Z, Grummer-Strawn LM, Thompson D, Dietz WH: Shifts in percentiles of growth during early childhood: analysis of longitudinal data from the California Child Health and Development Study. *Pediatrics* 2004, 113: e617–e627.

57. Olsen EM, Petersen J, Skovgaard AM, Weile B, Jorgensen T, Wright CM: Failure to thrive: the prevalence and concurrence of anthropometric criteria in a general infant population. *Arch Dis Child* 2007, 92: 109–114.

58. Bo S, Bertino E, Bagna R, Trapani A, Gambino R, Martano C, Mombro' M, Pagano G: Insulin resistance in pre-school very-low-birth weight pre-term children. *Diabetes Metab* 2006, 32: 151–158.

59. Clayton PE, Cianfarani S, Czernichow P, Johannsson G, Rapaport R, Rogol A: Management of the child born small for gestational age through to adulthood: a consensus statement of the International Societies of Pediatric Endocrinology and the Growth Hormone Research Society. *J Clin Endocrinol Metab* 2007, 92: 804–810.

60. Fisher D, Baird J, Payne L, Lucas P, Kleijnen J, Roberts H, Law C: Are infant size and growth related to burden of disease in adulthood? A systematic review of literature. *Int J Epidemiol* 2006, 35: 1196–1210.

61. Jain V, Singhal A: Catch up growth in low birth weight infants: striking a healthy balance. *Rev Endocr Metab Disord* 2012, 13: 141–147.

62. Lucas A: Programming by early nutrition: an experimental approach. *J Nutr* 1998, 128: 401S–406S.

63. Finken MJ, Keijzer-Veen MG, Dekker FW, Frolich M, Hille ET, Romijn JA, Wit JM: Preterm birth and later insulin resistance: effects of birth weight and postnatal growth in a population based longitudinal study from birth into adult life. *Diabetologia* 2006, 49: 478–485.

64. Ziegler EE: Meeting the nutritional needs of the low-birth-weight infant. *Ann Nutr Metab* 2011, 58 Suppl 1: 8–18.

65. Olsen IE, Richardson DK, Schmid CH, Ausman LM, Dwyer JT: Dietitian involvement in the neonatal intensive care unit: more is better. *J Am Diet Assoc* 2005, 105: 1224–1230.

66. Sullivan SA, Leite KR, Shaffer ML, Birch LL, Paul IM: Urban parents' perceptions of healthy infant growth. *Clin Pediatr (Phila)* 2011, 50: 698–703.

67. Ben-Joseph EP, Dowshen SA, Izenberg N: Do parents understand growth charts? A national, Internet-based survey. *Pediatrics* 2009, 124: 1100–1109.
68. Jain A: Where all the children are above average. *Pediatrics* 2009, 124: e803–e804.
69. Satter E: Eating competence: definition and evidence for the Satter Eating Competence model. *J Nutr Educ Behav* 2007, 39: S142–S153.
70. Hack M, Schluchter M, Cartar L, Rahman M, Cuttler L, Borawski E: Growth of very low birth weight infants to age 20 years. *Pediatrics* 2003, 112: e30–e38.
71. Carrascosa A, Vicens-Calvet E, Yeste D, Espadero RM, Ulied A: Children born small for gestational age (SGA) who fail to achieve catch up growth by 2–8 years of age are short from infancy to adulthood. Data from a cross-sectional study of 486 Spanish children. *Pediatr Endocrinol Rev* 2006, 4: 15–27.
72. Fewtrell MS, Cole TJ, Bishop NJ, Lucas A: Neonatal factors predicting childhood height in preterm infants: evidence for a persisting effect of early metabolic bone disease? *J Pediatr* 2000, 137: 668–673.
73. Lucas A, Brooke OG, Baker BA, Bishop N, Morley R: High alkaline phosphatase activity and growth in preterm neonates. *Arch Dis Child* 1989, 64: 902–909.

2 Assessment of Short- and Medium-Term Outcomes in Preterm Infants

Nicholas D. Embleton, Matthew J. Hyde, and Claire Wood

INTRODUCTION

Survival rates for preterm infants have increased dramatically in the last few years, and in most developed countries. Infants born at 24 weeks gestation have a greater than 50% chance of survival. This has led to a greater focus on long-term outcomes and the need to assess how early nutritional interventions can optimize them.

The ultimate goal of care is to enhance survival both in quantitative and qualitative terms. This includes optimizing growth, cardio-metabolic and neuro-cognitive phenotypes in later life, and maximizing long-term Health-Related Quality of Life (HRQoL).

Nutrition is a key to improving health status and should be seen as the bedrock on which good neonatal care can be delivered. Auxological measures are the most commonly measured nutritionally related outcomes in neonatal care. However, their relationship to longer-term outcomes remains to be determined. In addition, a range of other short- and medium-term outcomes and biomarkers deserve consideration when assessing the effects of nutritional exposures.

Nutritional interventions are complex and assessing their effects is not straightforward. Although most high-quality nutritional trials now use a pharmacological approach, for example, randomization to either high or low intakes, nutrients do not function in isolation. For example, additional protein may only be functionally available if sufficient additional energy is available for lean tissue accretion. Nutrition is undoubtedly a complex intervention, so any assessment of short- and medium-term outcomes requires an appreciation of confounding, interacting, and modulating influences. It is likely that responses to nutritional interventions will differ between populations, so an intervention that appears beneficial in one setting might not be associated with similar effects elsewhere.

HOW DOES NUTRITION MODULATE OUTCOMES IN PRETERM INFANTS?

There is likely to be a range of mechanisms linking nutrition to later outcomes. These include:

1. Structural effects whereby inadequate nutritional substrate may result in decreased cell number, for example, nephrons or pancreatic beta cells, that lead to an increased risk of renal disease or decreased insulin sensitivity.
2. Programming effects that include epigenetic or hormonal mechanisms.
3. Altered cellular aging such as effects on telomere length.

Preterm infants may be affected by several of these processes, which themselves are likely to interact and overlap. It is now increasingly apparent that short-term measures of "nutritional adequacy," such as a weight gain trajectory that follows a percentile line on a growth reference, are insufficient on their own to predict or optimize longer-term outcomes.[1] Nutritional status might be difficult to precisely define, but it is the combination of nutritional and other past history (e.g., prematurity, previous growth, etc.), ongoing demands (e.g., illness, recovery from chronic lung disease, etc.), and current nutrient intakes (e.g., parenteral nutrition, breast milk fortification, etc.). Nutritional status is a more complex concept than dietary intake alone.

CHOICE OF OUTCOMES FOR ASSESSMENT

There is a potentially inexhaustible list of assessments that might be worthy of consideration in both the short and longer term. In this chapter, we will focus on short-term assessments, defined as parameters (both exposures and outcomes) that are measured prior to routine hospital discharge, and medium-term outcomes that can be assessed in infancy and early childhood and are used as clinical or research assessments (Table 2.1). It is important to consider whether outcomes are functional, and whether they are likely to have an impact on HRQoL. For example, neuro-cognitive functioning is of considerable relevance to health, and economic and social status, whereas being of any specific weight or height may not be of such functional relevance, unless the measures are well outside the normal range.

TABLE 2.1

Examples of Short- and Medium-Term Outcomes Affected by Nutritional Status

Measures	Examples
Auxological	Length, weight, OFC, skin-folds
Biochemical	Electrolytes, serum proteins, plasma amino acids
Body composition	Bone mineral density, fat and lean mass, fat mass index
Neurological function	Developmental status, visual evoked potentials
Novel biomarkers	Metabonomics, proteomics and DNA methylation

---

WHY ASSESS NUTRITIONAL OUTCOMES?

Clinicians can only determine optimal nutritional management if the outcomes are clearly defined. Health practitioners are trained to assess growth, and the longer-term relevance and interpretation of this is rarely questioned. However, the long-term relevance of short-term growth outcomes is open to interpretation.

In the past, it was universally assumed that higher rates of growth were "good" and that these inevitably led to better health outcomes.[2] In most societies, bigger and typically fatter babies are considered to be healthier, and feeding regimes seemed to encourage growth promotion. This view was compounded by the use of growth charts based on references of both breast- and formula-fed babies. Breast-fed babies gain weight more slowly perhaps leading practitioners to incorrectly assume that they are not growing adequately.

A series of studies published by Barker et al. and by other groups in the 1990s suggested that poor fetal growth was associated with worse long-term outcomes, specifically cardiovascular disease and other markers of the metabolic syndrome.[3-6] The risk appeared to be greatest in those born small and thin (i.e., lower ponderal index), but there was also an inverse relationship between weight at 1 year of age and later risk. Closer examination of this epidemiological data (the "Fetal Origins of Adult Disease" hypothesis) also demonstrated that the greatest risk was in those not only born small and thin, but in whom there was poor early weight gain in the first few months.[7] Although, now there is evidence that growth acceleration in term infants in the first few weeks is likely to be harmful.[8]

Growth in preterm infants is often sub-optimal.[9,10] Most authorities continue to recommend that postnatal growth should approximate that of the *in utero* fetus.[11] However, there are few data to show that this necessarily results in the "best" outcomes. Despite this, it is difficult to identify a reference that is more valid, and clinicians must use some sort of reference on which to make a pragmatic assessment of growth.[12,13] Regardless of the reference, most preterm infants grow poorly in the first few weeks, and move down percentile positions on a growth chart.

There is a close relationship between this early growth failure and inadequate nutrient intakes. Studies have shown that in preterm infants born before 30 weeks gestation, the cumulative deficits at the end of the first week are approximately 400 Kcal/kg and 14 g/kg of protein.[10] The true protein deficit is likely to be significantly higher as these figures were calculated assuming a recommended protein intake of 3 g/kg/day. Newer recommendations are for approximately 4 g/kg/day meaning the likely first week protein deficit would be closer to 21 g/kg, compared to a "recommended" intake of approximately 28 g/kg.[11] Providing only 25% of protein needs is equivalent to the fetus receiving his or her required protein intake in just 2 days each week. This data might then argue that a key assessment of short-term outcomes should be that of nutrient intake, that is, "inputs."

An inadequate balance of nutrients compounds growth failure in preterm infants. While protein needs are frequently not met, it is generally easier to meet energy requirements. Indeed, many preterm infants may receive excess energy and demonstrate excess fat mass deposition.[14] Protein deficiency and a high-fat, high-carbohydrate diet via either the parenteral or the enteral route are typical of preterm nutrition in the first few weeks. Low protein-to-energy ratios are associated with decreases in lean mass accretion and increased deposition of adipose tissue. Weight gain per se may not be as important as weight gain composition. Low-protein, high-carbohydrate diets may also be associated with adverse programming. However, the effects of growth on later insulin sensitivity are limited and conflicting. In one study in preterm infants,[15] there appeared to be no association between growth (defined in this study as change in weight SD score) between birth and discharge and later insulin sensitivity. There were relationships between nutritional intakes in the first 3 months and weight SD score, but no relationships between total calorie intake, protein, lipid, and carbohydrate, and subsequent insulin sensitivity.

BENEFITS OF ASSESSING SHORT-TERM NUTRITIONAL OUTCOMES

The principal reasons for assessment of outcomes prior to hospital discharge are so that clinicians can maximize quality and minimize harm. The old management adage "you can't manage what you can't measure" is relevant. The principles guiding assessments are similar for both nutritional (e.g., growth) and non-nutritional (e.g., respiratory) exposures and include:

1. Direct clinical care: improved ability to direct follow-up programs and target early intervention to those at greatest risk, for example, dietetic follow-up for those with poor growth, or high-risk neuro-developmental follow-up for those who developed necrotizing enterocolitis (NEC).
2. Informing parents: providing parents with a better understanding of potential longer-term outcomes, for example, likely long-term growth outcomes of extremely in utero growth-restricted (IUGR) infants.
3. Audit, service review, and clinical governance: measurable outcomes of neonatal care provide quality assurance and contribute to identifying "potentially better practices."
4. Research: retrospective and prospective studies require robust assessments in the short and medium term in order to improve understanding of nutritional management and how to improve future outcomes.

Although there are strong associations between nutritionally related neonatal morbidities (e.g., NEC) and worse neuro-developmental outcome,[16] prediction at the individual level is poor. Parents deserve the right to information, but should not be subject to unnecessary tests or provided with "predictions" that are often inaccurate. Audit is a vital component of clinical care, and assessment of both exposures (e.g., breast milk intake) and outcomes (e.g., weight gain) can improve care. Several studies have shown the development and implementation of multidisciplinary evidence-based guidelines and subsequent appraisal focusing on both intakes and outcomes ("potentially better practices") leads to better nutritional care.[17]

In general, our current state of knowledge is such that we are better at explaining outcomes than predicting them. Our understanding and prediction for individual babies is poor. From the perspective of providing good clinical care, assessment of nutritional exposures (i.e., inputs such as use of parenteral nutrition, or duration and amount of breast milk), growth, and biochemical outcomes (i.e., *outputs*) appears to be the minimum required for good clinical care. At present, based on our current understanding, there is little to argue for more assessments that are complex.

BIOCHEMICAL MEASURES AS ASSESSMENTS OF SHORT-TERM NUTRITIONAL MANAGEMENT

ELECTROLYTES

Biochemical monitoring is an important component of neonatal care, but obsessive monitoring of serum parameters as a means of assessing nutritional adequacy is frequently misplaced. Measurement of electrolytes is an important guide to determining nutritional needs at that point in time, but rarely reflects total body stores. While it is important to maintain serum sodium, a normal value does not necessarily indicate sufficiency, and urinary sodium levels may be a better indicator of adequacy. Serum phosphate levels are extremely useful in determining needs especially for infants receiving breast milk,[18] whereas assessment of serum calcium is generally not useful in determining nutritional adequacy as most body calcium is present in bone, and only a tiny, highly regulated, fraction is present in the serum.[19]

SERUM PROTEINS

Measurement of plasma proteins might be a useful means of assessing nutritional adequacy over the short term[20,21] and a wide range of different plasma proteins have been considered as markers of protein status in preterm infants.[20,22] The most commonly used proteins are albumin and transthyretin (pre-albumin).

Albumin has a long circulating half-life (21 days) and a large volume of distribution as it exists in both the intra-vascular and extra-vascular compartments. Serum albumin concentration is considerably lower in preterm than in term infants, as is true for many other serum proteins.[23] There is little data to support the notion that the lower levels seen in well preterm babies are associated with harm or cause the peripheral edema commonly observed in otherwise well infants.

Transthyretin (pre-albumin) and retinol binding proteins (RBPs) have much shorter half-lives and are more reflective of nutritional adequacy over the preceding few days.[23] Pre-albumin is available in many clinical biochemistry laboratories, but the use of RBP protein measurement is largely restricted to research settings.

Serum concentrations of transthyretin (pre-albumin), RBP, and transferrin are correlated with protein (but not energy) intake in preterm infants.[20] Serum pre-albumin is also correlated with other possible markers of protein sufficiency such as pre-prandial amino acid levels, urine urea, and blood urea nitrogen (BUN),[20] and with relevant short-term outcomes such as weight and length growth.[20,24] Changes in pre-albumin concentration may precede accelerations in growth in preterm infants.[24] Investigations of these potential markers are likely to continue, in part due to a renewed interest in using the serum protein mass (the product of the serum protein concentration, the blood volume, and 1-hematocrit), rather than the serum protein concentration, as a marker of protein sufficiency. [22,25]

Whichever serum protein one considers, there is no evidence that manipulations of protein intake in response to the serum protein level alter clinically relevant short- or long-term outcomes.

SERUM UREA/BLOOD UREA NITROGEN (BUN)

BUN is widely used as a marker of protein adequacy in the NICU, although its use is confounded by its relationship to renal function.[23] BUN seems to perform much better as a marker of sufficiency of protein intake when preterm infants are being enterally fed than when they are receiving parenteral feeds.[26] Generally, BUN does not appear to correlate with enteral amino acid intake in early life.[27] For example, in a randomized controlled trial of high and low parenteral amino acid intakes in preterm infants, the higher intake was associated with improved nitrogen balance, increased leucine flux, increased leucine oxidation, and increased non-oxidative leucine disposal.[28] Despite this, BUN did not differ between the high and low amino acid groups.[28] The failure of BUN to respond to changes in protein intake at this age may be due to immaturity of urea synthesis in preterm infants, especially those with *in utero* growth retardation[29] or the confounding effects of maturing renal function.

The situation may be different with respect to enteral nutrition. Higher enteral protein intakes in hospital lead to higher BUN (and also with higher retinol binding protein concentrations).[30] Similarly, increased enteral protein intakes after hospital discharge lead to higher BUN concentrations, but do not affect either serum albumin concentration or the total serum protein concentration.[31]

The most compelling evidence to support the assessment of BUN during enteral feeds is the study by Arslanoglu et al.[32] In this controlled study, preterm infants were randomized to a standardized enteral regimen or one where human milk fortification was individualized based on the BUN concentration.[32] When the fortification of human milk was adjusted to maintain the BUN in the range of 9 to 14 mg/dL (3.2 to 5 mmol/L) preterm infants had significantly higher growth of weight and length than in the standard fortification group.[32]

SERUM CALCIUM AND PHOSPHATE

Serum calcium is under tight homeostatic control, and very little of the total body calcium is present in the serum.[19] Although serum phosphate does correlate with dietary phosphate intake, serum calcium is poorly responsive to changes in calcium intake.[19]

ALKALINE PHOSPHATASE

Alkaline phosphatase is often used in neonatal units as a marker of mineral bone disease, and both total and bone-specific alkaline phosphatase levels can be measured.[18] One reason for the widespread use of alkaline phosphatase measurements is probably the finding from a 1989 study that a serum alkaline phosphatase concentration greater than 1200 was associated with reduced long-term linear growth.[33]

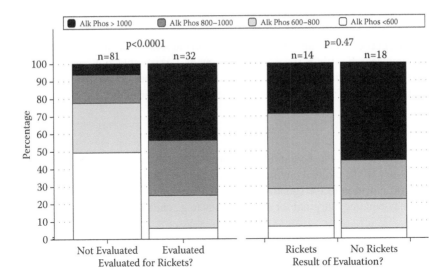

FIGURE 2.1   Distribution of serum alkaline phosphatase values in ELBW infants evaluated for rickets and those not evaluated for rickets (left panel), and in those who were evaluated and found to either have rickets or not have rickets (right panel). (From Reference 35.)

Alkaline phosphatase levels may relate to bone mineral turnover and are indicative of mineral and vitamin D intakes; however, it is not particularly useful on its own in terms of determining management.[18,19,34] For example, Mitchell et al. assessed alkaline phosphatase levels in 113 extremely low birthweight (ELBW) infants and found elevated levels to be common, especially in more preterm infants.[35] Thirty-two of these infants had knee radiographs taken to assess for rickets based on a variety of criteria. Those infants who were assessed for rickets had significantly higher alkaline phosphatase levels than those who did not (Figure 2.1), in part because persistently high alkaline phosphatase levels were a frequent *reason* for radiological evaluation.[35] However, among the infants assessed for rickets, there was no difference in peak alkaline phosphatase level between those who did and did not have rickets (1078 ± 356 vs. 943 ± 346) (Figure 2.1).

Another study in preterm infants less than 34 weeks gestation found an alkaline phosphatase level of greater than 700 to be a predictor of later osteopenia[36] with a sensitivity of 73% and a specificity of 73%.[36] However, the area under the receiver operator characteristic curve was only 0.74 for alkaline phosphatase and 0.72 for bone-specific alkaline phosphatase.[36] This would usually be considered only "fair" agreement.[*]

Alkaline phosphatase does not seem to predict later functional outcomes such as rickets or bone mineral density.[18,34,37] Some have suggested benefits to combining alkaline phosphatase measurements with the measurement of serum phosphorus,[18] but further data is needed.

---

[*] The usual convention for the area under the ROC curve is to consider areas between 0.6 and 0.7 as "poor" test, between 0.7 and 0.8 as "fair," between 0.8 and 0.9 as "good," and between 0.9 to 1.0 as an "excellent" test.

SERUM LIPIDS

Measurement of serum lipids is not a useful clinical marker of short-term adequacy, except in research settings specifically looking at, for example, polyunsaturated lipids. High levels of cholesterol and LDL in the neonatal period may relate to longer-term harm,[38] but optimal serum levels have yet to be determined.

VITAMIN LEVELS

Serum measures of most vitamins and growth factors are generally unhelpful or unnecessary in the clinical environment except in complex cases such as prolonged parenteral nutrition usage (greater than 3 to 4 weeks) or where fat soluble vitamin status may become marginal for other reasons (e.g., cholestasis).

NEURO-DEVELOPMENTAL ASSESSMENTS OF NUTRITIONAL MANAGEMENT

While optimizing neuro-cognitive outcome by careful nutritional management is an important goal, there are no studies that show any short-term developmental assessment (i.e., pre-discharge) to be useful in routine clinical practice. In addition, the predictive value of early developmental assessments appears limited. In one study, there was little evidence that a commonly used tool—the Neurobehavioral Assessment of the Preterm Infant (NAPI)—prior to discharge was of any use in predicting later neuro-developmental outcomes determined using Bayley Scales of Infant Development (BSID).[39]

In the immediate post-discharge period, neuro-developmental outcome is a key parameter, with use of BSID being the most widely used measure. Classic studies conducted by Lucas and others demonstrated that BSID at 18 months corrected age was sensitive to early nutrient intakes.[40–43] BSID might be considered as a key outcome for nutritional trials comparing group differences but it lacks precision and predictive value at the individual level. A low score on the BSID is an indication of delayed development but does not necessarily predict cognitive impairment. Most children with scores <2 SDs below the mean will still end up with a good HRQoL.

PREDICTIVE VALUE OF EARLY DEVELOPMENTAL ASSESSMENTS

In a recent follow-up study, rates of moderate and severe cognitive impairments were much lower at 5 years than at 18 months.[44] Less than 20% of the children who had a BSID score <70 (2 SDs below the mean) at 18 months had an IQ <70 at 5 years of age.[44]

Several other studies have found similarly disappointing predictive value for early assessments of development. Assessments made at early ages seem to over-identify impaired infants. For example, in a cohort of over 300 ELBW infants the rates of cognitive impairment fell from 39% at age 20 months to 16% at age 8 years.[45] In ELBW infants, the Bayley score at 2 years and at 3 years explains only 44% and 57% of the variation in full-scale IQ at 8 years, respectively.[46]

When data is expressed as nominal categories, the tests do not perform substantially better. A geographically defined cohort of ELBW infants was classified as have either no disability, or mild, moderate, or severe disability at 2 years of age, and again at 8 years.[47] The concordance between the two assessments was evaluated using Cohen's Kappa.[47] A kappa statistic less than 0 indicates no agreement between the two time points, a kappa of 0 to 0.20 is slight agreement, 0.21 to 0.40 is fair, 0.41 to 0.60 is moderate, 0.61 to 0.80 is substantial, and 0.81 to 1 is almost perfect agreement.[48] In this cohort, kappa was 0.20 (slight agreement) for ELBW and 0.37 (fair agreement) for term infants.[47] A similar study compared 18-month and 24-month Bayley scores with 8- to 9-year IQ in ELBW infants.[49] The 24-month Bayley performed better as an assessment of 8-year IQ (kappa = 0.43, "moderate" agreement) than did the 18-month Bayley (kappa = 0.25, "fair" agreement).[49]

In one large cohort, a marital development index (MDI) score <70 at 20 months had a positive predictive value of 37% for identifying a mental processing composite less than 70 at 8 years.[45] For scores of <85 at both time points, sensitivity was 91% and specificity 71%.[45] The likelihood ratio for a positive test was 3.7 (i.e., infants with an MDI < 70 at 20 months, had a 3.7-fold higher mental processing composit (MPC) < 70 at 8 years than those with an MDI > 70), and the likelihood ratio for a negative test was 0.19 (i.e., infants with a normal test at 20 months were 0.19 times more likely to have an abnormal test at 8 years).

This suggests that both short- and medium-term neuro-developmental assessments might be of limited usefulness, particularly in relation to nutritional management. Although BSID at 18 to 24 months is viewed by many as the gold standard outcome for both assessment/audit of clinical outcomes and for neonatal trials, it was designed to detect developmental delay and not school age cognitive attainment— the outcome most practitioners (and perhaps parents) are interested in. As recently stated, ". . . the BSID is not an adequate indicant of specific cognitive skills that may be differentially affected by interventions or exposures, nutritional or otherwise, and so its use to evaluate the construct of infant cognition is seriously deficient in the context of recent advances in developmental science."[50]

CNS IMAGING

Cranial ultrasound and magnetic resonance imaging (MRI) are specific markers of brain injury, but neither has sufficient sensitivity using current methodologies to be useful as measures of nutritional adequacy prior to discharge. While the negative predictive value of MRI at discharge for later delay (BSID MDI or PDI <70) is as high as 95%, the positive predictive value is only around 30%.[51] Even when used for the presence of brain injury, MRI is poorly predictive, so it is unlikely to be useful in assessment of nutritional adequacy. Most authors now agree that neuro-developmental assessment of extremely preterm infants requires a follow-up period of at least 6 years in order to make reliable statements.[52] More detailed neuro-imaging techniques, for example, volumetric analysis of specific brain areas such as the caudate, are useful in later childhood in a research setting,[53] but have not been examined in relation to nutritional management in the short and medium term.

NOVEL NEUROPHYSIOLOGICAL MARKERS

In recent years more specific assessments of potential neurological function have started to be developed, and might be considered valid measures of short- and medium-term nutritional adequacy, for example, the use of electro-retinograms as a marker of fatty acid or vitamin A status.[54,55] Event-related potentials (ERP) have been used to compare the response of infants to their own mothers' voices and a stranger's voice.[56] These techniques have been used to demonstrate evidence of CNS iron deficiency in infants of diabetic mothers[56] and to demonstrate function correlations with more simple measures of iron status such as serum ferritin.[57] Although such novel methods are largely restricted to research settings, they are intriguing and point to the development of function assessments of brain development and the effect of nutrition on them. Functional MRI imaging may provide similar insights in the future.

DO EARLY GROWTH PATTERNS PREDICT WEIGHT AND HEIGHT IN LATER LIFE?

Early postnatal growth of preterm children is almost inevitably compromised, although approximately 80% demonstrate catch-up growth.[58] Catch-up growth occurs mainly within the first two years after birth,[59,60] but also during childhood and through adolescence into adulthood.[61–64] Preterm born children continue to lag behind; most individuals born preterm remain shorter and lighter than term-born peers at all time points during childhood, adolescence, and adulthood (see Figure 2.2).

One prediction model for growth in a cohort of very low birth weight (VLBW) survivors found that mid-parental height SD score, birth weight SD score, and height and weight SD scores at 1 year could predict height SD score at 5 years,[60] but the model remains untested for tracking growth through to adulthood. A further study suggested that infants who reach a length within the normal range by 3 months of age display a virtually normal growth pattern in childhood, adolescence, and adulthood, but infants who do not catch up show a similar growth pattern as term-born small-for-gestational-age (SGA) babies.[59]

Being preterm and SGA (likely to be a marker for IUGR) appears to be associated with reduced catch-up growth; in one study, only 46% of VLBW SGA showed complete height catch-up by adulthood, again with worse outcomes for the males.[63] Specific genetic polymorphisms have also been implicated, including polymorphisms of the growth hormone receptor gene[65] and glucocorticoid receptor genes.[66]

ACCURACY, PRECISION, AND USEFULNESS OF SHORT- AND MEDIUM-TERM ASSESSMENTS

When assessing outcomes of clinical relevance, it is important that the parameter be measured accurately. Accuracy tells us how close to the real value the measurement is, whereas precision indicates repeatability or reproducibility. Most weighing scales are both accurate and precise, whereas many length measures tend to lack precision. If a parameter is to be measured repeatedly and used to guide clinical decisions, it is important it is precise. A descriptive study examined intra- and inter-examiner reliability of four techniques: crown-heel, supine, paper barrier, and neo-infantometer length. Measurements were undertaken by nurses blind to their own and to the other nurse's measurements.[67] Intra- and inter-examiner differences were significantly larger when examiners used the crown-heel measurement technique. Although the intra- and inter-examiner reliability of length measurements obtained with the other techniques did not differ significantly, the amount of error in these measurements was large. Similar work has examined the intra- and inter-examiner reliability of weight, occipitofrontal circumference (OFC), and other auxological measures.[100] Intra-examiner differences tended to be smaller than inter-examiner differences for all measures except weight, which remained stable for intra- and inter-examiner comparisons. The findings also suggested that weight and OFC were the most reliable measures, whereas length and mid-arm circumference were the least reliable measures.

RELATIONSHIP OF MEDIUM-TERM GROWTH AND FINAL ADULT SIZE

Several longitudinal studies of growth in extremely preterm or ELBW infants have been published since 2000[61,64,68–71] (Figure 2.2A–C). By 2 years of age, catch-up in height for age z-score is largely complete. An assessment of body length at age 2 years should be relatively well correlated with height as an adult. If groups on different nutritional protocols are to be compared, then at 2–3 years seems a reasonable age at which

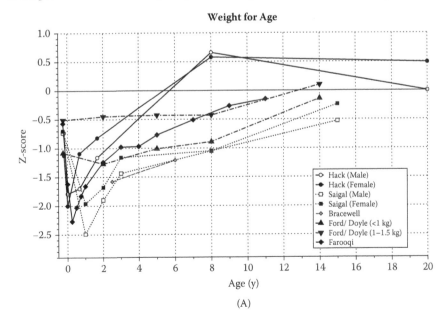

FIGURE 2.2 Longitudinal measurements of weight (A), length/height (B), and head circumference (C) in extremely low birth weight (ELBW) infants between birth and 20 years of age. (Data are from References 61, 64, 68–71.) *(continued)*

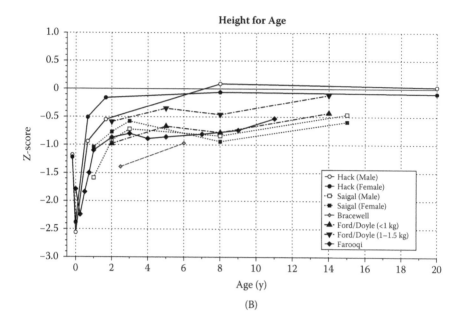

(B)

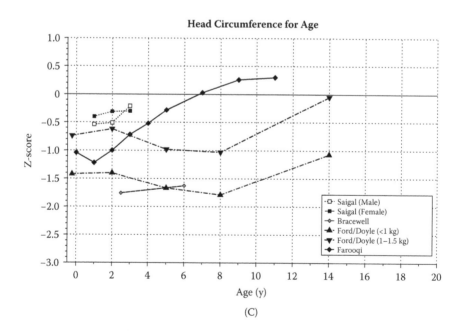

(C)

FIGURE 2.2 (CONTINUED) Longitudinal measurements of weight (A), length/height (B), and head circumference (C) in extremely low birth weight (ELBW) infants between birth and 20 years of age. (Data are from References 61, 64, 68–71.)

to assess height/length achievement. After this age, subjects will continue to grow, but as a group, their place within the population distribution is fairly well set (Figure 2.2B).

The situation for weight is very different (Figure 2.2A) where catch-up growth relative to the general population continues into the teenage years and for head circumference (Figure 2.2C) where little catch-up growth is seen in ELBW infants.

BODY COMPOSITION

While the quantity of growth (i.e., how much weight or length babies accrue) is clearly relevant, the quality of growth in terms of the relative balance of lean and fat mass, that is, body composition, may be more important for longer-term cardio-metabolic phenotype. Although measures of body composition are largely research tools, accuracy and precision are important considerations. Dual X-ray Absorptiometry (DXA) provides precise measures of fat and lean mass, and accurate and precise measures of bone mineral content. However, the technique involves many assumptions and it is virtually impossible to determine accuracy especially for fat and lean mass, as no gold standard exists.[72] Furthermore, because DXA provides a 2-dimensional assessment of body tissues (which are 3-dimensional) additional difficulties in interpretation arise, especially when comparing groups of different body size.

While DXA appears to provide reasonably accurate measures of fat mass, it does not measure adipose tissue directly and therefore is unable to determine partitioning between subcutaneous and intra-abdominal stores. This is important, as it appears that the abnormal partitioning of fat stores, rather than the total fat mass, is the key component determining cardio-metabolic risk. MRI provides an accurate measure of intra-abdominal fat and measures lipid deposition within metabolically important tissues such as liver and muscle, but it remains a research tool.[73] Air-displacement plethysmography provides a precise measure of body volume from which fat mass can be estimated. Comparison against stable isotope studies suggests it might be accurate.[74] As it is non-invasive, quick, and low cost (after initial capital investment), it might provide for repeated measures over time.

The usefulness of any parameter is determined by whether it enables better decision making in clinical practice, and whether it promotes interpretation in a research setting. Auxological measures are generally useful in clinical settings, whereas most imaging techniques currently fail to provide data of direct relevance for clinical care. Overall, while there is a range of robust data on short-term group outcomes, their validity for predicting long-term outcomes for individuals remains limited. Better measures in the short and medium term are needed in order to provide a more reliable assessment of nutritional adequacy, as well as to give a better indication of longer-term outcomes at the individual level.

NOVEL METHODS OF SHORT- AND MEDIUM-TERM ASSESSMENT: THE "OMICS" AND BIOMARKERS

Identifying validated biomarkers with high specificity and sensitivity for long-term outcomes is a "needle-in-a-haystack" search. To expedite the process, researchers have turned to high-throughput technologies that are non-invasive, utilize small sample volumes, and allow screening of large numbers of potential biomarkers simultaneously. The development of analytical platforms capable of measuring multiple analytes in a single sample simultaneously has enabled the proliferation of "omic" technologies. The suffix "–ome" implies a degree of totality: an ability to measure and describe all attributes of an entity. A number of distinct, yet complimentary "omic" fields, (e.g., lipidomics, proteomics, genomics, and metabonomics; each respectively setting out to describe the global characteristics of the lipid, protein, genetic material, and metabolites within a biological system) have developed individually, although in tandem, each employing distinct modalities, but also with considerable overlap of analytical and bio-informatic platforms. The use of "omic" technologies in searching for biomarkers of long-term outcomes of preterm birth is gathering pace. However, to date, no high-specificity and high-sensitivity biomarkers have been published and validated.

METABONOMICS

The terms *metabonomics* and *metabolomics* are often used interchangeably, although they were respectively originally defined as: "the quantitative measurement of the dynamic multi-parametric metabolic response of living systems to pathophysiological stimuli or genetic modification"[75] and "a comprehensive and quantitative analysis of all metabolites"[76] in a given system. Because metabonomics measures chemical phenotypes that are a net result of genomic, transcriptomic, and proteomic variability, it provides the most integrated profile of biological status. Metabonomic analysis can be applied to samples of urine and stool water, collection of which is minimally invasive, and open to serial sampling. The metabolic profile of urine may accentuate the changes in response to disease-induced stress, because of the body's attempt to maintain homeostasis[77] while metabonomic analysis of stool water is a useful tool for obtaining some idea of microflora colonization of the infant.[78] Similarly, there is a range of rapidly developing *in vivo* metabonomic technologies that could be utilized within clinic settings, although current knowledge is mainly limited to the field of oncology.[79, 80]

It is important to appreciate when carrying out any "omic" analysis in preterm infants that body organ systems follow two broad trajectories postbirth. The first tracks postconceptual age and is largely genetically defined. This includes aspects of renal and brain development. The second tracks postpartum age, and is followed by organ systems that mainly mature postpartum, for example, the skin and the gut. Consequently, it is important to compare within groups, or control data analysis, independently for both postconceptual and postpartum age. Metabonomic studies of urine from preterm compared to term infants have unsurprisingly shown large differences in their metabonome at both birth and term-corrected age.[81, 82] Such studies are complicated by the presence of large differences of creatine and creatinine. Indeed, a recent study reporting differences in the metabonome of intrauterine growth-restricted neonates, compared to normal birth weight controls, reported creatine and creatinine to be two of the major metabolites differing between the groups.[83] It is likely these metabolites are noninvasively measurable biomarkers of lean muscle mass with limited use as biomarkers for long-term outcomes. Consequently, it remains an ongoing issue as to whether metabolite profiles should be normalized to these metabolite peaks (in essence correcting the metabonome for muscle mass), or whether they should be discarded from the final analysis.

To date, the most promising potential biomarkers for long-term outcome identified from urinary metabonomics have been identified in the urine of asphyxiated babies.[84] Work comparing the metabonome of urine samples from infants who went on to develop type 1 diabetes and those who did not has also located putative biomarkers for early determination of risk of developing type 1 diabetes, with elevated concentrations of glutamic acid preceding the production of glutamic acid decarboxylase antibodies.[85] The use of metabonomics in neonatal studies has been recently reviewed.[86–88]

One of the difficulties with all these techniques is that large numbers of metabolites from multiple subjects generate complex datasets, the analysis and interpretation of which relies on statistical software and multivariate data analysis to classify subjects into groups by common metabolites.[89,90] Complex modeling seeks the optimal discrimination between groups. Discriminant metabolites can be considered as biomarkers for the phenotype of interest, or by matching metabolites with specific enzymes and metabolic pathways using databases, thus determining the underlying metabolic mechanisms potentially driving the phenotype of interest. Biomarkers essentially fall into three categories:

1. Direct measures, which arise from an actual disease or aberrant physiological process; for example, retinol-binding protein is a measure of protein status.
2. Indirect measures, which are a surrogate for a disease or aberrant physiological process; for example, growth as a marker of nutritional status.
3. Indicators of risk or benefit, which are associated with an outcome but may not be causally linked; for example, presence or absence of a specific gene may correlate with disease risk.

GENETIC AND EPIGENETIC PROFILING

Of the other "omic" technologies, genomic and epigenetic profiling are probably key for perinatal research. In terms of genomics, telomere length has possibly been one of the potential biomarkers that have received most interest. Telomeres are lengths of non-coding DNA at the ends of the chromosome, which help prevent loss of coding DNA during the life of a cell. Loss of telomeres is thought to increase risk of teratogenesis and mutagenesis, and has been considered as a marker of the aging process, although there remains doubt as to how good a marker of aging telomere length really is.[91] It has been suggested that the increased presence of oxidative stress in preterm infants may reduce their telomere length during infancy, and may explain why young adults born preterm manifest symptoms associated with aging.[92] A few studies have shown reduced telomere length in low birth weight infants compared to normal birth weight infants.[93]

Recent work has highlighted that early life events program later life outcomes via epigenetic mechanisms.[94] There is a range of epigenetic mechanisms that involve chemical alterations to DNA without changing the DNA sequence. The most commonly researched of these are DNA methylation and histone acetylation, and it seems likely that these then affect gene expression and subsequent transcription. Data has shown correlations between DNA methylation in early life biological samples and later obesity phenotype.[95] Studies have also determined relationships between patterns of early catch up growth in preterm infants and DNA methylation of certain candidate genes, although determining direction of causality is complicated.[96,97] In the future, it might be possible to predict later life risks of health and disease phenotype based on epigenetic modifications present at the time of initial hospital discharge.

These techniques using samples from preterm babies only identify biomarkers that discriminate the infants at the time of sampling, based on their known phenotype. How these biomarkers may project as predictors of future outcome is difficult to determine, and requires work from both ends, with tandem studies to identify biomarkers in children and adults born preterm, with a range of long-term outcomes. The only way to accurately identify and determine the specificity and sensitivity of biomarkers during the perinatal period for long-term outcomes is the establishment and full "omic" characterization of a large prospective cohort of preterm and term-born infants, who can be then be tracked over the life-course. While the costs of "omic" analyses are decreasing on a per sample basis, the analytical platforms are unlikely to become easily accessible to most clinicians in the near future. Instead, once biomarkers have been identified, the next race will be to produce cot-side technology for their immediate measurement.

CONCLUSIONS

Promoting good nutritional status is a key to improving short- and long-term outcomes in preterm infants. When assessing these outcomes though, it is important to consider who the key stakeholders are. For neonatal nutrition there are likely to be many: babies and parents, because "better" outcomes mean something to them; society, because the burden of sub-optimal health status is associated with significant costs; health care systems that need to provide quality assurance; and research that might improve outcomes for future generations. All these groups may have different priorities, and it is all too easy to allow the intellectual curiosity of health professionals cloud what might be best for their patients. Brain MRI has become a standard component of care in many units but there is scant evidence it really helps parents or provides better information to plan individual care over and above that which could be ascertained from a good history and examination.[98]

The personalized long-term growth potential for each preterm child remains to be elucidated and growth patterns at early ages may not predict later growth trajectories. Ongoing research into the control of growth and factors that influence later growth attainment is required. Whether it really matters to preterm born adults that they are slightly smaller than their peers is uncertain. Most individuals would not want to be more than 2 to 3 SDs from the mean, but whether being on, for example, the 10th height percentile long term for ex-preterm adults really matters is questionable. Assessments that predict later metabolic disease, for example, insulin resistance or hypertension, are likely of greater importance.

Biochemical assessments in general do not predict later outcomes. Body composition is a key to interpretation of growth, but virtually no data allow prediction at the individual level. Clinicians and researchers must work with parents to determine which outcomes matter. Neuro-cognitive outcome is likely to be of major interest, and while we know that the presence of risk factors such as NEC dramatically increase the risk, there are no good short-term assessments that predict outcome at the individual level. The new "omics" may ultimately provide an insight into better understanding nutritional exposures and their relationships to meaningful long-term outcomes, but prediction at the individual level seems a long way off. Determining novel biomarkers in adults that explain the effects of early life exposures is important, but relate to neonatal care practices and populations 20 to 30 years ago and may not be relevant today. It could be argued that what matters most is HRQoL.[99] This reflects total well being and includes aspects of emotional, social, and physical functioning, and how it is impacted over time by health, disease, and disability. Current short- and medium-term assessments of nutrition in early life currently tell us only a little about long-term HRQoL.

REFERENCES

1. Vasu V, Modi N. Assessing the impact of preterm nutrition. *Early Hum Develop* 2007;83:813–818.
2. Jain V, Singhal A. Catch up growth in low birth weight infants: striking a healthy balance. *Rev Endo Metabol Dis* 2012;13:141–147.
3. Barker DJ, Winter PD, Osmond C, Margetts B, Simmonds SJ. Weight in infancy and death from ischaemic heart disease. *Lancet* 1989;2:577–580.
4. Barker DJ. The fetal and infant origins of adult disease. *BMJ* 1990;301:1111.
5. Hales CN, Barker DJ, Clark PM, et al. Fetal and infant growth and impaired glucose tolerance at age 64. *BMJ* 1991;303:1019–1022.
6. Barker DJ. The effect of nutrition of the fetus and neonate on cardiovascular disease in adult life. *Proc Nutr Soc* 1992;51:135–144.
7. Eriksson JG, Forsen T, Tuomilehto J, Winter PD, Osmond C, Barker DJ. Catch-up growth in childhood and death from coronary heart disease: longitudinal study. *BMJ* 1999;318:427–431.
8. Stettler N. Nature and strength of epidemiological evidence for origins of childhood and adulthood obesity in the first year of life. *Int J Obes (Lond)* 2007;31:1035–1043.
9. Ehrenkranz RA, Younes N, Lemons JA, et al. Longitudinal growth of hospitalized very low birth weight infants. *Pediatrics* 1999;104:280–289.
10. Embleton NE, Pang N, Cooke RJ. Postnatal malnutrition and growth retardation: an inevitable consequence of current recommendations in preterm infants? *Pediatrics* 2001;107:270–273.
11. Agostoni C, Buonocore G, Carnielli VP, et al. Enteral nutrient supply for preterm infants: commentary from the European Society of Paediatric Gastroenterology, Hepatology and Nutrition Committee on Nutrition. *J Pediatr Gastroenterol Nutr* 2010;50:85–91.
12. Sauer PJ. Can extrauterine growth approximate intrauterine growth? Should it? *Am J Clin Nutr* 2007;85:608S–613S.
13. Cooke RW. Conventional birth weight standards obscure fetal growth restriction in preterm infants. *Arch Dis Child Fetal Neo Ed* 2007;92:F189–192.
14. Embleton ND. Optimal protein and energy intakes in preterm infants. *Early Hum Develop* 2007;83:831–837.

15. Regan FM, Cutfield WS, Jefferies C, Robinson E, Hofman PL. The impact of early nutrition in premature infants on later childhood insulin sensitivity and growth. *Pediatrics* 2006;118:1943–1949.
16. Soraisham AS, Amin HJ, Al-Hindi MY, Singhal N, Sauve RS. Does necrotising enterocolitis impact the neurodevelopmental and growth outcomes in preterm infants with birthweight < or = 1250 g? *J Paediatr Child Health* 2006;42:499–504.
17. Kuzma-O'Reilly B, Duenas ML, Greecher C, et al. Evaluation, development, and implementation of potentially better practices in neonatal intensive care nutrition. *Pediatrics* 2003;111:e461–470.
18. Tinnion RJ, Embleton ND. How to use…alkaline phosphatase in neonatology. *Arch Dis Child Ed Pract Ed* 2012;97:157–163.
19. Atkinson SA, Tsang RC. Calcium, magnesium, phosphorus and vitamin D. In: Tsang RC, Uauy R, Koletzko B, Zlotkin SH, Eds. *Nutrition of the Preterm Infant: Scientific Basis and Practical Guidelines.* Cincinnati, OH: Digital Eductation Publishing; 2005:245–277.
20. Polberger SK, Fex GA, Axelsson IE, Raiha NC. Eleven plasma proteins as indicators of protein nutritional status in very low birth weight infants. *Pediatrics* 1990;86:916–921.
21. Georgieff MK, Sasanow SR. Nutritional assessment of the neonate. *Clin Perinatol* 1986;13:73–89.
22. Raubenstine DA, Ballantine TV, Greecher CP, Webb SL. Neonatal serum protein levels as indicators of nutritional status: normal values and correlation with anthropometric data. *J Pediatric Gastroenterol Nutr* 1990;10:53–61.
23. Moyer-Mileur LJ. Anthropometric and laboratory assessment of very low birth weight infants: the most helpful measurements and why. *Sem Perinatol* 2007;31:96–103.
24. Giacoia GP, Watson S, West K. Rapid turnover transport proteins, plasma albumin, and growth in low birth weight infants. *JPEN* 1984;8:367–370.
25. Cardoso LE, Falcao MC. Nutritional assessment of very low birth weight infants: relationships between anthropometric and biochemical parameters. *Nutricion Hospitalaria* 2007;22:322–329.
26. Roggero P, Gianni ML, Morlacchi L, et al. Blood urea nitrogen concentrations in low-birth-weight preterm infants during parenteral and enteral nutrition. *J Pediatr Gastroenterol Nutr* 2010;51:213–215.
27. Ridout E, Melara D, Rottinghaus S, Thureen PJ. Blood urea nitrogen concentration as a marker of amino-acid intolerance in neonates with birthweight less than 1250 g. *J Perinatol* 2005;25:130–133.
28. Thureen PJ, Melara D, Fennessey PV, Hay WW, Jr. Effect of low versus high intravenous amino acid intake on very low birth weight infants in the early neonatal period. *Pediatric Res* 2003;53:24–32.
29. Boehm G, Teichmann B, Jung K, Moro G. Postnatal development of urea synthesis capacity in preterm infants with intrauterine growth retardation. *Biol Neonate* 1998;74:1–6.
30. Embleton ND, Cooke RJ. Protein requirements in preterm infants: effect of different levels of protein intake on growth and body composition. *Pediatric Res* 2005;58:855–860.
31. Cooke RJ, Griffin IJ, McCormick K, et al. Feeding preterm infants after hospital discharge: effect of dietary manipulation on nutrient intake and growth. *Pediatric Res* 1998;43:355–360.
32. Arslanoglu S, Moro GE, Ziegler EE. Adjustable fortification of human milk fed to preterm infants: does it make a difference? *J Perinatol* 2006;26:614–21.
33. Lucas A, Brooke OG, Baker BA, Bishop N, Morley R. High alkaline phosphatase activity and growth in preterm neonates. *Arch Dis Child* 1989;64:902–909.
34. Visser F, Sprij AJ, Brus F. The validity of biochemical markers in metabolic bone disease in preterm infants: a systematic review. *Acta Paediatr* 2012;101:562–568.

35. Mitchell SM, Rogers SP, Hicks PD, Hawthorne KM, Parker BR, Abrams SA. High frequencies of elevated alkaline phosphatase activity and rickets exist in extremely low birth weight infants despite current nutritional support. *BMC Pediatrics* 2009;9:47.

36. Hung YL, Chen PC, Jeng SF, et al. Serial measurements of serum alkaline phosphatase for early prediction of osteopaenia in preterm infants. *J Paediatr Child Health* 2011;47:134–139.

37. Faerk J, Peitersen B, Petersen S, Michaelsen KF. Bone mineralisation in premature infants cannot be predicted from serum alkaline phosphatase or serum phosphate. *Arch Dis Child Fetal Neo Ed* 2002;87:F133–136.

38. Lewandowski AJ, Lazdam M, Davis E, et al. Short-term exposure to exogenous lipids in premature infants and long-term changes in aortic and cardiac function. *Arteriosclerosis Thrombosis Vascular Biol* 2011;31:2125–2135.

39. Harijan P, Beer C, Glazebrook C, et al. Predicting developmental outcomes in very preterm infants: validity of a neonatal neurobehavioral assessment. *Acta Paediatr* 2012;101:e275–281.

40. Lucas A, Fewtrell MS, Morley R, et al. Randomized outcome trial of human milk fortification and developmental outcome in preterm infants. *Am J Clin Nutr* 1996;64:142–151.

41. Lucas A, Morley R, Cole TJ, Gore SM. A randomised multicentre study of human milk versus formula and later development in preterm infants. *Arch Dis Child Fetal Neo Ed* 1994;70:F141–146.

42. Lucas A, Morley R, Cole TJ, et al. Early diet in preterm babies and developmental status in infancy. *Arch Dis Child* 1989;64:1570–1578.

43. Lucas A, Morley R, Cole TJ, et al. Early diet in preterm babies and developmental status at 18 months. *Lancet* 1990;335:1477–1481.

44. Schmidt B, Anderson PJ, Doyle LW, et al. Survival without disability to age 5 years after neonatal caffeine therapy for apnea of prematurity. *JAMA* 2012;307:275–282.

45. Hack M, Taylor HG, Drotar D, et al. Poor predictive validity of the Bayley Scales of Infant Development for cognitive function of extremely low birth weight children at school age. *Pediatrics* 2005;116:333–341.

46. Potharst ES, Houtzager BA, van Sonderen L, et al. Prediction of cognitive abilities at the age of 5 years using developmental follow-up assessments at the age of 2 and 3 years in very preterm children. *Develop Med Child Neurol* 2012;54:240–246.

47. Roberts G, Anderson PJ, Doyle LW. The stability of the diagnosis of developmental disability between ages 2 and 8 in a geographic cohort of very preterm children born in 1997. *Arch Dis Child* 2010;95:786–790.

48. Landis JR, Koch GG. The measurement of observer agreement for categorical data. *Biometrics* 1977;33:159–174.

49. Doyle LW, Davis PG, Schmidt B, Anderson PJ. Cognitive outcome at 24 months is more predictive than at 18 months for IQ at 8-9 years in extremely low birth weight children. *Early Hum Develop* 2012;88:95–98.

50. Belfort MB, Rifas-Shiman SL, Sullivan T, et al. Infant growth before and after term: effects on neurodevelopment in preterm infants. *Pediatrics* 2011;128:e899–906.

51. Woodward LJ, Anderson PJ, Austin NC, Howard K, Inder TE. Neonatal MRI to predict neurodevelopmental outcomes in preterm infants. *New Eng J Med* 2006;355:685–694.

52. Voss W, Neubauer AP, Wachtendorf M, Verhey JF, Kattner E. Neurodevelopmental outcome in extremely low birth weight infants: what is the minimum age for reliable developmental prognosis? *Acta Paediatr* 2007;96:342–347.

53. Isaacs EB, Gadian DG, Sabatini S, et al. The effect of early human diet on caudate volumes and IQ. *Pediatric Res* 2008;63:308–314.

54. Leaf A, Gosbell A, McKenzie L, Sinclair A, Favilla I. Long chain polyunsaturated fatty acids and visual function in preterm infants. *Early Hum Develop* 1996;45:35–53.

55. Mactier H, McCulloch DL, Hamilton R, et al. Vitamin A supplementation improves retinal function in infants at risk of retinopathy of prematurity. *J Pediatr* 2012;160:954–959 e1.

56. Deregnier RA, Nelson CA, Thomas KM, Wewerka S, Georgieff MK. Neurophysiologic evaluation of auditory recognition memory in healthy newborn infants and infants of diabetic mothers. *J Pediatr* 2000;137:777–784.

57. Siddappa AM, Georgieff MK, Wewerka S, Worwa C, Nelson CA, Deregnier RA. Iron deficiency alters auditory recognition memory in newborn infants of diabetic mothers. *Pediatric Res* 2004;55:1034–1041.

58. Euser AM, de Wit CC, Finken MJ, Rijken M, Wit JM. Growth of preterm born children. *Hormone Res* 2008;70:319–328.

59. Finken MJ, Dekker FW, de Zegher F, Wit JM. Long-term height gain of prematurely born children with neonatal growth restraint: parallelism with the growth pattern of short children born small for gestational age. *Pediatrics* 2006;118:640–643.

60. Trebar B, Traunecker R, Selbmann HK, Ranke MB. Growth during the first two years predicts pre-school height in children born with very low birth weight (VLBW): results of a study of 1,320 children in Germany. *Pediatric Res* 2007;62:209–214.

61. Saigal S, Stoskopf B, Streiner D, Paneth N, Pinelli J, Boyle M. Growth trajectories of extremely low birth weight infants from birth to young adulthood: a longitudinal, population-based study. *Pediatric Res* 2006;60:751–758.

62. Doyle LW, Faber B, Callanan C, Ford GW, Davis NM. Extremely low birth weight and body size in early adulthood. *Arch Dis Child* 2004;89:347–350.

63. Brandt I, Sticker EJ, Gausche R, Lentze MJ. Catch-up growth of supine length/height of very low birth weight, small for gestational age preterm infants to adulthood. *J Pediatr* 2005;147:662–668.

64. Hack M, Schluchter M, Cartar L, Rahman M, Cuttler L, Borawski E. Growth of very low birth weight infants to age 20 years. *Pediatrics* 2003;112:e30–38.

65. Schreiner F, Stutte S, Bartmann P, Gohlke B, Woelfle J. Association of the growth hormone receptor d3-variant and catch-up growth of preterm infants with birth weight of less than 1500 grams. *J Clin Endo Metabol* 2007;92:4489–4493.

66. Finken MJ, Meulenbelt I, Dekker FW, et al. The 23K variant of the R23K polymorphism in the glucocorticoid receptor gene protects against postnatal growth failure and insulin resistance after preterm birth. *J Clin Endo Metabol* 2007;92:4777–4782.

67. Johnson TS, Engstrom JL, Warda JA, Kabat M, Peters B. Reliability of length measurements in full-term neonates. *JOGNN* 1998;27:270–276.

68. Bracewell MA, Hennessy EM, Wolke D, Marlow N. The EPICure study: growth and blood pressure at 6 years of age following extremely preterm birth. *Arch Dis Child Fetal Neo Ed* 2008;93:F108–114.

69. Doyle LW, Davis PG, Morley CJ, McPhee A, Carlin JB. Outcome at 2 years of age of infants from the DART study: a multicenter, international, randomized, controlled trial of low-dose dexamethasone. *Pediatrics* 2007;119:716–721.

70. Ford GW, Doyle LW, Davis NM, Callanan C. Very low birth weight and growth into adolescence. *Arch Pediatr Adol Med* 2000;154:778–784.

71. Farooqi A, Hagglof B, Sedin G, Gothefors L, Serenius F. Growth in 10- to 12-year-old children born at 23 to 25 weeks' gestation in the 1990s: a Swedish national prospective follow-up study. *Pediatrics* 2006;118:e1452–1465.

72. Wells JC, Fewtrell MS. Measuring body composition. *Arch Dis Child* 2006;91:612–617.

73. Uthaya S, Thomas EL, Hamilton G, Dore CJ, Bell J, Modi N. Altered adiposity after extremely preterm birth. *Pediatric Res* 2005;57:211–215.

74. Roggero P, Gianni ML, Amato O, et al. Evaluation of air-displacement plethysmography for body composition assessment in preterm infants. *Pediatric Res* 2012;72:316–320.

75. Nicholson JK, Lindon JC, Holmes E. "Metabonomics": understanding the metabolic responses of living systems to pathophysiological stimuli via multivariate statistical analysis of biological NMR spectroscopic data. *Xenobiotica* 1999;29:1181–1189.

76. Fiehn O. Combining genomics, metabolome analysis, and biochemical modelling to understand metabolic networks. *Comparative Functional Genomics* 2001;2:155–168.

77. Lindon JC. *Metabonomics: Techniques and Applications.* Business Briefings Future Drug Discovery, South Kensington, UK: Metabometrix Ltd, 2004.

78. Martin FP, Collino S, Rezzi S, Kochhar S. Metabolomic applications to decipher gut microbial metabolic influence in health and disease. *Front Physiol* 2012;3:113.

79. Nicholson JK, Holmes E, Kinross JM, Darzi AW, Takats Z, Lindon JC. Metabolic phenotyping in clinical and surgical environments. *Nature* 2012;491:384–392.

80. Takats Z, Denes J, Kinross J. Identifying the margin: a new method to distinguish between cancerous and noncancerous tissue during surgery. *Future Oncol* 2012;8:113–116.

81. Atzori L, Antonucci R, Barberini L, et al. 1H NMR-based metabolomic analysis of urine from preterm and term neonates. *Front Biosci (Elite Ed)* 2011;3:1005–1012.

82. Hyde MJ, Beckonert OP, Yap IKS. The effect of preterm delivery on the urinary metabolome. In: *Neonatal Society Summer Meeting* 2010; 2010.

83. Dessi A, Ottonello G, Fanos V. Physiopathology of intrauterine growth retardation: from classic data to metabolomics. *J Matern Fetal Neo Med* 2012;25:13–18.

84. Chu CY, Xiao X, Zhou XG, et al. Metabolomic and bioinformatic analyses in asphyxiated neonates. *Clin Biochem* 2006;39:203–209.

85. Oresic M, Simell S, Sysi-Aho M, et al. Dysregulation of lipid and amino acid metabolism precedes islet autoimmunity in children who later progress to type 1 diabetes. *J Experiment Med* 2008;205:2975–2984.

86. Fanos V, Antonucci R, Barberini L, Noto A, Atzori L. Clinical application of metabolomics in neonatology. *J Maternal Fetal Neo Med* 2012;25 Suppl 1:104–109.

87. Fanos V, Van den Anker J, Noto A, Mussap M, Atzori L. Metabolomics in neonatology: fact or fiction? *Semin Fetal Neo Med* 2013;18:3–12.

88. Atzori L, Antonucci R, Barberini L, Griffin JL, Fanos V. Metabolomics: a new tool for the neonatologist. *J Matern Fetal Neo Med* 2009;22 Suppl 3:50–53.

89. Madsen R, Lundstedt T, Trygg J. Chemometrics in metabolomics: a review in human disease diagnosis. *Analytica Chimica Acta* 2010;659:23–33.

90. Trygg J, Lundstedt T. *Chemometric Techniques for Metabonomics.* Amsterdam, The Netherlands: Elsevier; 2007.

91. Mather KA, Jorm AF, Parslow RA, Christensen H. Is telomere length a biomarker of aging? A review. *J Gerontol Series A, Biol Sci Med Sci* 2011;66:202–213.

92. Hallows SE, Regnault TR, Betts DH. The long and short of it: the role of telomeres in fetal origins of adult disease. *J Pregnancy* 2012;2012:638476.

93. Entringer S, Epel ES, Kumsta R, et al. Stress exposure in intrauterine life is associated with shorter telomere length in young adulthood. *Proc National Acad Sci USA* 2011;108:E513–518.

94. Groom A, Elliott HR, Embleton ND, Relton CL. Epigenetics and child health: basic principles. *Arch Dis Child* 2011;96:863–869.

95. Relton CL, Groom A, St Pourcain B, et al. DNA methylation patterns in cord blood DNA and body size in childhood. *PloS one* 2012;7:e31821.

96. Groom A, Potter C, Swan DC, et al. Postnatal growth and DNA methylation are associated with differential gene expression of the TACSTD2 gene and childhood fat mass. *Diabetes* 2012;61:391–400.

97. Turcot V, Groom A, McConnell JC, et al. Bioinformatic selection of putative epigenetically regulated loci associated with obesity using gene expression data. *Gene* 2012;499:99–107.

98. Pearce R, Baardsnes J. Term MRI for small preterm babies: Do parents really want to know and why has nobody asked them? *Acta Paediatr* 2012;101.

99. Glinianaia SV, Embleton ND, Rankin J. A systematic review of studies of quality of life in children and adults with selected congenital anomalies. *Birth Defects Res Part A, Clin Mol Teratol* 2012;94:511–520.

100. Johnson TS, Engstrom JL, Gelhar DK. "Intra- and interexaminer reliability of anthropometric measurements of term infants. *J Pediatr Gastroenterol Nutr.* 1997;24(5):497–505.

3 Causes of Postnatal Growth Failure in Preterm Infants

Enrico Bertino, Paula Di Nicola, Luciara Occhi, Giovanna Prandi, and Giorgio Gilli

LIST OF ABBREVIATIONS

AGA: adequate for gestational age
BPD: bronchopulmonary dysplasia
ELBW: extremely low birth weight
EUGR: extrauterine growth restriction
GA: gestational age
LBW: low birth weight
LGA: large for gestational age
NICU: neonatal intensive care unit
PNGF: postnatal growth failure
SD: standard deviation
SDS: standard deviation score
SGA: small for gestational age
VLBW: very low birth weight

INTRODUCTION

The postnatal growth pattern of preterm infants is markedly different from that of full-term infants. The American Academy of Pediatrics suggested that the goal for nutrition of the preterm infant should be to achieve a postnatal growth rate approximating that of the normal fetus of the same gestational age (GA).[1] However, such a pattern is seldom attained in premature neonates, who almost always show a postnatal cumulative nutritional deficit and a so-called Post-Natal Growth Failure (PNGF) or Extra-Uterine Growth Restriction (EUGR).[2,3]

DEFINITION AND INCIDENCE

There is no consensus among neonatologists regarding the best way to define EUGR. Suggested definitions include a weight-for-age below the 10th percentile of the reference anthropometric charts at 36-weeks-corrected gestational age,[2,4–7] at the time of hospital discharge,[8] or at 28 days of postnatal life.[5,8] Such definitions are similar to the WHO definition of intra-uterine growth restriction (IUGR), that is a weight-for-age below the 10th percentile for the reference population.[9] Makoul et al. describe EUGR as weight standard deviation score (SDS) below –1.88 at discharge (which is equivalent to a weight-for-age below the 3rd percentile).[10]

In older children, the definition of failure to thrive often combines both a smaller body size and a reduced rate of weight gain.[11] One typical definition is a body weight below the 5th percentile for age, or downward crossing of two "major" percentile lines.[12] In some studies, EUGR is defined based on the decrease in weight SDS between birth and discharge.[13–15] Whereas Cooke et al.[13] did not exactly quantify their definition, others have defined EUGR as a fall in weight SDS of at least 1.0[14] or 2.0.[15] This negative difference between SDSs appears on distance charts as a downward percentile crossing.

At present, a definition based on the negative change of SDS from birth to term-corrected age is probably the most appropriate[16] because age at discharge could be biased by different discharge policies over time and between centers. These differences would affect the estimated prevalence of EUGR.

The heterogeneity of definitions, clinical interventions, and the populations involved in the various studies makes it difficult to establish the incidence of EUGR in preterm neonates. This explains why the reported incidence of EUGR for weight ranges from 11% to 97%[2,4,5,8,10,14,15,17,18] (Table 3.1).

Usually the term EUGR is used to define a failure in weight growth, but length and head circumference may be taken into account as well. An EUGR for length or

TABLE 3.1

Incidence of *Ex Utero* Growth Restriction by Various Definitions

Author	Population	Definition	Incidence (%)
Lemons et al.[4]	VLBW, GA <30 w	Weight < 10th percentile at 36 w PMA	97
Radmacher et al.[17]	ELBW, GA <29 w	Weight < 10th percentile at discharge	59
Clark et al.[2]	LBW, GA ≤34 w	Weight < 10th percentile at 36 w PMA	28
Marks et al.[15]	VLBW	Decrease in weight SDS score >2 from birth to discharge	11
Franz et al.[14]	VLBW, GA <26 w	Decrease in weight SDS score >2 from birth to discharge	50
Martin et al.[5]	ELBW	Weight < 10th percentile at age 28 d	75
Makhoul et al.[10]	VLBW	Weight < 10th percentile at discharge	26
Karagol et al.[8]	ELBW, non-SGA	Weight < 10th percentile at age 28 d	26
Karagol et al.[8]	ELBW, non-SGA	Weight < 10th percentile at discharge	17
Roggero et al.[18]	VLBW, AGA	Decrease in weight SDS score >2 from birth to discharge	13–30[a]

[a] Historical rate of 30%, which was reduced to 13% following institution of comprehensive range of nutritional interventions.

head circumference has been observed by various authors.[2,19–22] For example, Clark and co-workers have reported an incidence of EUGR of 34% based on changes in length, and 16% based on changes in head circumference.[2]

BODY COMPOSITION AND EUGR

Standard anthropometry alone is inadequate to fully assess the growth and nutritional status of preterm infants, and the evaluation of body composition would ideally be integrated into both clinical practice and research.[18] In several studies, it has been observed that preterm infants at term-corrected age show an increased adiposity compared with infants born at term.[23]

According to a recent systematic review,[24] preterm infants at term-equivalent age are shorter and lighter and have a smaller head circumference than neonates born at term. However, this review found that the higher percentage of total body fat was in large part explained by a lesser fat-free mass rather than a true increase in fat mass.[24] The increase of fat mass could reflect a physiological adaptation to postnatal life of these infants to provide storage of energy and to reduce heat loss (as also observed after birth in term infants). On the other hand, the relative paucity of lean tissue could be due to morbidities, hormonal influences (including the postnatal use of corticosteroids that can decrease protein accretion[25]), and inadequate protein and energy intakes.[3,26,27] Costa-Orvay et al. demonstrated greater weight gains in preterm infants receiving high protein and energy intakes compared with preterm infants receiving standard intakes.[28] The greater weight gains reflected a greater increase in fat-free mass assessed by total body electrical impedance analysis.[28] Other authors showed that, while increased energy and protein intakes improved the growth with regard to weight and head circumference, there was no significant effect on body composition at term-equivalent age when compared with historic controls.[18,29] Overall, these observations may suggest that the quality of proteins provided in the diet and the relative adequacy in terms of dietary essential amino acids should be considered as well.

The independent effect of EUGR on adiposity has still to be quantified. However, more rapid growth is associated with increased adiposity at hospital discharge, at term-expected age, and at 3, 6, 9, and 12 months corrected age.[23] The finding of a positive relationship between discharge weight and percentage adiposity does not suggest that EUGR leads to short-term changes in adiposity. However, whether these early changes are beneficial or harmful is not clear.

BIOLOGICAL VARIABLES AND THE ETIOLOGY OF EUGR

Gestational Age

The effect of gestational age on the incidence of EUGR has been stressed by several authors who observed that the percentage of infants with severe EUGR increased significantly with decreasing gestational age.[2,3,15] Other authors have confirmed this observation, reporting a marked downward percentile crossing from birth to term in groups with lower gestational age, even after adjustment for gender, gestational age-corrected size at birth, major morbidities, need for nutritional and respiratory support, and age at discharge. We, for example, have examined weight gain velocity in preterm infants born at different gestational ages: 23 to 28 weeks, 29 to 30 weeks, 31 to 32 weeks, or 33 to 38 weeks.[30] At term-corrected age, achieved body size was very different between the groups, but by 12 months of age the groups had approached each other. Growth velocities (i.e., weight gain in g/d) during the first 13 weeks of postnatal life also differ substantially, with more preterm babies having slower growth velocity than more mature infants.[30] However, after approximately 13 weeks of age, the growth velocities of the groups are indistinguishable.[30] This suggests that EUGR becomes established early in life, and that interventions in the first 2 to 3 months of life are required to prevent it.

GENDER

The physiological growth difference between males and females is also present in preterm infants. For example, the anthropometric data of Italian neonates[31] show that males are heavier than females are at all gestational ages (Figure 3.1).

We have also studied the growth velocity of 262 very low birth weight (VLBW) infants.[30] Growth velocity in both males and females was initially poor, with females having a lower growth velocity than males. The difference was highest at 13 weeks of postnatal age before gradually declining (Figure 3.2).[30]

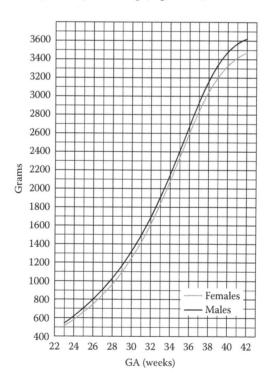

FIGURE 3.1   Mean birth weight for males and females at gestational ages from 23 weeks to 42 weeks, from the Italian Neonatal Anthropometric Charts.[31]

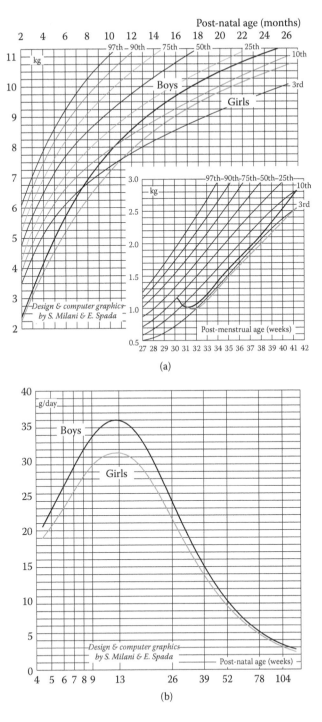

FIGURE 3.2 Body weight (g, upper panel) and growth rate (g/d, lower panel) in male and female VLBW infants. (Reproduced from Reference 30, with permission.)

The body weights of male and female preterm infants (expressed as weight-for-age SDS computed on gender-specific anthropometric charts) corrected for GA, major morbidities, and nutritional and respiratory support are similar in males and females at birth (−0.99 and −0.97) and at term-corrected age (−2.02 and −1.97).[30] Therefore, female gender does not appear to be a risk factor for EUGR per se.[30]

Other studies have not seen differences in weight gain between VLBW girls and boys,[32-34] perhaps because the higher morbidity in boys counterbalances their higher growth potential.[35] Hack et al. reported higher increase in weight SDS from term to 8 months in girls and ascribed this finding to the lower morbidity shown by girls during the neonatal period.[36]

PATHOLOGICAL CONDITIONS AND EUGR

Both nutritional and non-nutritional factors contribute to EUGR.[37] However, it is difficult to define the specific and independent role of each factor because most of them are intertwined. Embleton et al. have shown that only 45% of variation in postnatal growth can be attributed to energy intake and protein intake.[3] Non-nutritional factors affecting growth, such as illness severity and stress, are varied and operate across a wide temporal continuum. It is possible that critical illnesses and surgery occurring in preterm neonates alter metabolism and divert proteins and energy from growth to tissue repair.[38]

Moreover, in a recent retrospective study, it has been demonstrated that the influence of critical illnesses on the risk of adverse outcomes and poor growth in extremely low birth weight (ELBW) infants is mediated by early nutrition, particularly by energy intake in the first week of life.[7]

SMALL-FOR-GESTATIONAL-AGE (SGA) INFANTS

We have observed a slight divergence in weight growth up to term between appropriate for gestational age (AGA) and small-for-gestational-age (SGA) babies, suggesting a greater risk of EUGR in SGA babies.[30]

In contrast, Ehrenkranz et al. reported that, from birth to discharge, VLBW infants of the same birth weight grow faster if they are SGA;[33] however, this finding could be ascribed to the confounding effects of GA and GA-related morbidities. It is of note that, in several studies, the weight growth impairment in SGA VLBW infants has been observed to persist even after term.[36,39,40]

Lower postnatal weight loss and shorter time required to regain birth weight have been reported in SGA VLBW infants[33] and in SGA ELBW infants.[32] But Diekmann et al.[32] observed that the growth curves of AGA and SGA ELBW infants diverge between 15 and 98 days of life, due to slightly slower growth velocity of SGA infants, and Radmacher et al. noted that SGA ELBW infants have significantly higher incidence of EUGR at discharge.[17]

The analysis of growth kinetics is revealing. The weight gain of SGA is initially similar to that of AGA infants.[41] However, between 4 and 26 weeks of age, weight gain is slower in SGA infants. After 26 weeks of age, through to 104 weeks, the growth rates of the two groups are virtually identical. The largest differences in growth rate occur between the 2nd and 4th months of life.[41] This implies that there is a critical period of postnatal age, when SGA babies grow more slowly. This is not immediately after birth when infants might be expected to be sicker and less stable, but begins 4 to 8 weeks later. The growth impairment that occurs in this period is still apparent at 2 years of age.[41] This may suggest either an intrinsic lower growth potential, or a persistent postnatal effect of the growth restriction experienced *in utero*. This difference in growth velocity emerges during a period when, according to Boehm,[42] an improvement of the ability to utilize or metabolize proteins occurs in preterm SGA; this fact should be considered when planning more appropriate nutritional strategies.

Bronchopulmonary Dysplasia (BPD)

Failure to thrive is frequent in bronchopulmonary dysplasia (BPD) infants.[3,43] Such growth failure is multifactorial. Among the various causes, increased energy expenditure consequent to the shunting of energy toward respiratory needs, and suboptimal nutritional intake including fluid restriction play a major role.[44,45]

Further difficulties in nutritional management of these infants, for example due to swallowing dysfunction of gastro-esophageal reflux, may also worsen BPD by compromising lung growth.[44,45]

Hypoxia per se can be related to growth failure in BPD infants. The mechanism responsible for the effect of oxygen on growth is not precisely known. However, animal studies have documented decreased protein synthesis rates and DNA synthesis under experimental conditions of hypoxia.[46,47]

Medications such as methylxanthines, β-sympathomimetics, and steroids can interfere with growth by increasing energy expenditure.[44] Dexamethasone administration produces a state of protein catabolism, and numerous animal and human studies have confirmed both transient and long-term negative effects of steroids on growth.[44,45]

We have examined the effect of BPD in a cohort of Italian VLBW infants (Figure 3.3).[30] The growth pattern of the BPD group is interesting. The group that will develop BPD is more preterm and appears at first to be relatively better grown *in utero*. However, the large differences in birth weight disappear after adjusting for gestational age and the other covariates, indicating that most of this difference depends on the difference in gestational age, which emerges as the most important risk factor for BPD. During the neonatal period, the adjusted difference in growth pattern between the two groups is negligible; therefore, the growth deficit during the first month, reported in neonates who will develop BPD, is likely due to inadequate nutrition as a consequence of major morbidities (Figure 3.3).[30] Subsequently, babies with BPD suffer from a more severe EUGR and their growth impairment increases through the first year, mainly because of the lower growth velocity. The nutritional strategies required to contrast such a complex impairment should consider this critical period (from the second to fourth month) when most of the growth impairment in BPD neonates occurs.[30]

To date, few evidence-based recommendations exist for the nutritional management of infants with BPD. However, early enteral feeding[48] as well as a higher intake

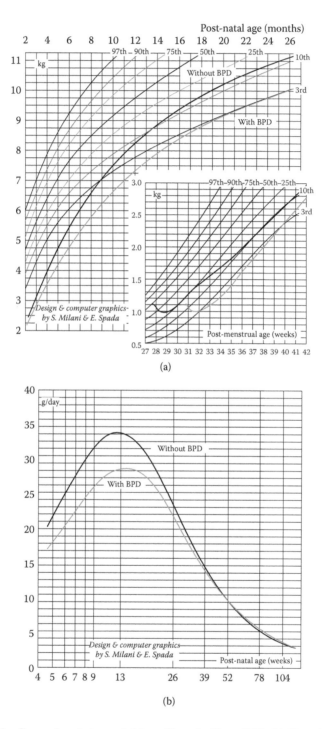

FIGURE 3.3 Comparison between babies with and without BPD. (a) Growth curves. (b) Weight velocity curves (log scale). (Reproduced from Reference 30, with permission.)

of proteins and calories has been suggested to reduce EUGR and to decrease the incidence of BPD.[22,44,48]

SEPSIS

Some studies have shown an association between neonatal infections and EUGR in preterm infants,[17,49] but the precise responsible mechanisms for this growth impairment have not yet been clarified. Studies in adults have shown that the metabolic response to sepsis is characterized by hypermetabolism and by increased tissue catabolism.[38,50] In neonates with sepsis, there are increases in oxygen consumption and a negative effect on nitrogen balance, proportional to the severity of illness.[51] Moreover, sepsis has been reported to be associated with gastrointestinal symptoms, that is, anorexia, vomiting, and abdominal distention, which can contribute to reduce nutrient intake and EUGR.[52]

OTHER MEDICAL CONDITIONS

Many other morbidities can be involved in the pathogenesis of EUGR, such as respiratory disorders, neurological complications (i.e., severe intraventricular hemorrhage or periventricular leukomalacia), necrotizing enterocolitis, kidney failure, and any condition requiring surgery (i.e., patent ductus arteriosus). However, the role of most morbidities in the etiology of EUGR has not been yet precisely defined.

NUTRITION AND EUGR

Although not all variations in growth can be attributed to nutrient intakes, insufficient nutritional support is certainly one of the most important factors to be considered in the etiology of EUGR, and it may even be the factor that explains the poor growth of critically ill patients.[7]

Embleton et al. reported a large cumulative deficit in energy and protein intakes in preterm infants during the first weeks of life.[3] These deficits explained approximately one-half of the variability in in-hospital growth.[3]

In recent years, the recommended range of protein and energy supplies for preterm infants has been increased, for which the term "aggressive nutrition" has become widely used.[53–57] The aim of this approach is to prevent a catabolic state in the first few days after birth and later to ensure appropriate growth.[58] Some of these approaches have been shown to improve short-term growth outcomes[53,57,59,60] and may reduce the rate of EUGR at 36 weeks corrected age[59] or at hospital discharge.[54]

Given the heterogeneity of these newborns and the complexity of their morbidities, optimal nutrition strategies for preterm infants are still debated. Nevertheless, several studies reported that aggressive regimens of early parenteral and enteral nutritional support can be safely provided to critically ill VLBW infants and that the use of these regimens is associated with improved growth, without an increased risk of adverse clinical outcomes.[14,61,62]

As regards parenteral nutrition, studies confirmed that preterm infants who received parenteral nutrition enriched with higher supplies of energy and proteins soon after birth show an improvement of postnatal growth and a reduction in the cumulative deficits of both energy and protein.[63-65]

However, various questions still have not been solved. For instance, the time of the initiation of parenteral lipid infusion to VLBW infants varies widely among different neonatal intensive care units (NICUs). A recent review showed that the addition of lipids within the first 2 days of life in VLBW infants appears to be safe and well tolerated; however, according to Vlaardingerbroek et al. this treatment or the type of lipid emulsion did not have any beneficial effect on growth.[66]

As for enteral nutrition, early postnatal feeding with small amounts of human milk or formula and the rapid advancement of enteral feeding[8] can decrease the incidence of EUGR.[27,67]

Human milk, adequately fortified, is the best choice for feeding of preterm infants.[62,68-71]

However, according to current standard methods, infants fed with fortified human milk show a consistently lower postnatal growth when compared with infants receiving apparently isocaloric volumes of preterm formula. This fact appears mainly due to inadequate protein intake as a consequence of the wide inter-individual variability of the protein content in human milk.[71-75]

To deal with this problem, two different approaches have been suggested:

1. Standardized feeding regimen using new fortifiers with protein content higher than conventional human milk fortifiers.[47,76] New fortifiers have been shown to improve growth in weight,[47,76] length,[47,76] and head circumference,[76] thereby reducing EUGR.
2. Individualized fortification. Currently, two methods have been proposed: the first, "targeted fortification," is depending on analyses of human milk composition; the second, "adjustable fortification," is depending on the metabolic response of each infant.[62,75,77,78]

A combination of these two methods, based on the evaluation of growth and metabolic parameters of preterm infants, performing human milk analyses and tailoring fortification only when growth or blood urea nitrogen deviate from the ranges of normality, has been also suggested.[78]

When human milk is not available, enriched preterm formulas have been developed to meet preterm infants' high nutritional requirements. The optimum composition of these preterm formulas is still debated[79,80]. In 2010, guidelines developed from the European Society of Pediatric Gastroenterology, Hepatology and Nutrition have suggested major changes in protein and energy requirements. These recommendations are useful to define preterm milk formula composition and to optimize nutritional intakes and postnatal growth. As to protein and energy intakes, at present, the use of formula milk with a protein/energy ratio of 3.3 to 3.5 g/100 kcal appears to be safe and could represent a possible choice for these infants.[81] It has been observed that the variation in nutrition explains much of the difference in growth among different NICUs.[37]

Recent reviews have demonstrated that there is still a marked variation in nutritional practices within and among centers in both enteral[82] and parenteral nutrition.[55,67] The standardization of nutritional protocols in NICUs has been shown to allow better growth and a reduction of EUGR during hospital stays.[29,65,78,83]

ENVIRONMENTAL FACTORS AND EUGR

The reduction of stressful environmental stimuli may allow the potential benefits of nutritional strategies to be realized. In animals, early environmental stressors have been shown to reduce body weight gain.[84,85] Reduced weight gain has also been reported in rat pups exposed to repetitive pain in the first seven days of life.[86] A recent study on human preterm neonates has shown that procedural pain in the NICU was associated with decreased early postnatal body weight and head growth, independently of other medical confounders.[87] These observations suggest that appropriate nursing care and a reduction of stressful stimuli may have a positive influence on incidence and severity of EUGR.

SYSTEM FACTORS AND EUGR

Embleton et al.[3] reported a cumulative deficit in energy and protein intakes in preterm infants during the first weeks of life. They calculated the difference between the intakes the infant actually received from that recommended. Deficits in energy intake developed rapidly. By the end of the first week of life, infants of GA ≥31weeks had received a mean of 355 kcal/kg less energy than recommended, and those of GA ≤30 weeks, a mean of 406 kcal/kg less. Deficits continued to increase during hospitalization and, by the end of 5 weeks, were, as mean, 382 kcal/kg and 813 kcal/kg in those ≥31 weeks and ≤30 weeks, respectively. Variations in nutrient intake accounted for almost half the variation in growth.

These deficits can be tackled in two ways: (1) ensuring that what is prescribed is the same as what is recommended and (2) ensuring what is ordered is actually given.

Providing prescribers (usually but not always physicians) with clear visual feedback of how closely their nutritional orders correspond to recommended intakes, for example, using a "traffic light" system (see Chapter 12), can help to improve prescribing practices. This leads to significant improvements in nutrient intake and in growth (see Chapter 12).

Ensuring that prescribed intakes are received is difficult. There are multiple reasons why nutrition may be delayed or held; for example, parenteral nutrition infusions cannot be given without intravenous (IV) lines, so if an IV needs replacing, nutrition must be held while this is done. Although it would be possible to account for this by increasing the infusion rate of parenteral nutrition over the next 4 to 6 h or longer, this is time-consuming and rarely done. Enteral feeds may also be given at amounts less than prescribed. For example, during the establishment of oral feeds, if the infant takes "almost all" of a feed by mouth, there may be reluctance to place a gastric tube to give the remaining small amount of feed, or even a reluctance to a gavage tube feeding even if it is present. The effect of this decision on each individual feed may be small, but as we will see later, small systematic changes can make a large difference over time.

As an example, let us imagine a preterm infant who is enteral fed and grows along the 50th percentile line of 2003 Fenton growth curves[88] and who is prescribed to receive

120 kcal/kg/d. Each day, on rounds, the feeding prescription is written, based on the infant's reported weight. However, in some units the weight is measured by the night shift (often 8 to 12 hours earlier), to be ready to be presented by the day shift on rounds. The weight used for calculations is therefore between 12 hours out-of-date (immediately after rounds) and 36 hours out-of-date (immediately before rounds the next morning). Figure 3.4 shows the cumulative energy intake of the hypothetical infant if ordered using the actual weight of the baby on rounds, and the dotted line shows the cumulative energy intake if feeds are based on a weight that was measured 12 hours before rounds. The absolute daily error is small, but by 36 weeks post-menstrual age, these small errors have accumulated and reduced the cumulative energy intake by over 100 kcal/kg (Figure 3.4). Furthermore, in some units, feed orders for more stable

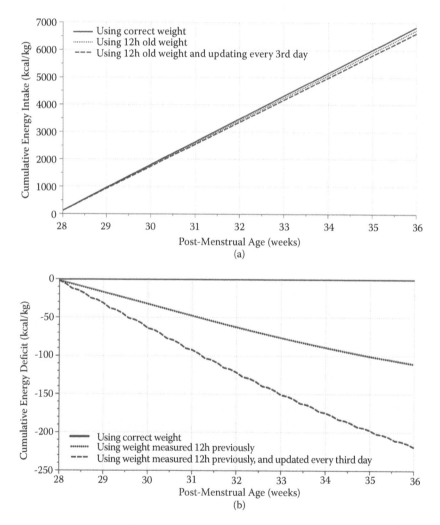

FIGURE 3.4   (a) Cumulative energy intake according to the intake is on the weight immediately before rounds, or 12 h earlier (b), and whether the weight is updated every day or every third day.

"feeder grower" babies are not re-written every day, sometimes only twice a week (for example, every Monday and Thursday). This practice worsens the unplanned reduction in calorie intake, so that by 36 weeks post-menstrual age over 200 kcal/kg less energy have been prescribed than would otherwise be the case.

Other, apparently inconsequential, decisions can also significantly affect nutrient intake. For example, imagine that our hypothetical infant is receiving 24 kcal/oz (80 kcal/dL) formula-fed every 3 hours. The desired energy intake is converted to a volume to be fed every 3 hours. A very common practice would be to round up or round down the calculated amount to the nearest 1 ml. The seeming trivial, probably subconscious, decision can also significantly affect nutrient intake. The difference between rounding up and rounding down leads to a small daily difference in energy intake, but repeated over the entire period between 28 weeks and 36 weeks post-menstrual age equates to a difference of over 200 kcal/kg in the energy prescribed (Figure 3.5).

There are multitudes of other potential "small" decisions that can accumulate and quickly become important. A few milliliters of a feed can easily be lost if feeding syringes contain inadequate overfill to flush the extension tubes, if feeds are left in extension tubes and discarded rather than being flushed to the baby, if the "last few" milliliters of an oral feed are not gavage-fed in a baby working on oral feeds, etc. Similarly, the "occasional" feed being held for procedures or for blood transfusions can lead to surprising large effects if these procedures are common in the infant (which they can be, especially in the sickest infants).

Caregiver behaviors can also reduce the amount of parenteral nutrition: new orders for parenteral nutrition are written in the morning but not started until that

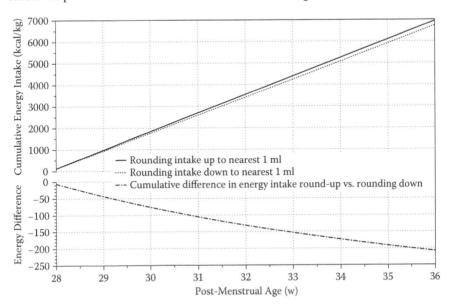

FIGURE 3.5 Cumulative energy deficit according to the intake is on the weight immediately before rounds, or 12 h earlier, and whether the weight is updated every day or every third day.

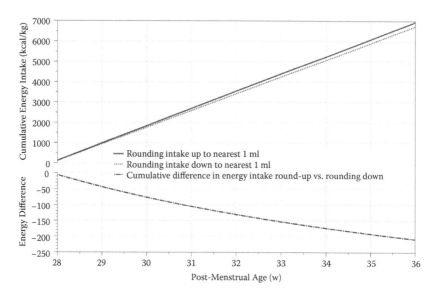

FIGURE 3.6   Cumulative energy intake according to the practice of rounding-up or rounding-down feeding amount (upper portion of figure), and the cumulative difference in energy intake between the two methods of rounding (lower portion of figure).

afternoon or evening, changes in parenteral nutrition rates are delayed until the new bags of parenteral nutrition (TPN) are delivered, the time that parenteral nutrition is held for line changes, reinsertion of IVs, for medication infusions, etc.

When repeated frequently, or even systematically day after day, these "small" or "unimportant" system/process issues can lead to effects that are neither small nor unimportant.

CONCLUSIONS

The causes of EUGR are multiple and varied. Therefore, the strategies to contrast EUGR must take into account nutritional factors, as well as environmental factors and morbidities. Improvements in perinatal care should have reduced the incidence of EUGR, but at present, given the heterogeneity of the published studies it is difficult to detect changes in incidence and severity of EUGR over the years.

The fact is that the ideal model of postnatal growth of preterm infants has not yet been defined. The increased metabolic risk associated with over-nutrition and rapid catch-up growth needs to be balanced against the risk of impaired neurodevelopmental deficit observed in cases of postnatal under-nutrition with concurrent EUGR.[89] The difficult question that remains is how to optimize neurodevelopment and appropriate extrauterine growth in this population. In this sense, the optimal postnatal growth of preterm infants has to be considered not only in quantitative terms (i.e., anthropometry), but also in qualitative terms (i.e., body composition).

What is the future direction? As suggested by Vasu and Modi, "the systematic documentation of nutritional intakes coupled to standardized clinical variables, in powerful electronic database should be promoted as a means to explore variations in practice and outcome, to generate hypotheses and to facilitate clinical trials."[90] Necessarily, such trials have to consider a long-term follow-up evaluating auxological, metabolic, and neurodevelopmental outcomes.

REFERENCES

1. American Academy of Pediatrics–Committee on Nutrition. Nutritional needs of low-birth-weight infants. *Pediatrics* 1985; 75(5): 976–986.
2. Clark RH, Thomas P, Peabody J. Extrauterine growth restriction remains a serious problem in prematurely born neonates. *Pediatrics* 2003; 111(5 Pt 1): 986–990.
3. Embleton NE, Pang N, Cooke RJ. Postnatal malnutrition and growth retardation: an inevitable consequence of current recommendations in preterm infants? *Pediatrics* 2001; 107(2): 270–273.
4. Lemons JA, Bauer CR, Oh W, Korones SB, Papile LA, Stoll BJ, et al. Very low birth weight outcomes of the National Institute of Child health and human development neonatal research network, January 1995 through December 1996. NICHD Neonatal Research Network. *Pediatrics* 2001; 107(1): E1.
5. Martin CR, Brown YF, Ehrenkranz RA, O'Shea TM, Allred EN, Belfort MB, et al. Nutritional practices and growth velocity in the first month of life in extremely premature infants. *Pediatrics* 2009; 124(2): 649–657.
6. Mestan K, Yu Y, Matoba N, Cerda S, Demmin B, Pearson C, et al. Placental inflammatory response is associated with poor neonatal growth: preterm birth cohort study. *Pediatrics* 2010; 125(4): e891–e898.
7. Ehrenkranz RA, Das A, Wrage LA, Poindexter BB, Higgins RD, Stoll BJ, et al. Early nutrition mediates the influence of severity of illness on extremely LBW infants. *Pediatr Res* 2011; 69(6): 522–529.
8. Karagol BS, Zenciroglu A, Okumus N, Polin RA. Randomized controlled trial of slow vs rapid enteral feeding advancements on the clinical outcomes of preterm infants with birth weight 750–1250 g. *JPEN* 2013; 37(2): 223–228.
9. Committee WE. *Physical Status: The Use and Interpretation of Anthropometry.* Geneva, Switzerland: WHO; 1995.
10. Makhoul IR, Awad E, Tamir A, Weintraub Z, Rotschild A, Bader D, et al. Parental and perinatal factors affecting childhood anthropometry of very-low-birth-weight premature infants: a population-based survey. *Acta Paediatr* 2009; 98(6): 963–969.
11. Griffin IJ. Failure to thrive in the NICU graduate. In: Malcolm WF, Ed. *Beyond the NICU: Comprehensive Care of the High-Risk Infant.* New York: McGraw-Hill; 2013.
12. Bithoney WG, Dubowitz H, Egan H. Failure to thrive/growth deficiency. *Pediatr Rev* 1992; 13: 453–460.
13. Cooke RJ, Ainsworth SB, Fenton AC. Postnatal growth retardation: a universal problem in preterm infants. *Arch Dis Child Fetal Neonatal Ed* 2004; 89(5): F428–F430.
14. Franz AR, Pohlandt F, Bode H, Mihatsch WA, Sander S, Kron M, et al. Intrauterine, early neonatal, and postdischarge growth and neurodevelopmental outcome at 5.4 years in extremely preterm infants after intensive neonatal nutritional support. *Pediatrics* 2009; 123(1): e101–e109.
15. Marks KA, Reichman B, Lusky A, Zmora E. Fetal growth and postnatal growth failure in very-low-birthweight infants. *Acta Paediatr* 2006; 95(2): 236–242.

16. Costeloe KL, Hennessy EM, Haider S, Stacey F, Marlow N, Draper ES. Short term outcomes after extreme preterm birth in England: comparison of two birth cohorts in 1995 and 2006 (the EPICure studies). *BMJ* 2012; 345: e7976.

17. Radmacher PG, Looney SW, Rafail ST, Adamkin DH. Prediction of extrauterine growth retardation (EUGR) in VVLBW infants. *J Perinatol* 2003; 23(5): 392–395.

18. Roggero P, Gianni ML, Orsi A, Amato O, Piemontese P, Liotto N, et al. Implementation of nutritional strategies decreases postnatal growth restriction in preterm infants. *PloS One* 2012; 7(12): e51166.

19. Carroll J, Slobodzian R, Steward DK. Extremely low birthweight infants: issues related to growth. *Am J Mat Child Nurs* 2005; 30(5): 312–318; quiz 9–20.

20. Bracewell MA, Hennessy EM, Wolke D, Marlow N. The EPICure study: growth and blood pressure at 6 years of age following extremely preterm birth. *Arch Dis Child Fetal Neo Ed* 2008; 93(2): F108–114.

21. Funkquist EL, Tuvemo T, Jonsson B, Serenius F, Nyqvist K. Preterm appropriate for gestational age infants: size at birth explains subsequent growth. *Acta Paediatr* 2010; 99(12): 1828–1833.

22. Theile AR, Radmacher PG, Anschutz TW, Davis DW, Adamkin DH. Nutritional strategies and growth in extremely low birth weight infants with bronchopulmonary dysplasia over the past 10 years. *J Perinatol* 2012; 32(2): 117–122.

23. Griffin IJ, Cooke RJ. Development of whole body adiposity in preterm infants. *Early Hum Dev* 2012; 88 Suppl 1: S19–24.

24. Johnson MJ, Wootton SA, Leaf AA, Jackson AA. Preterm birth and body composition at term equivalent age: a systematic review and meta-analysis. *Pediatrics* 2012; 130(3): e640–e649.

25. Leitch CA, Ahlrichs J, Karn C, Denne SC. Energy expenditure and energy intake during dexamethasone therapy for chronic lung disease. *Pediatr Res* 1999; 46(1): 109–113.

26. Cooke RJ, Griffin I. Altered body composition in preterm infants at hospital discharge. *Acta Paediatr* 2009; 98(8): 1269–1273.

27. Leaf A, Dorling J, Kempley S, McCormick K, Mannix P, Linsell L, et al. Early or delayed enteral feeding for preterm growth-restricted infants: a randomized trial. *Pediatrics* 2012; 129(5): e1260–e1268.

28. Costa-Orvay JA, Figueras-Aloy J, Romera G, Closa-Monasterolo R, Carbonell-Estrany X. The effects of varying protein and energy intakes on the growth and body composition of very low birth weight infants. *Nutr J* 2011; 10: 140.

29. Rochow N, Fusch G, Muhlinghaus A, Niesytto C, Straube S, Utzig N, et al. A nutritional program to improve outcome of very low birth weight infants. *Clin Nutr* 2012; 31(1): 124–131.

30. Bertino E, Coscia A, Boni L, Rossi C, Martano C, Giuliani F, et al. Weight growth velocity of very low birth weight infants: role of gender, gestational age and major morbidities. *Early Hum Dev* 2009; 85(6): 339–347.

31. Bertino E, Spada E, Occhi L, Coscia A, Giuliani F, Gagliardi L, et al. Neonatal anthropometric charts: the Italian neonatal study compared with other European studies. *J Pediatr Gastroenterol Nutr* 2010; 51(3): 353–361.

32. Diekmann M, Genzel-Boroviczeny O, Zoppelli L, von Poblotzki M. Postnatal growth curves for extremely low birth weight infants with early enteral nutrition. *Eur J Pediatr* 2005; 164(12): 714–723.

33. Ehrenkranz RA, Younes N, Lemons JA, Fanaroff AA, Donovan EF, Wright LL, et al. Longitudinal growth of hospitalized very low birth weight infants. *Pediatrics* 1999; 104(2 Pt 1): 280–289.

34. Guo SS, Roche AF, Chumlea WC, Casey PH, Moore WM. Growth in weight, recumbent length, and head circumference for preterm low-birthweight infants during the first three years of life using gestation-adjusted ages. *Early Hum Dev* 1997; 47(3): 305–325.
35. Stevenson DK, Verter J, Fanaroff AA, Oh W, Ehrenkranz RA, Shankaran S, et al. Sex differences in outcomes of very low birthweight infants: the newborn male disadvantage. *Arch Dis Child Fetal Neo Ed* 2000; 83(3): F182–F185.
36. Hack M, Schluchter M, Cartar L, Rahman M, Cuttler L, Borawski E. Growth of very low birth weight infants to age 20 years. *Pediatrics* 2003; 112(1 Pt 1): e30–e38.
37. Olsen IE, Richardson DK, Schmid CH, Ausman LM, Dwyer JT. Intersite differences in weight growth velocity of extremely premature infants. *Pediatrics* 2002; 110(6): 1125–1132.
38. McHoney M, Eaton S, Pierro A. Metabolic response to surgery in infants and children. *Eur J Pediatr Surgery* 2009; 19(5): 275–285.
39. Bardin C, Piuze G, Papageorgiou A. Outcome at 5 years of age of SGA and AGA infants born less than 28 weeks of gestation. *Sem Perinatol* 2004; 28(4): 288–294.
40. Jordan IM, Robert A, Francart J, Sann L, Putet G. Growth in extremely low birth weight infants up to three years. *Biol Neonate* 2005; 88(1): 57–65.
41. Bertino E, Coscia A, Mombro M, Boni L, Rossetti G, Fabris C, et al. Postnatal weight increase and growth velocity of very low birthweight infants. *Arch Dis Child Fetal Neo Ed* 2006; 91(5): F349–F356.
42. Boehm G, Teichmann B, Jung K, Moro G. Postnatal development of urea synthesis capacity in preterm infants with intrauterine growth retardation. *Biol Neonate* 1998; 74(1): 1–6.
43. Huysman WA, de Ridder M, de Bruin NC, van Helmond G, Terpstra N, Van Goudoever JB, et al. Growth and body composition in preterm infants with bronchopulmonary dysplasia. *Arch Dis Child Fetal Neo Ed* 2003; 88(1): F46–F51.
44. Biniwale MA, Ehrenkranz RA. The role of nutrition in the prevention and management of bronchopulmonary dysplasia. *Sem Perinatol* 2006; 30(4): 200–208.
45. Reynolds RM, Thureen PJ. Special circumstances: trophic feeds, necrotizing enterocolitis and bronchopulmonary dysplasia. *Sem Fetal Neonatal Med* 2007; 12(1): 64–70.
46. Green LR, Kawagoe Y, Hill DJ, Richardson BS, Han VK. The effect of intermittent umbilical cord occlusion on insulin-like growth factors and their binding proteins in preterm and near-term ovine fetuses. *J Endocrinol* 2000; 166(3): 565–577.
47. Miller J, Makrides M, Gibson RA, McPhee AJ, Stanford TE, Morris S, et al. Effect of increasing protein content of human milk fortifier on growth in preterm infants born at <31 wk gestation: a randomized controlled trial. *Am J Clin Nutr* 2012; 95(3): 648–655.
48. Wemhoner A, Ortner D, Tschirch E, Strasak A, Rudiger M. Nutrition of preterm infants in relation to bronchopulmonary dysplasia. *BMC Pulmonary Med* 2011; 11: 7.
49. Stoll BJ, Hansen NI, Adams-Chapman I, Fanaroff AA, Hintz SR, Vohr B, et al. Neurodevelopmental and growth impairment among extremely low-birth-weight infants with neonatal infection. *JAMA* 2004; 292(19): 2357–2365.
50. Thureen P, Hay WW. *Neonatal Nutrition and Metabolism.* Cambridge: Cambridge University Press; 2006.
51. Mrozek JD, Georgieff MK, Blazar BR, Mammel MC, Schwarzenberg SJ. Effect of sepsis syndrome on neonatal protein and energy metabolism. *J Perinatol* 2000; 20(2): 96–100.
52. Bonocore G, Bracci R, Weindling M. *Neonatology: A Practical Approach to Neonatal Diseases.* Milan, Italy: Springer; 2012.
53. Can E, Bulbul A, Uslu S, Comert S, Bolat F, Nuhoglu A. Effects of aggressive parenteral nutrition on growth and clinical outcome in preterm infants. *Pediatr Int* 2012; 54(6): 869–874.

54. Dinerstein A, Nieto RM, Solana CL, Perez GP, Otheguy LE, Larguia AM. Early and aggressive nutritional strategy (parenteral and enteral) decreases postnatal growth failure in very low birth weight infants. *J Perinatol* 2006; 26(7): 436–442.

55. Ehrenkranz RA. Early, aggressive nutritional management for very low birth weight infants: what is the evidence? *Sem Perinatol* 2007; 31(2): 48–55.

56. Ibrahim HM, Jeroudi MA, Baier RJ, Dhanireddy R, Krouskop RW. Aggressive early total parental nutrition in low-birth-weight infants. *J Perinatol* 2004; 24(8): 482–486.

57. Wilson DC, Cairns P, Halliday HL, Reid M, McClure G, Dodge JA. Randomised controlled trial of an aggressive nutritional regimen in sick very low birthweight infants. *Arch Dis Child Fetal Neo Ed* 1997; 77(1): F4–F11.

58. Ziegler EE, Thureen PJ, Carlson SJ. Aggressive nutrition of the very low birthweight infant. *Clin Perinatol* 2002; 29(2): 225–244.

59. Maggio L, Cota F, Gallini F, Lauriola V, Zecca C, Romagnoli C. Effects of high versus standard early protein intake on growth of extremely low birth weight infants. *J Pediatr Gastroentero Nutr* 2007; 44(1): 124–129.

60. Tan M, Abernethy L, Cooke R. Improving head growth in preterm infants: a randomised controlled trial II: MRI and developmental outcomes in the first year. *Arch Dis Child* 2008; 93(5): F342–F346.

61. Poindexter BB, Langer JC, Dusick AM, Ehrenkranz RA. Early provision of parenteral amino acids in extremely low birth weight infants: relation to growth and neurodevelopmental outcome. *J Pediatr* 2006; 148(3): 300–305.

62. Senterre T, Rigo J. Optimizing early nutritional support based on recent recommendations in VLBW infants and postnatal growth restriction. *J Pediatri Gastroenterol Nutr* 2011; 53(5): 536–542.

63. Riskin A, Shiff Y, Shamir R. Parenteral nutrition in neonatology: to standardize or individualize? *Israel Med Assoc J* 2006; 8(9): 641–645.

64. Eleni-dit-Trolli S, Kermorvant-Duchemin E, Huon C, Mokthari M, Husseini K, Brunet ML, et al. Early individualised parenteral nutrition for preterm infants. *Arch Dis Child Fetal Neo Ed* 2009; 94(2): F152–F153.

65. Senterre T, Rigo J. Reduction in postnatal cumulative nutritional deficit and improvement of growth in extremely preterm infants. *Acta Paediatr* 2012; 101(2): e64–70.

66. Vlaardingerbroek H, Veldhorst MA, Spronk S, van den Akker CH, van Goudoever JB. Parenteral lipid administration to very-low-birth-weight infants: early introduction of lipids and use of new lipid emulsions: a systematic review and meta-analysis. *Am J Clin Nutr* 2012; 96(2): 255–268.

67. Uhing MR, Das UG. Optimizing growth in the preterm infant. *C Perinatol* 2009; 36(1): 165–176.

68. De Curtis M, Rigo J. The nutrition of preterm infants. *Early Hum Dev* 2012; 88 Suppl 1: S5–7.

69. American Academy of Pediatrics–Section on breast-feeding. Breastfeeding and the use of human milk. *Pediatrics* 2012; 129(3): e827–e841.

70. Schanler RJ. Outcomes of human milk-fed premature infants. *Sem Perinatol* 2011; 35(1): 29–33.

71. Schanler RJ, Shulman RJ, Lau C. Feeding strategies for premature infants: beneficial outcomes of feeding fortified human milk versus preterm formula. *Pediatrics* 1999; 103(6 Pt 1): 1150–1157.

72. Carlson SJ, Ziegler EE. Nutrient intakes and growth of very low birth weight infants. *J Perinatol* 1998; 18(4): 252–258.

73. Pieltain C, De Curtis M, Gerard P, Rigo J. Weight gain composition in preterm infants with dual energy X-ray absorptiometry. *Pediatr Res* 2001; 49(1): 120–124.

74. O'Connor DL, Jacobs J, Hall R, Adamkin D, Auestad N, Castillo M, et al. Growth and development of premature infants fed predominantly human milk, predominantly premature infant formula, or a combination of human milk and premature formula. *J Pediatr Gastroenterol Nutr* 2003; 37(4): 437–446.

75. Arslanoglu S, Moro GE, Ziegler EE. Adjustable fortification of human milk fed to preterm infants: does it make a difference? *J Perinatol* 2006; 26(10): 614–621.

76. Moya F, Sisk PM, Walsh KR, Berseth CL. A new liquid human milk fortifier and linear growth in preterm infants. *Pediatrics* 2012; 130(4): e928–e935.

77. Arslanoglu S, Ziegler EE, Moro GE. Donor human milk in preterm infant feeding: evidence and recommendations. *J Perinatal Med* 2010; 38(4): 347–351.

78. Corvaglia L, Aceti A, Paoletti V, Mariani E, Patrono D, Ancora G, et al. Standard fortification of preterm human milk fails to meet recommended protein intake: bedside evaluation by near-infrared-reflectance-analysis. *Early Hum Dev* 2010; 86(4): 237–240.

79. Klein CJ. Nutrient requirements for preterm infant formulas. *J Nutr* 2002; 132(6 Suppl 1): 1395S–1577S.

80. Agostoni C, Buonocore G, Carnielli VP, De Curtis M, Darmaun D, Decsi T, et al. Enteral nutrient supply for preterm infants: commentary from the European Society of Paediatric Gastroenterology, Hepatology and Nutrition Committee on Nutrition. *J Pediatri Gastroenterol Nutr* 2010; 50(1): 85–91.

81. Fanaro S, Ballardini E, Vigi V. Different pre-term formulas for different pre-term infants. *Early Hum Dev* 2010; 86 Suppl 1: 27–31.

82. Klingenberg C, Embleton ND, Jacobs SE, O'Connell LA, Kuschel CA. Enteral feeding practices in very preterm infants: an international survey. *Arch Dis Child Fetal Neo Ed* 2012; 97(1): F56–61.

83. Street JL, Montgomery D, Alder SC, Lambert DK, Gerstmann DR, Christensen RD. Implementing feeding guidelines for NICU patients <2000 g results in less variability in nutrition outcomes. *JPEN* 2006; 30(6): 515–518.

84. Bhatnagar S, Vining C, Iyer V, Kinni V. Changes in hypothalamic-pituitary-adrenal function, body temperature, body weight and food intake with repeated social stress exposure in rats. *J Neuroendocrin* 2006; 18(1): 13–24.

85. Gamallo A, Villanua A, Beato MJ. Body weight gain and food intake alterations in crowd-reared rats. *Physiol Behav* 1986; 36(5): 835–837.

86. Anand KJ, Coskun V, Thrivikraman KV, Nemeroff CB, Plotsky PM. Long-term behavioral effects of repetitive pain in neonatal rat pups. *Physiol Behav* 1999; 66(4): 627–637.

87. Vinall J, Miller SP, Chau V, Brummelte S, Synnes AR, Grunau RE. Neonatal pain in relation to postnatal growth in infants born very preterm. *Pain* 2012; 153(7): 1374–1381.

88. Fenton TR. A new growth chart for preterm babies: Babson and Benda's chart updated with recent data and a new format. *BMC Pediatr* 2003; 3: 13.

89. Wiedmeier JE, Joss-Moore LA, Lane RH, Neu J. Early postnatal nutrition and programming of the preterm neonate. *Nutr Rev* 2011; 69(2): 76–82.

90. Vasu V, Modi N. Assessing the impact of preterm nutrition. *Early Hum Dev* 2007; 83(12): 813–818.

Section I Conclusions

Well-constructed growth references are available to assess the growth of preterm infants (Chapter 1). They clearly show that the growth of preterm infants is much slower than the *in utero* reference, both in the short-term (Chapter 2) and in the long term (Chapter 3). This should not be a surprise. The growth rate of the fetus during the last trimester is more rapid than at any other time in life, and at its peak (in g/d) is almost three times that seen during the adolescent growth spurt (Figure I.1). When fractional growth rates (g/kg/d) are considered, this is even more striking. For much of the third trimester, the fetus gains 15 to 20 g/kg every day. This rate decreases rapidly, and after 2 years of age growth rates are below 1 g/kg/d (Figure I.2).

Growth among preterm infants is typically far lower than this, and *ex utero* growth restriction (EUGR) is the rule rather than the exception. By 36 weeks corrected age, the average weight of preterm infants born at 26 to 27 weeks is approximately 1.8 to 1.9 kg,[1] only 70% of that expected had they continued to grow at *in utero* rates. There is some subsequent catch-up growth in preterm infants after hospital discharge, but the average weights, heights, and head circumferences of former preterm infants remain below their peers through to late childhood and beyond.

We will now consider what, if any, are the long-term consequences of such slow early growth.

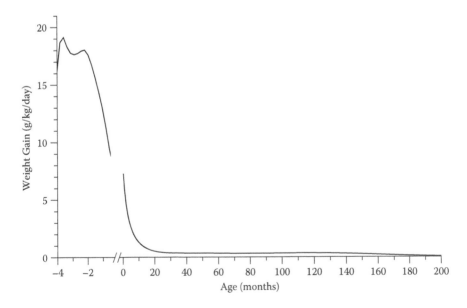

FIGURE I.1 Growth rate in g/day of the female (prenatal data from Reference 2 and postnatal data from Reference 3) from approximately 24 weeks gestation to 200 months.

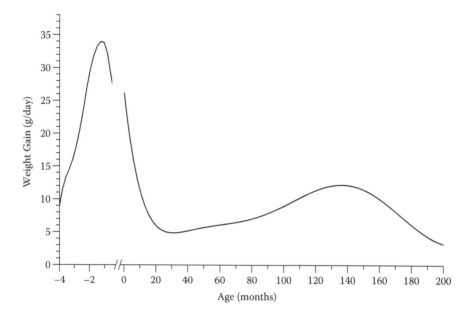

FIGURE I.2 Growth rate in g/kg/day of the female (prenatal data from Reference 2 and postnatal data from Reference 3) from approximately 24 weeks gestation to 200 months.

REFERENCES

1. Ehrenkranz, R.A., Younes, N., Lemons, J.A., et al. Longitudinal growth of hospitalized very low birth weight infants. *Pediatrics* 104: 280–289, 1999.
2. Fenton T.R., Nasser, R., Eliasziw, M., Kim, J.H., Bilan, D., and Sauve, R. Validating the weight gain of preterm infants between the reference growth curve of the fetus and the term infant. *BMC Pediatr.* 13(1): 92, 2013.
3. WHO. The WHO Child Growth Standards. http://www.who.int/childgrowth/standards/en/, 2013.

Section II

The Effects of In Utero and Ex Utero Growth in Term and Preterm Infants

INTRODUCTION

The high incidence of *ex utero* growth restriction seen in preterm infants, and the partial catch-up growth that occurs later should lead us to question the effect this abnormal growth pattern has on long-term outcomes. The so-called *Barker Hypothesis* is now over 30 years old. There is now strong epidemiological data in humans, and experimental data in animal models, linking early growth patterns with the long-term risk of insulin resistance, type II diabetes, hypertension, and coronary heart disease. In this section, we will examine the evidence supporting a relationship between *in utero* growth and postnatal growth with these metabolic disorders in term infants (Chapter 4), small-for-gestational-age infants (Chapter 4), and large-for-gestational-age infants (Chapter 5). We will also examine the effect of preterm birth, and of *ex utero* growth restriction and subsequent catch-up growth in preterm infants on these outcomes (Chapter 6). Finally, we will assess the effect of *in utero* and *ex utero* growth on cognitive and neurodevelopmental outcomes in term and preterm infants (Chapter 7).

4 Fetal and Postnatal Growth, and the Risks of Metabolic Syndrome in the AGA and SGA Term Infant

Ian J. Griffin

INTRODUCTION

The widespread appreciation that the *in utero* environment may have long-term effects on the risk of adult diseases is now over 30 years old.[1,2] The idea has been called the *Barker hypothesis* or the *fetal (or developmental) origins of adult diseases.*[2–4] It is hypothesized that the fetus has *developmental plasticity*, and that the final phenotype depends on environmental exposure during critical periods.[5] For example, exposure to nutritional restriction *in utero* may shift the phenotype toward one that is better adapted to tolerate lower nutrition intake. These adaptations may be beneficial and increase the survival of the fetus, albeit at reduced body weight. Subsequently, however, this plasticity is lost and those phenotypic changes become fixed or *programmed.*[5] If the individual is now exposed to conditions of nutritional excess, those same adaptations that were advantageous *in utero* may become maladaptive and increase the risk of adult diseases such as coronary heart disease (CHD), type 2 diabetes, and hypertension.

Although it is now widely accepted that the heart attack suffered by an elderly man or the diabetes mellitus affecting his wife may be partly due to events that occurred before they were born, it is informative to review some of the classic cohort studies that have contributed to this understanding, and to other possible explanations for the possible link between poor *in utero* growth and chronic adult diseases.

HERTFORDSHIRE COHORT

In the late 1980s, David Barker and colleagues published the first of a series of papers on a cohort of predominantly human-milk-fed infants born in Hertfordshire between 1911 and 1930. Birth weights had been collected and recorded by the midwife

65

attending the delivery, and the infant's weight and mode of feeding recorded at 1 year of age.[6] Almost 6000 men were identified and their mortality from CHD was determined from centralized records. Of the 5654 men, 1186 had died between age 20 years and age 74 years[6] and death from CHD was related to lower birth weight and to lower weight at age 1 year.[6] The highest-risk population were those in the lowest weight tertile at birth and at age 1 year (Figure 4.1). The authors concluded, "measures that promote prenatal and postnatal growth may reduce deaths from ischaemic heart disease. Promotion of postnatal growth may be especially important in boys who weigh below 7.5 pounds (3.4 kg) at birth."

Subsequently, the authors revisited the cohort and reported cardiovascular mortality in over 15,000 subjects of both genders.[7] This confirmed the inverse relationship between birth weight and premature cardiovascular mortality in both men and women (Figure 4.2).[7] Lower weight at 1 year of age was also a risk factor for cardiac mortality, but only in men (Figure 4.3). The highest-risk groups were males who were light at birth and light at 1 year, and females who were light at birth, but heavy by 17 years of age.[7]

The associations of low birth weight were not limited to cardiovascular mortality. A subgroup of men from the cohort had oral glucose tolerance tests.[8] The odds of having an abnormal glucose tolerance test were inversely related to birth weight, and to weight at age 1 year (Figure 4.4).[8]

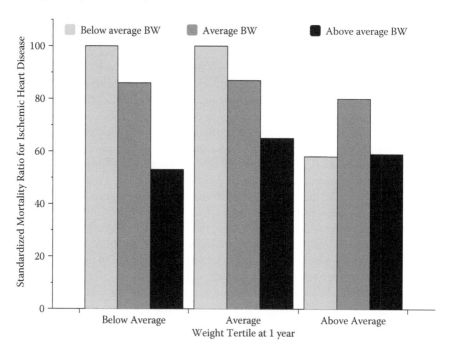

FIGURE 4.1 Standardized mortality ratios for coronary heart disease in men depending on their weight tertile at 1 year of age (below average, average, or above average) and their birth weight (BW) tertile (below average, average, or above average). The highest mortality is seen in men who were below average weight at birth and at 1 year of age. (Data from Reference 6.)

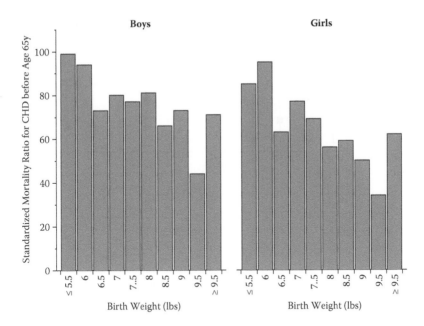

FIGURE 4.2 Standardized mortality ratios for coronary heart disease in males and females depending on their birth weight. Highest mortality rates are seen in those with the lowest birth weight. (Data from Reference 7.)

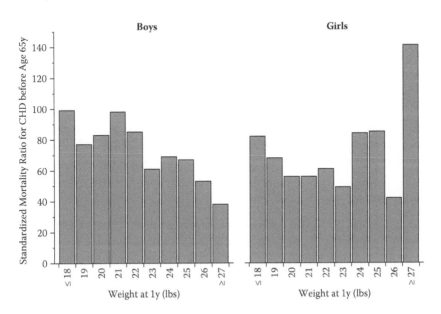

FIGURE 4.3 Standardized mortality ratios for coronary heart disease in males and females depending on their weight at age 1 year. Highest mortality rates in males are seen in those with the lowest weight at 1 year. There is no significant relationship between weight at 1 year and mortality in females. (Data from Reference 7.)

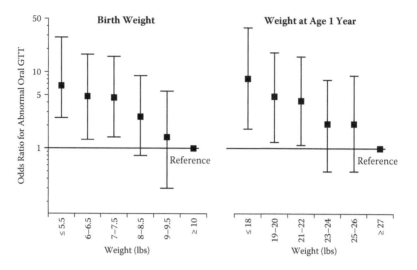

FIGURE 4.4   Odds ratio (and 95% confidence interval) for abnormal glucose tolerance test depending on birth weight and weight at age 1 year. Lower weight at either age is associated with an increased risk for abnormal glucose tolerance. (Data from Reference 8.)

OTHER EARLY RETROSPECTIVE COHORT STUDIES

Similar findings were reported by the authors in unrelated cohorts. For example, systolic blood pressure (BP) in two separate adult cohorts was highest in those born at lower birth weight.[2,9] In 10-year-olds, systolic BP is higher in those with higher current weight. However, within each weight tertile, lower birth weight is associated with higher blood pressure.[2]

POSTNATAL COHORT STUDIES

Although Barker and colleagues were not the first to suggest a relationship between low birth weight and later metabolic or cardiovascular diseases,[10] their results sparked a wave of epidemiological studies examining a variety of other cohorts.

TYPES OF STUDIES

These studies can be divided generally into four main types: (1) retrospective cohort studies, (2) prospective cohort studies, (3) case-control studies that typically compare small-for-gestational-age (SGA) infants to appropriate for gestational age (AGA) infants, and (4) famine studies.

Retrospective Population-Based Cohort Studies

The studies described previously[2,6–9] are typical examples of retrospective population-based, or geographically defined, cohort studies.

In these studies, data is usually collected for administrative or bureaucratic reasons, rather than for research purposes. Many years later, the subjects may be traced and their long-term health outcomes compared to measurements of growth made many years previously. In some cases, the birth details can be combined with other records, such as school records, military conscription records, or centralized records of the cause of death.

These retrospective records can be supplemented by prospectively collected data. For example, a subset of the cohort may be recruited for assessment of body composition, insulin sensitivity, IQ, or biochemical outcomes.

The strengths of such cohorts are that data on thousands, or tens of thousands of subjects may be available. However, the quality control of the historical data is unclear, although in many cases it seems to be very good. In addition, the long-term health outcomes are available without waiting for a prospectively enrolled cohort of newborns to age 60 or 70 years.

The main weaknesses of these designs are that they are observational and unable to prove a cause and effect relationship. The association between poor growth in the first year of life and later mortality from heart disease (for example) may indeed be a causally one, so measures to improve growth during this vulnerable period might reduce the risk of later cardiovascular mortality. However, it is also possible that a separate condition, for example an unfavorable genotype (see later), leads to both slower postnatal growth and to later mortality from heart disease. In this case, interventions that change to the rate of postnatal growth would not be expected to affect later mortality.

The most productive of the retrospective studies are probably the Helsinki Birth Cohort studies,[5,11,12] which are reviewed later.

Prospective Population-Based Cohort Studies

In prospective cohort studies, a large population of pregnant women, or newborn infants, is identified and enrolled. The populations are typically geographically or administratively related—for example, all being born in the same hospital or in the same administrative region of a country. Subjects are followed prospectively and data collected as they age. This allows greater quality control of data collection, but is more burdensome for study participants, so retention rates may fall as patients withdraw their consent for ongoing participation with time. The studies are also more expensive, time consuming, and involved for researchers.

As is the case with retrospective studies, they examine the effects of naturally occurring variability in birth weight and its relationship to subsequent outcomes. They are, therefore, able to identify associations, but cannot prove cause and effect.

An example of such a study is the Avon Longitudinal Study of Parents and Children (ALSPAC),[13,14] which is reviewed later.

Case-Control Studies of SGA Infants

Some of these studies have a prospective, longitudinal design. Subjects born small for gestational age (SGA, cases) and those born appropriate for gestational age (AGA, controls) are recruited at birth, and outcomes assessed prospectively at predetermined intervals. Cases may be matched to controls (e.g., by gender or current body size). These studies are typically much smaller than many cohort studies, but the outcome measures may be more intensive. Other case-control studies are cross-sectional. For example, SGA and AGA infants are recruited based on their attendance at a specific health care facility, or by public enrollment, sometime after birth.

These studies are most useful for assessing whether being SGA is a risk factor for later disease, so that high-risk subjects can be identified earlier and interventions provided. It is not clear, however, how applicable they are to the case of *ex utero* growth restriction in preterm infants (see later).

Famine Studies

These can be considered as "natural experiments." They take advantage of historical events that led to periods of profound nutritional deprivation for identifiable cohorts.[15, 16] Subjects can be recruited as adults and their exposure to famine conditions determined from the date and place of birth, from their own recollection, or from historical records. Subjects with famine exposure can then be compared to controls without famine exposure. In some such famines, for example the Dutch Hungerwinter (see later), the exposure to severe malnutrition was relatively short so the effect of the timing of famine exposure on outcomes can also be examined.[15, 16]

RETROSPECTIVE POPULATION-BASED COHORTS

HELSINKI BIRTH COHORTS

The Helsinki Birth Cohorts are two related population-based cohorts born at the Helsinki University Central Hospital.[11, 12] The first cohort of 7086 individuals was born between 1924 and 1933,[11, 12, 17, 18] and the second cohort of 8760 between 1934 and 1944.[11, 12, 19, 20] In 1971, adults from the cohorts were traced and 92% of the first cohort were found and were still living in Finland, as were 83% of the second cohort.[11] Both cohorts contain birth data and data on childhood growth (more for the second cohort than the first). Individuals have been linked to child welfare records, school records (which included such data as father's occupation, apartment size, number of siblings, diet, etc.), records collected in early adulthood when men presented for military service (which includes anthropometric assessments and standardized cognitive assessments), and national registries of mortality.[11, 12]

Coronary Heart Disease

Small body size at birth is a risk factor for later CHD in both Helsinki cohorts, and in both genders.[17-19, 21-24] In males, thinness at birth (i.e., a low body weight) appears to be more important than being short at birth (i.e., a low birth length),[17, 19] while in females, birth length seems more important than birth weight.[18, 22]

Slower weight gain in the first year of life was also a risk factor for later CHD[19, 25] as was smaller body size at 1 to 2 years of life.[19, 21, 25]

Although smaller body size at age 2 years was generally associated with higher cardiac risk, the effect may be modified by size at birth. For example, in one study, increasing body mass index at 2 years was only associated with cardiac risk in infants born at lower birth weight.[21]

Although more rapid growth in infancy (until 1 to 2 years) reduced the risk of CHD, more rapid growth after 3 years (especially in BMI) increased it.[22] For example, among women in the 1934–1944 cohort, an increase in BMI Z-score between 3 years and 11 years was a significant risk factor for CHD, particularly in the women with lower birth lengths.[22] Similarly, higher BMI at 6 years was associated with CHD, but only in individuals who were thin at birth (Ponderal Index < 26).[19] Lower BMI remained a risk factor in infants who were larger at birth.[19] By 11 years of age, BMI was associated with increased risk especially in those who were already at higher risk due to a lower BMI at 2 years.[21]

Summary of High-Risk Growth Pattern

The growth pattern most associated with an increased risk of CHD from the Helsinki cohorts is one of:

- Low body size at birth (especially weight in males, and length in females)
- Slow growth during the first 1 to 2 years
- Small body size (especially BMI) at 2 years
- Rapid growth (especially BMI) between 3 and 11 years

Obesity

In both the 1924–1933[26] and the 1934–1944[27] cohorts, approximately one-third of adults were obese (based on BMI), and *larger* body size at birth was associated with a higher adult BMI. In males, both birth weight[26,27] and birth ponderal index[26,27] were positively associated with adult BMI, while in females only birth ponderal index was associated with adult BMI.[27] As subjects progressed through infancy and childhood, the positive association between size (either the ponderal index or the BMI) and the incidence of adult obesity (based on adult BMI) increased (Figure 4.5).[27]

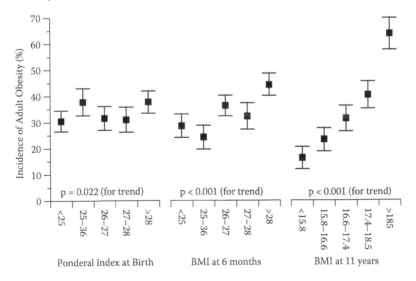

FIGURE 4.5 Incidence of obesity (percent, and 95% confidence interval) depending on ponderal index at birth (left panel), BMI at 6 months (middle panel), and 11 years (right panel). The effect of body size (PI or BMI) increases at increasing age. (Date from Reference 27.)

The relationship between birth size and adult CHD, and between birth size and adult obesity (based on the BMI) is, therefore, very different. However, BMI is not an ideal proxy for body adiposity or for percentage body fat.

Yliharsila et al.[28] recruited over 2000 subjects from the 1934–1944 cohort at age 56 to 70 years and assessed their weight, height, and BMI, and their body composition using bioelectrical impedance.[28] Consistent with prior reports,[26, 27] higher body size at birth (in this case birth weight) was associated with a higher adult BMI in males, and less significantly in females as well. However, higher birth weight was associated with a greater lean body mass in adulthood. In males, each additional 1 kg birth weight equated to an additional 4.1 kg of adult lean mass; in females, there was an additional 2.9 kg of adult lean mass for each additional 1 kg birth weight.[28] Fat mass also increased with higher birth weight in males, but not in females.[28] The result was a significant decrease in percentage body fat as birth weight increased (Figure 4.6).[28]

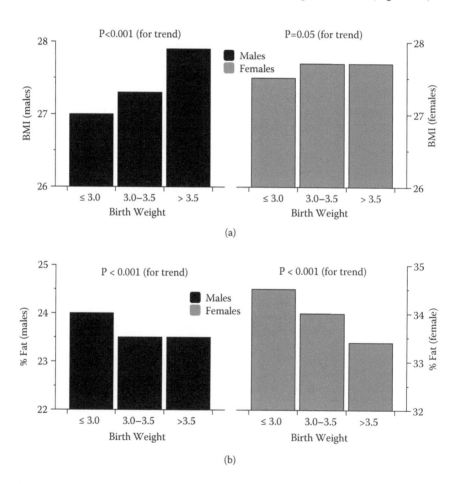

FIGURE 4.6 Effect on birth weight on the adult BMI (A, upper panel) and percentage body fat (B, lower panel) in males and females. Increasing birth weight is associated with higher adult BMI but lower adult percentage body fat. (Data from Reference 28.)

Summary of High-Risk Growth Pattern

The growth pattern most associated with increased obesity (based on adult BMI) from the Helsinki cohorts is one of:

- Higher body size at birth
- Higher body size after 6 months of age and throughout childhood

Type 2 Diabetes

In both cohorts, small size at birth (either weight, length, or ponderal index) and small placental size were associated with increased risk of type 2 diabetes.[24, 29] Each 1 kg fall in birth weight increased the odds ratio for the development of types II diabetes by 38% (95% confidence interval 15% to 66%).[29] The effect of birth weight appeared to be due to an increase in insulin resistance and a decrease in insulin secretion.[30] These findings are consistent with other retrospective cohorts born in the 1920s.[31]

Slower growth in the first 2 years was a significant risk factor for the development of type 2 diabetes.[32] Slower growth during the first 6 months of life appears to be particularly detrimental,[32] growth between 6 months and 12 months was less important, and growth between 12 months and 24 months was least important of all.[32] The effect of growth rate during the first 24 months was most significant for subjects with the lowest birth weight (i.e., at the highest initial risk of type 2 diabetes).[32]

Although slower infantile growth was a risk factor for type 2 diabetes,[32] more *rapid* growth in childhood also increased the risk of type 2 diabetes.[32] In the 1924–1933 cohort, a 1-SD gain in weight Z-score between 7 and 15 years of age was associated with an odds ratio for the development of type 2 diabetes of 1.39 (95% confidence interval 1.21 to 1.61),[29] and a similar effect has been seen in the 1934–1944 cohort.[32] The effect of rapid childhood growth is more marked in those with lower birth weights.[29, 32] For example, if birth weight was less than 3 kg, a 1-SD gain in weight Z-score between 7 and 15 years was associated with an odds ratio (OR) of 1.83 (95% confidence interval 1.37 to 2.45) for the development of diabetes,[29] compared to an odds ratio of 1.25 (95% confidence interval 1.06 to 1.48) if birth weight was greater than 3 kg.[29]

In the two cohorts combined, type 2 diabetes, CHD, and hypertension are associated with a smaller body size at birth and during the first year of life, and an increase in BMI Z-score between 3 and 11 years.[24]

BMI usually reaches a nadir in early childhood before steadily increasing. This nadir is called the BMI rebound. An early age of BMI rebound was associated with increased risks of development of type 2 diabetes,[25, 33] as was a higher BMI at age 11 years.[29]

Summary of High-Risk Growth Pattern

The growth pattern most associated with an increased risk of type 2 diabetes from the Helsinki cohorts is one of

- Low body size at birth
- Slow growth during the first 1 to 2 years

- Small body size at 2 years
- Rapid growth starting between 3 and 7 years of age
- An earlier age of BMI (or adiposity) rebound
- Higher body size (BMI) by age 11 years

Hypertension

Once again, small body size at birth was associated with the development of hypertension, and this is true whether birth weight, length, or ponderal index was considered.[34] As seen for CHD and type 2 diabetes, slower size during the first 1 to 2 years of life, and accelerated growth between 3 and 11 years were risk factors,[24] particularly if subjects were above average size by 8 years of age.[20]

Summary of High-Risk Growth Pattern

The growth pattern most associated with an increased risk of hypertension from the Helsinki cohorts is one of

- Low body size at birth
- Slow growth during the first 1 to 2 years
- Small body size at 2 years
- Rapid growth starting after 3 years

Mortality

Both greater birth weight and greater birth length are significantly associated with lower mortality prior to the age of 55 years in males and females[35] (Table 4.1). The only beneficial effect of lower birth weight on mortality was a significantly reduced mortality from cancer.[35] Mortality is also associated with weight at 1 year of age, and this effect is more significant that the effect of birth weight[36] (Figure 4.7).

Cognition

Raikkonen et al.[37] examined the results of standardized cognitive scores in men aged 20 years. Three separate scales were measured. Higher birth weight and higher birth BMI were associated with significantly higher scores on at least one of the scales.[37] Birth length had no such effect.[37] Greater weight, length, or BMI growth between birth and 6 months, and greater weight, length, or BMI growth between 6 and 24 months were also associated with improved scores.[37]

The same investigators also measured IQ in a subset of this cohort at age 68 years and compared it to measures of body size taken at birth, 2 years, 7 years, 11 years, 20 years, and 68 years.[38] Once again, cognitive scores at age 20 years were directly correlated with body size at birth. Each 1 SD increase in birth weight, birth length, or birth head circumference was associated with a 1 to 1.5 point increase in IQ.[38]

IQ at 68 years was positively associated with weight at birth, 2 years, 7 years, and 20 years, but not 11 years or 68 years; with length or height at birth, 2 years, 20 years, and 68 years (not at 7 years or 11 years); and with ponderal index or BMI at 2 years, 7 years, and 68 years (not at birth, 11 years, or 20 years). Head circumference was

TABLE 4.1

Odds Ratio (95% Confidence Interval) for the Effect of 1 kg Change in Birth Weight or 1 cm Change in Birth Length on All Causes of Mortality at Any Age, All Causes of Mortality before 55 Years, Non-Cardiovascular Mortality, and Mortality from Cancer in Males and Females

	Effect of 1 kg Change in Birth Weight		Effect of 1 cm Change in Birth Length	
	Males	Females	Males	Females
All causes of mortality at any age	1.08	**1.25**	1.01	**1.10**
	(0.96–1.19)	**(1.05–1.49)**	(0.98–1.02)	**(1.05–1.15)**
All causes of mortality before 55 years	**1.23**	**1.45**	**1.05**	**1.15**
	(1.06–1.45)	**(1.09–1.92)**	**(1.01–1.10)**	**(1.08–1.23)**
All causes of mortality after 55 years	0.94	1.16	0.97	**1.06**
	(0.82–1.10)	(0.93–1.45)	(0.83–1.02)	**(1.00–1.12)**
Non-cardiovascular mortality	0.93	**1.25**	0.99	**1.09**
	(0.81–1.06)	**(1.01–1.54)**	(0.95–1.03)	**(1.03–1.15)**
Mortality from cancer	**0.76**	1.09	0.97	1.06
	(0.61–0.95)	(0.82–1.43)	(0.91–1.03)	(0.99–1.14)

Note: Odds ratios significantly different from 1 are shown in bold.
Source: Data from Reference 35.

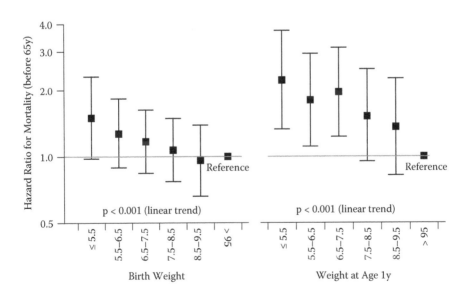

FIGURE 4.7 Hazard ratio (and 95% confidence interval) for mortality before age 65 years depending on birth weight (left panel) and weight at age 1 year (right panel) for males and females. Higher weight at birth and at age 1 year is associated with higher hazard ratios for mortality before age 65 years. (Data from Reference 36.)

only measured at birth and at 68 years; at both time points it was positively associated with IQ at 68 years.[38]

Finally, higher birth weight, length, and head circumference were associated with a reduced decline in test scores between 20 and 68 years. Each 1 SD increase in birth weight, length, or head circumference reduced the decline in cognitive scores by 0.1 SD.

In other words, larger size at birth was associated with improved cognitive scores at 20 years and at 68 years, and with reduced cognitive declines between the ages of 20 years and 68 years.[38]

Other Effects

Lower birth size increased the risk for

- hyperlipidemia,[39]
- thrombotic strokes (birth weight more significant than birth head circumference),[40]
- hemorrhagic strokes (birth head circumference more significant than birth weight),[40] and
- poorer physical function in the elderly.[41]

Similarly, slower growth in the first 2 years of life increased the risk of

- lower non-LDL cholesterol and higher LDL cholesterol,[39]
- strokes,[42] and
- poorer physical function in the elderly.[41]

Interactions between Growth and Other Risk Factors

High-risk growth patterns may have their largest impact in combination with other risk factors for CHD, including socioeconomic, dietary, or behavioral risk factors.

Social Factors

Men in the 1924–1933 cohort were at increased risk of CHD if they were of lower social class and this effect was most marked in men who were thin at birth.[43] A similar interaction was seen with ponderal index at birth and household income (Figure 4.8).[43] Lower social class also worsened the adverse effect a rapid weight gain between 1 and 12 years had on CHD risk.[43] Unmarried men have a higher risk of CHD, but this is only seen in males with lower birth weight.[44]

Social class also modifies the risk of hypertension in men in the 1934–1944 cohort. Lower birth weight significantly increased the incidence of hypertension, but this effect was only seen in those of lower social class and not in those of higher social class.[20] Conversely, higher IQ reduced later mortality in the 1934–1944 cohort. However, this effect was only seen in higher-social-class men and not in lower-social-class men.[45] Men with increased risk of CHD or hypertension due to small size at birth were therefore most affected by adverse social risk factors.[20, 43–45]

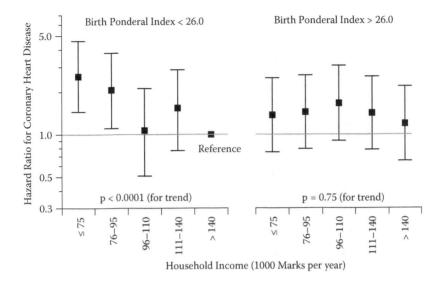

FIGURE 4.8 Effect of household income of hazard ratio for coronary heart disease (and 95% confidence interval) in subjects with a ponderal index at birth <26 (left panel) or >26 (right panel). Lower household income is associated with higher risk of coronary heart disease in subjects with low birth PI, but not in those with higher birth PI. (Data from Reference 43.)

Other Factors

Salt intake is known to affect the rates of hypertension, but in the 1934–1944 cohort, salt intake was not correlated with systolic blood pressure at age 62 years.[46] However, in the highest-risk individuals (birth weight < 3.05 kg), a significant positive correlation was seen—1g/day additional salt intake increased systolic blood pressure by an average of 2.5 mmHg.[46] In other words, low birth weight predisposed to the adverse effects of high dietary salt intakes[46] just as it did to adverse social risk factors.[20, 43–45]

Exercise is known to reduce the risk of metabolic syndrome, and adults who were small at birth appear to exercise more than those who were larger at birth.[47] They may also benefit more from the exercise than their higher birth weight peers do. Exercising more than three times a week significantly reduced the risk of type 2 diabetes in subjects born below 3 kg, but has little effect on those born weighing more than 3 kg. Similarly, it benefited those with a lower ponderal index at birth more than those with a higher ponderal index (Figure 4.9).[47]

Summary of High-Risk Growth Pattern from Retrospective Cohort Studies

The Hertfordshire cohort,[6-8] the other early Barker cohorts,[2, 9] and the Helsinki cohort studies[11, 12, 17–25, 29, 32, 34–41, 43] broadly agree that risk factors for a wide range of adult diseases including hypertension, hyperlipidemia, CHD, strokes, type 2 diabetes, mortality, and impaired cognitive function are:

- Small size at birth
- Slow growth between birth and 1 to 2 years

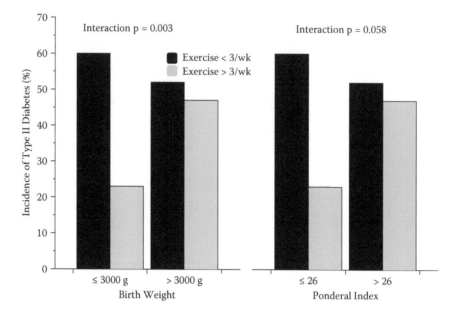

FIGURE 4.9   Effect on exercise (<3/wk or >3/wk) on the incidence of type 2 diabetes in subjects with higher or lower birth weights (left panel), and higher or lower ponderal index at birth (right panel). More exercise reduces the incidence of type 2 diabetes in subjects with low size at birth (weight or ponderal index), but not those with higher weight or ponderal index at birth. (Data from Reference 47.)

- Small body size at 1 to 3 years
- Faster growth after about 3 years of age
- Larger body size in later childhood

These high-risk group patterns are summarized in Figure 4.10.

The exception appears to be obesity, whose risk is increased by larger body size at birth than at any time afterward, and with more rapid postnatal growth.

PROSPECTIVE COHORT STUDIES

THE AVON LONGITUDINAL STUDY OF PREGNANCY AND CHILDHOOD

The Avon Longitudinal Study of Pregnancy and Childhood is an ongoing prospective study. Pregnant women were recruited from a geographically defined area and they and their children were followed longitudinally.[14, 48] Detailed prenatal and postnatal information was collected via questionnaires, and linked to medical records.[14] Physical examination and blood sampling were carried out in a subset.[14] A total of 14,541 pregnant women who delivered infants between April 1, 1991 and December 31, 1992 were enrolled from a socially diverse area of Avon, in the West of England.[13] This represented approximately 85% of the eligible population.[13]

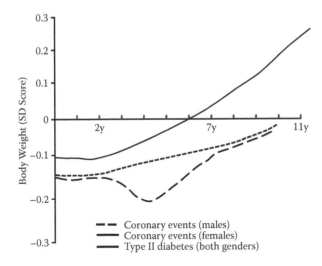

FIGURE 4.10 Diagrammatic representation of high-risk growth pattern associated with adverse coronary events and the development of type 2 diabetes, as described in retrospective cohort studies. (Modified from Reference 21 [coronary events] and Reference 33 [type 2 diabetes].)

The study has several advantages over the Helsinki cohorts including the prospective design, the more intensive early data collection, and early physical examinations and blood samples in a subset of children.

Obesity

The effect of growth rate between birth and 3 years was assessed by dividing the cohort into three groups:

- "Catch-up": weight Z-score increased at least by 0.67 units between birth and 3 years (≈31% of the sample)
- "Catch-down": weight Z-score decreased at least by 0.67 units between birth and 3 years (≈25% of the sample)
- "Normal growth": weight Z-score changed less than 0.67 units between birth and 3 years (≈ 44% of the sample)

The catch-up group had higher weight/height Z-scores and BMI at 2 years and 5 years of age,[49] and higher percentage body fat at 5 years[49] and at 8 years[50] (Figure 4.11).

Cohorts from Germany,[51], the United States,[52] and the Seychelles[53] also reported a positive association between rapid weight gain in the first 1 to 2 years and the later risk of adiposity, as does a recent systematic review.[54]

Insulin Sensitivity

Using a similar catch-up/catch-down/normal classification as used for obesity, Ong et al. demonstrated that more rapid early weight gain was associated with poorer insulin sensitivity and increased insulin secretion[55] (Figure 4.12).

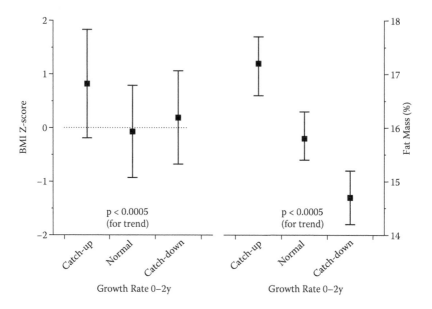

FIGURE 4.11 Effect of growth rate between birth and 2 years of age ("catch-up," "normal," or "catch-down") and BMI Z-score (mean and 95% confidence interval; left panel) and percent fat mass (mean and 95% confidence interval; right panel) at age 5 years. Catch-up growth is associated with higher BMI and higher percentage body fat. (Data from Reference 49.)

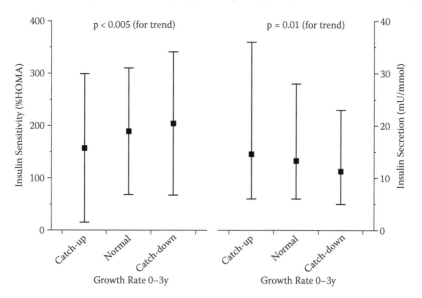

FIGURE 4.12 Effect of growth rate between birth and 3 years of age ("catch-up," "normal," or "catch-down") and insulin sensitivity (%HOMA and 95% confidence interval; left panel) and insulin secretion (mean and 95% confidence interval; right panel). Catch-up growth is associated with increased insulin resistance and reduced insulin secretion. (Data from Reference 55.)

Not all studies agree, however. In a prospective cohort study of almost 1500 subjects from India, adult insulin resistance or diabetes was associated with *lower* BMI at age 2 years of life, an early age of adiposity rebound, and upward percentile crossing *after* age 2 years.[56]

Blood Pressure

Birth weight showed a significant inverse relationship with blood pressure at 3 years[57] and 10 years.[58] The effect is seen in males and in females, but is stronger for systolic blood pressure than for diastolic blood pressure.[57,58]

Faster postnatal weight gain was also associated with higher blood pressure. A 1-kg increase in weight gain between birth and 3 years of age was associated with an increase in systolic blood pressure of 1.6 mmHg and an increase of 0.5 mmHg in diastolic blood pressure.[57] Both infantile (0 to 2 years) and childhood (2 to 10 years) weight gains were significantly positively associated with blood pressure at age 10 years.[58]

Greater height after age 4 months or greater weight-for-height after 3 years was associated with higher systolic blood pressure.[58] Only weight-for-height after 3 years was associated with higher diastolic blood pressure.[58]

Cognition

Larger head circumference at birth and more rapid head circumference growth between 0 and 1 year were associated with higher full-scale IQ, verbal IQ, and performance IQ at 4 years.[59] A 1 SD difference in birth head circumference was associated with a 2.4-point benefit in full-scale IQ, a 1.7-point benefit in verbal IQ, and a 2.5-point benefit in performance IQ.[59] A 1 SD increase in head circumference growth between birth and 1 year was associated with increases of 2.0 points (full-scale IQ, and verbal IQ) and 1.4 points (performance IQ).[59] The rate of head circumference growth between 1 and 4 years had no effect on IQ at 4 years.[59] Effects were less marked at 8 years.[59]

Early growth faltering (between birth and 9 months of age) was associated with a significant reduction in IQ at age 8 years.[60] When this time period was examined in more detail, there was a significant linear association between gain in weight Z-score between 0 and 8 weeks and IQ at 8 years, but not between weight Z-score gain between 8 weeks and 9 months and IQ[60] (Figure 4.13).

In a modern cohort (born in the 1980s) recruited in Helsinki, larger size at birth and faster growth after birth were significantly associated with improved cognitive scores at 4.5 years.[61] For example (Table 4.2), a 1 SD increase in birth weight was associated with a 1.85-point increase in general reasoning and a 3.23-point increase in visual motor score (both significant), but no significant change in verbal or language competences.[61] Growth between birth and 5 months of age appears to be most important than at later periods, and gains in length or head circumference seem more important than gains in weight or BMI.[61] This is broadly consistent with the ALSPAC data showing that early weight gains (birth to 8 weeks) were significantly positively associated with cognitive outcomes, but later growth rates (8 weeks to 9 months) were not.[60]

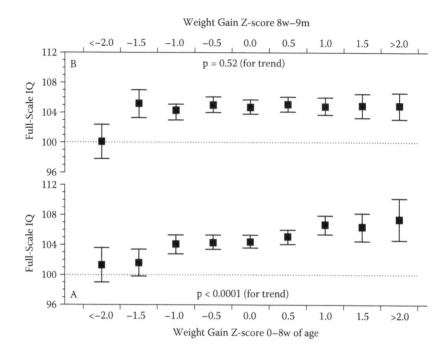

FIGURE 4.13   Effect of growth rate between birth and 8 weeks of age (expressed as change in weight Z-score [A, lower panel]) and 8 weeks and 9 months of age (B, upper panel) on full-scale IQ (mean, 95% confidence interval). Increasing catch-up growth between 0 and 8 weeks, but not between 8 weeks and 9 months is associated with higher full-scale IQ. (Data from Reference 60.)

THE STOCKHOLM WEIGHT DEVELOPMENT STUDY

In the prospective Stockholm Weight Development Study, weight was measured at birth, and at 6 months, 3 years, 6 years, and 17 years of age.[62, 63] The effects of infantile weight gain (between birth and 6 months) and childhood weight gain (between 3 years and 6 years) were examined for a range of measurements of body size, body composition, and metabolic risk (using a cluster metabolic risk score) at age 17.[62,63]

Weight gain during infancy (0–6 months) and weight gain during childhood (3 to 6 years) was positively associated with BMI, waist circumference, absolute fat mass (kg), and relative fat mass (%) at 17 years.[92] In each case, the ß-coefficient was higher for childhood weight gain than for infantile weight gain, suggesting a stronger correlation.[63] Height at age 17 years was significantly associated with infantile but not childhood weight gain.[62]

When the cohort was divided into those who gained weight rapidly (an increase of >0.67 SD), slowly (decrease of >0.67 SD), or normally (Z-score did not change >0.67 SD), two different patterns were seen. Fat mass, waist circumference, and BMI at 17 years were highest in the rapidly growing group, but similar in the other two groups.[62] In contrast, height and fat-free mass were highest in the groups that grew more quickly or grew at a normal rate, and lowest in the group that lost more than

TABLE 4.2

Effect of 1-SD Difference in Body Size (Weight, Length/Height, Head Circumference, and BMI) and Growth Rate (0–5 months, 5–20 months, and 20–56 months) on General Reasoning, Visual-Motor, Verbal Competence, and Language Competency Score

		General Reasoning	Visual Motor	Verbal Competence	Language Competence
Weight	At birth	**1.85**	**3.23**	ns	ns
	0–5 m	**1.08**	**1.93**	ns	ns
	5–20 m	ns	ns	ns	ns
	20–56 m	ns	ns	ns	ns
Length/height	At birth	**0.58**	**0.84**	**0.77**	**0.55**
	0–5 m	ns	ns	ns	ns
	5–20 m	ns	**1.29**	ns	ns
	20–56 m	ns	ns	**1.57**	**1.03**
Head circumference	At birth	**0.78**	**1.34**	**1.47**	ns
	0–5 m	ns	**1.46**	ns	ns
	5–20 m	ns	**1.29**	ns	**1.17**
	20–56 m	ns	ns	ns	ns
BMI	At birth	ns	**0.86**	ns	ns
	0–5 m	**0.97**	**2.20**	ns	ns
	5–20 m	ns	ns	ns	ns
	20–56 m	ns	ns	ns	ns

Note: Significant differences are shown in bold, non-significant differences are shown as ns.
Source: Data from Reference 61.

0.67 SD.[62] The same patterns were seen for weight gain in infancy and for weight gain in childhood.

In other words, the optimum growth pattern between birth and 6 months and between 3 years and 6 years was for subjects to grow along their percentile line. Upward percentile crossing (weight SD-score increasing more than 0.67) was associated with adverse changes in measures of body fatness (BMI, waist circumference, and fat mass). Downward percentile crossing (weight SD decreasing more than 0.67) was associated with adverse changes in height and lean body mass.[62]

More rapid infantile (birth to 6 months) growth was associated with an increase in the clustered metabolic risk at 17 years, and this remained true even adjusting for birth weight Z-score, gestational age, gender, current height, maternal height, and social class (none of which were significant).[63] Higher weight gain between birth and 6 months was also associated with higher waist circumference, higher blood pressure, higher serum triglycerides, higher HDL cholesterol, and a trend toward lower serum insulin (P = 0.08), but no effect on blood glucose.[63]

Summary of Effects of Early Growth from Prospective Cohort Studies

Lower birth weight was associated with:

- No difference in blood pressure at age 3 years[57]
- Lower systolic and diastolic blood pressure at 10 years[58]
- Reduced insulin secretion at 8 years[55]
- Decreased cardiovascular fitness at 8 years[64]
- Increased optimality deviance and retinal tortuosity at 12 years (a possible marker for early endothelial dysfunction)[65]
- Lower full-scale, performance, and verbal IQ at 4 years of age (head circumference)[59]
- No effect on full-scale, performance, and verbal IQ at 8 years of age (head circumference)[59]

Faster growth between birth and 3 years of age was associated with:

- Higher BMI at 5 years and 8 years (49,50,55), and at 17 years[62]
- Higher fat mass (%) at 5 years (49) and 17 years[62]
- Lower insulin sensitivity at 8 years[55]
- Higher systolic and diastolic blood pressure at age 3 years[57]
- Higher systolic blood pressure at 10 years[58]
- Higher full-scale, performance, and verbal IQ at 4 years of age (head circumference growth 0 to 1 year)[59]
- Higher full-scale and performance IQ at 4 years of age (head circumference growth 0 to 1 year)[59]

Larger body size at 3 years was associated with:

- Higher BMI in later childhood[49,50]
- Higher systolic and diastolic blood pressure at age 3 years (height and BMI)[57]

Faster childhood growth (after 3 years) is associated with:

- Higher BMI at 17 years[62]
- Higher fat mass (kg or %) at 17 years[62]

CASE-CONTROL COHORTS

One limitation of the large retrospective or prospective cohort studies is that they contain a relatively small proportion of SGA infants. An alternative study design is to recruit SGA infants and compare them to AGA infants (a case-control design).

In one series of papers from Barcelona, Spain,[66,67] small groups (n = 20–30) of SGA and AGA infants were followed prospectively. The SGA group, as expected, was of significantly lower birth weight than the AGA group (2.1 [SD 0.5] vs. 3.3 kg [SD 0.5], P < 0.001) but of similar gestation age.[66] The SGA caught-up with the AGA group by 2 years of age and the groups were of similar weight, length, and BMI at 2 years, 3 years, and 4 years of age.[66]

At 2 years, the SGA group had significantly lower fasting insulin levels and significantly higher insulin sensitivity than the AGA group.[66] These differences were lost by 3 years of age, and by 4 years of age the situation had reversed—the SGA group now had significantly higher fasting insulin levels and significantly lower insulin sensitivity than the AGA group.[66]

There were no significant differences between groups in lean body mass, percentage body fat, or abdominal fat mass at 2 years or 3 years of age, but by 4 years of age the SGA group had significantly higher percentage body fat, higher abdominal fat mass, and lower lean mass.[66] The major determinant of either abdominal fat mass or percentage body fat in the SGA children at 4 years was the rate of weight gain between 0 and 2 years.[66] Weight gain between 2 and 4 years was significantly related to percentage body fat, but not to abdominal fat mass.[66]

When the cohort was re-studied at age 6 years, the SGA infants now had higher BMI than the AGA infants[67] and greater visceral fat mass by X-ray absorptiometry (DXA).[67] The previous differences in total fat mass, abdominal fat mass, percentage body fat, and fasting insulin were even more marked at 6 years than they had been at age 4 years.[67] In other words, markers of adiposity and insulin resistance continued to diverge between 4 years and 6 years,[67] even though the groups gained similar amounts of weight between 4 years and 6 years.[67]

In a comparison of 32 SGA and 32 AGA children matched for weight, height, and BMI at 6 years of age, the SGA infants had significantly higher fasting insulin, higher subcutaneous fat, higher visceral fat, and higher visceral-to-subcutaneous fat ratio.[68] At 8 years of age, the differences in fasting insulin were maintained but the differences in body composition had diverged further.[69] Between 6 years and 8 years, the SGA children gained approximately 25% less lean mass than the AGA children ($p = 0.01$) and 33% more fat mass ($p < 0.05$).[69] The SGA infants also had a larger increase in BMI between 6 years and 8 years than the AGA infants did.[69]

The effect of catch-up growth among SGA infants has been examined in a number of studies. Soto et al. compared 23 AGA infants and 85 SGA infants.[70] Approximately 75% of the SGA infants had rapid weight gain in the first year of life (an increase in weight Z-score >0.67) and approximately 50% had rapid length gain. At age 1 year, rapid weight gain was associated with a higher BMI, but rapid length gain was not.[70] SGA infants with rapid weight or length gains had higher fasting insulin levels than SGA infants without rapid gains and AGA infants. Rapid length gain was also associated with poorer glucose tolerance.[70]

When this cohort was re-examined at age 3 years[71] the SGA infants still had significantly lower weight, height, and BMI than the AGA infants. Despite this, the SGA infants had higher fasting insulin levels, worse insulin resistance, and lower glucose disposal index (a measure of beta-cell function).[71] Increased weight gain during the first 3 years of life was associated with significantly higher insulin resistance.[71] Of note, this relationship *did not differ whether subjects were SGA or AGA*. In other words, the higher insulin resistance in SGA infants was not due to their SGA-status itself, but was instead due to the more rapid growth rate seen in SGA infants. Therefore, early growth rate may mediate the apparent relationship between

SGA and insulin resistance. When glucose disposal rates were examined in the AGA and SGA infants combined, a higher glucose disposal rate (i.e., improved beta-cell function) was positively associated with both birth weight and postnatal growth rate.[71] Lower birth weight, therefore, reduces glucose disposal rate, but faster postnatal growth (including catch-up growth) improved it.[71]

Ibanez et al. compared 32 AGA infants, 32 SGA infants with catch-up in height, and 24 SGA infants who remained short[72] at approximately 6 to 7 years of age. The short SGA infants had significantly lower fasting insulin, lower insulin resistance, lower fat and lean mass (by DXA), and lower subcutaneous fat mass (by MRI) than the other two groups. The short SGA children also had higher visceral fat mass than the SGA group with catch-up, and higher visceral-to-subcutaneous fat ratio than the AGA infants.[72] Similarly, in a Chinese cohort, SGA infants with catch-up growth had higher fasting insulin and worse insulin resistance at age 6 years than AGA infants, or than SGA infants without catch-up growth.[73]

In a diverse cohort of adults with short stature (SGA n = 25, AGA n = 23) or with normal height (SGA n = 23, AGA n = 26), faster weight gains between 0 and 3 months appear to affect later adiposity and insulin resistance more than growth between 3 and 6 months, 6 and 9 months, or 9 and 12 months.[74] Higher gains in weight Z-score between 0 and 3 months were associated with higher waist circumference, lower insulin sensitivity, higher acute insulin response, higher total-to-HDL cholesterol ratio, and higher serum triglycerides.[74] Growth between 3 and 6 months was positively associated with acute insulin response but not to BMI, percentage body fat, trunk-to-total fat ratio, waist circumference, waist-to-hip ratio, insulin sensitivity, glucose disposal index, serum cholesterol, serum triglycerides, or blood pressure. Growth between 6 to 9 months and 9 to 12 months had no detectable effect on these outcomes.[74]

CASE-CONTROL COHORTS—SUMMARY

Case-control cohorts are consistent in demonstrating that SGA status at birth is associated with improved insulin sensitivity and reduced adiposity in early life, but this situation is soon reversed and SGA infants are at long-term risk of increase adiposity, increased visceral adiposity, and poorer glucose tolerance. More rapid postnatal "catch-up" growth appears to further worsen the situation and increases the risk of both insulin resistance and increased adiposity.

FAMINE STUDIES

Episodes of famine, from failure of harvests, social upheaval, or war, constitute what have been called "natural experiments" in which to study the effect of maternal (and hence fetal) malnutrition.[15] Many such cohorts have been reported, dating from 19th century crop failures in Sweden, to seasonal famines in Bangladesh from 1970 to the 2000s.[15] Two of the more widely studied famines are the Dutch Famine of 1944 (the Hunger Winter) and the Siege of Leningrad (1941–1944), both of which resulted from human actions at the end of World War II.

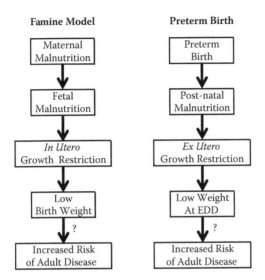

FIGURE 4.14   Conceptual model of the similarities between maternal famine exposure and preterm birth. EDD = expected date of delivery.

Superficially, the famine model is reminiscent of what happens to preterm infants (Figure 4.14). Similar to fetal malnutrition during a famine, preterm birth leads to a reduced body weight at the expected date of delivery (EDD, term corrected age). By comparing subjects exposed and not exposed to famine conditions, we may gain insight into the metabolic risks that preterm babies with *ex utero* growth restriction may be exposed to.

DUTCH FAMINE (THE HUNGER WINTER)

In 1944, toward the end of World War II, large parts of the Netherlands were blockaded by German forces leading to a widespread, severe famine (the Hunger Winter, *Hongerwinter*). As the nutritional insult was relatively short, this has allowed researchers to examine the effects of nutritional deprivation at different stages of gestation as well as at different ages during postnatal life.[5, 15] Several different cohorts have been examined and published that may differ in their degree and duration of famine exposure.[15]

Obesity

One of the first follow-up studies of adults affected by the Hunger Winter prenatally was published in 1976, pre-empting the later work of Barker and colleagues by more than 20 years.[10] Approximately 300,000 men who presented for military service at age 20 years were examined.[10] Rates of obesity depended on the timing of famine exposure, with those exposed in early pregnancy being at *increased* risk of adult obesity, while those exposed later in pregnancy being at *reduced* risk.[10]

Subsequent studies showed that at 50 years of age, women with early gestational famine exposure had increased BMI and waist circumference compared to non-exposed women,[75] but there was no such effect in men.[75] Exposure to famine in mid- or late gestation had no effect in either gender at age 50 years.[75]

Mortality

One closely followed cohort is that born in Amsterdam at the Wilhelmina Gasthuis Hospital, who have had their mortality rates assessed at multiple times.

At age 50 years, mortality rates were 11.5% for those exposed in early pregnancy, 11.2% for those exposed in mid-pregnancy, 14.2% for those exposed in late pregnancy, 15.2% for those exposed postnatally, and 7.2% for those who were not exposed to the famine.[76] However, this difference in mortality was entirely explained by differences in mortality in the first week of life.[76] There were no differences in adult mortality rates depending on famine exposure either at age 50 years[76] or at age 57 years.[77] However, by age 60 to 64 years, women exposed to famine in early pregnancy had significantly increased adult mortality rates than non-exposed subjects.[78] Significant differences were identified both for adult mortality from cancer, and from cardiovascular disease, as well as overall mortality.[78] No differences were apparent in males.[78] The dominant effect on cancer appears to be an increase in breast cancer.[79] Mid- or late pregnancy exposure had no effect on mortality.[78]

Summary of Outcomes at Different Exposure Times

The effect of the Dutch Famine appears to depend on the time of exposure.

Periconceptional exposure is associated with:

- Decreased fertility[16]
- Increased neural tube defects[16]

Exposure during early pregnancy is associated with:

- Increased stillbirths[16]
- Normal birth weight[5]
- Increased mortality in first week of life[16]
- Increased obesity at 19 years[10]
- Adverse blood lipid profile[80]
- Increased CHD[80]
- Schizophrenia[81]
- Personality disorders[81]

Exposure in late pregnancy is associated with:

- Preterm birth[16]
- Low birth weight birth[81]
- Increased mortality in the first week of life[16]
- Reduced obesity at 19 years[10] but no difference at age 50 years[75]
- Poorer glucose tolerance[80–82]
- Increased hypertension[81]

Postnatal exposure is associated with:

- Early menopause[81]
- Increased breast cancer rates[81]

In general, famine exposure during early pregnancy significantly increased still-birth rates, but those who survived were of normal birth weight, had higher early neonatal mortality, and developed later obesity, atherogenic lipid profiles, and CHD.[5, 16, 80] Exposure later in pregnancy increased the risk of preterm birth and low birth weight birth and reduced rates of adult obesity, but was associated with insulin resistance and hypertension as an adult.[16, 80, 81]

LENINGRAD SIEGE

The Siege of Leningrad began on September 8, 1941 and continued until January 27, 1944, a total of 874 days. At least 1.5 million people died and as many as another 1.4 million were evacuated (many of whom also died). The survivors suffered dramatic, profound, and sustained starvation. In contrast to the Dutch Famine, fetuses who were malnourished prenatally usually also suffered prolonged postnatal starvation as well. Catch-up growth was much less common than seen in the Dutch Famine.

One of the first published medical reports of the neonatal effects of the Siege was in 1947.[83] The Siege led to dramatic increases in the stillbirth rate, reduced average birth weight by 500 to 600 g, and greatly increased neonatal mortality (to as high as 32%).[83] Despite this, adults who experienced the Siege prenatally showed no dramatic changes in adult weight, height, or BMI.[84] Nor were blood pressure, glucose tolerance, lipid profiles, or CHD significantly different.[84] It has been speculated that this may be because the prolonged duration of the Siege ($\approx$ 900 days) meant that subjects were exposed pre- and postnatally to starvation, and there was no "mismatching" between *in utero* and postnatal nutritional availability.[84]

Exposure to the Siege and the resultant famine conditions as children *does* have detectable long-term consequences. For example, adult blood pressure is increased with exposure between 6 and 8 years in females, and between 9 and 15 years in males.[85] Mortality from CHD is increased in men exposed between 6 and 8 years of age, or between 9 and 15 years of age.[85]

OTHER FAMINES

In an extensive review of the diverse famine literature, Lumey et al. conclude that the best evidence for an effect of prenatal famine is on adult obesity, glucose intolerance, and schizophrenia.[15]

One confounding effect of all famine studies is that the stillbirth rate is usually high during famine conditions.[15] It is possible that the newborns who survive to be born alive during severe famines are not representative of all fetuses, or of the fetuses born in non-famine conditions. Famine, therefore, may select for a population of fetuses able to withstand nutrition deprivation *in utero*, perhaps through genetic differences. It is possible that the same genotype modifies the later risk of insulin resistance (see "Thrifty Genotype").

The same, of course, may be true of preterm infants as well. Subjects that deliver prematurely may have genotypic differences from those who are not born preterm, and those who survive extremely preterm birth may have genotypic from those who do not. In theory, at least, these differences could be related to differences in long-term outcomes between preterm infants and those born at term.

CONFOUNDING FACTORS IN COHORT STUDIES

In Utero (Fetal) Studies

One major limitation of these studies is the use of birth weight as an assessment of adequacy of the fetal nutritional environment. A neonate may be born below the third percentile at birth for a variety of reasons. For example, the fetus may have (1) suffered a sustained nutritional insult through much or all of pregnancy, (2) suffered a brief nutritional deficiency immediately before birth, (3) suffered a short-term nutritional insult early in pregnancy that they have partially (but incompletely) caught-up by the time of delivery, or (4) been genetically "predetermined" to be below the third percentile and have grown appropriately *in utero* and been born at his or her genetically optimal body size. Some SGA infants, therefore, may be growth restricted, but not all. One way to overcome the difficulty in using body weight as a proxy measure of *in utero* growth is to directly measure growth in the fetus before delivery. As growth is a dynamic process, serial measurements of *in utero* size can identify true fetal growth restriction from an adequate rate of weight gain between two timed assessments.

Birth Size as a Proxy for Fetal Growth

Cross-sectional studies of fetuses with a diagnosis of *in utero* growth restriction (IUGR) have demonstrated decreased fetal fat deposition at 30 to 31 weeks of gestation[86] and at 33 to 34 weeks gestation.[87] However, to really assess the effect of *in utero* growth rates, serial, longitudinal, assessments are required.

Hemachandra et al.[88] used serial ultrasounds to diagnose IUGR, and then measured body size at birth. Fetuses with growth restriction during the third trimester had lower weight and ponderal index at birth.[88] However, fetuses with first trimester growth retardation "caught-up" and had similar body weight to controls at birth[88] (Figure 4.15).

Ay et al. estimated weight of fetuses at 20 weeks of gestation and at 30 weeks of gestation by ultrasound, and measured body weights at birth, 6 weeks, and 6 months postnatal age in the same subjects. Body composition was assessed at 6 months.[89] The association between weight and later measures of adiposity increased with advancing age. Neither estimated fetal weight at 20 weeks or 30 weeks was significantly related to total percent fat, truncal fat percent, or peripheral fat percent at 6 months.[89] However, birth weight was significantly positively associated with total fat percent and peripheral fat percent, and weight at 6 weeks was significantly positively

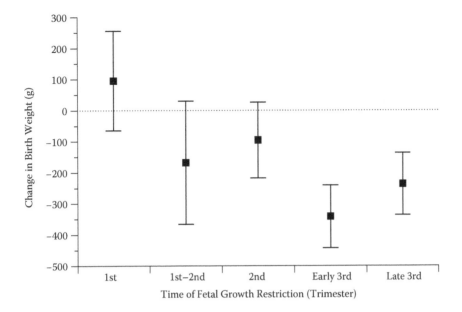

FIGURE 4.15 Effect on birth weight (mean and 95% confidence interval) of fetal growth restriction at different times during gestation. Fetal growth restriction during the third trimester, not at other times, is associated with lower birth weight. (Data from Reference 88.)

correlated with total fat percent, peripheral fat percent, and truncal fat percent.[89] Growth rates between 20 and 30 weeks of gestation were positively correlated with fat mass, lean mass, and percentage fat at 6 months of age. Growth rate between 30 weeks gestation and birth had no such effects. Postnatal growth between birth and 6 weeks, and between 6 weeks and 6 months, were both positively associated with fat mass and fat mass percent, but not with lean mass at 6 months.[89]

Subjects were then classified into those with catch-up growth (an increase in weight Z-score of >0.67 between two sequential measurements), catch-down growth (a fall in weight Z-score of >0.67 between two sequential measurements), and "non-changers" (sequential measurements of weight did not differ by more than 0.67 SD)[89] (similar to that described in the postnatal ALSPAC[49,55] and the Stockholm Weight Development Study[62,63] cohorts). At each time interval (20 to 30 weeks gestation, 30 weeks gestation to term, term to 6 weeks, 6 weeks to 6 months), catch-up growth tended to be associated with higher percentage fat at 6 months of age compared to non-chargers. Catch-down was similarly associated with a lower percentage fat mass at 6 months with the exception of the period between 30 weeks and term. Over this time, both catch-up and catch-down growth were associated with increased body fat percentage at 6 months.[89]

Beltrand et al. used fetal ultrasound examinations at 22, 26, 32, and 36 weeks to identify a cohort of fetuses with and without fetal growth restriction.[90] Postnatal body size was followed at birth, 4 months, and 12 months of age. At birth, the fetal growth-restricted subjects had lower BMI, lower BMI Z-score, lower sum of skin folds, and lower upper arm muscle circumference than the subjects without fetal growth restriction. There were no differences in any of these four outcomes at 4 months or 12 months of age.[90] Among the subjects diagnosed with fetal growth restriction, sum of skin folds at 4 months was significantly associated with change in weight Z-score between 22 weeks and term, with birth weight (p = 0.06), and with change in BMI Z-score between birth and 4 months.[90] Similarly, the sum of skin folds at 12 months in the subjects with fetal growth restriction was significantly associated with change in weight Z-score between 22 weeks and term, with birth weight (p = 0.10) and with change in BMI Z-score between birth and 4 months, and between 4 and 12 months.[90] Significant effects of fetal growth on sum of skin folds at 4 months or at 12 months was not seen for those subjects who had not been diagnosed with fetal growth restriction, but the effects of postnatal changes in BMI Z-score did remain significant.[90]

Summary of Effects of Fetal Growth Rate

Fetal growth during the first 20 weeks of gestation is associated with no effect on birth weight.[88]

Fetal growth rate during the second 20 weeks of gestation may be associated with:

- lower birth weight[88]
- lower BMI, lower BMI Z-score, lower sum of skin folds, and lower upper arm muscle circumference at birth[90]
- lower sum skin folds at 4 and 12 months (only if diagnosed with fetal growth restriction [FGR])[90]
- lower fat mass, lean mass, and percentage body fat at 6 months (only for growth 20 to 30 weeks, not growth 30 weeks to birth)[89]

DIET AND EXERCISE AS CONFOUNDING VARIABLES

Diet and exercise are known to affect the risk of long-term cardiovascular mortality and the risk of type 2 diabetes. However, in the 1934–1944 Helsinki cohort, size at birth was also associated with nutritional intakes in later life.[91] For example, lower ponderal index at birth and lower birth weight are associated with a significantly lower intake of fruits and berries, rye and rye products, a trend toward higher intakes of potatoes and potato products, and a trend toward higher intakes of processed meats in adults.[91]

One can ask why these different food preferences are seen.

- Are they "programmed" by the different nutritional exposures *in utero*?
- Are the results of learned food preferences in childhood reflecting the different foods offered due to differences in factors (social or lifestyle) that were associated with lower body size at birth?
- Are the results of learned food preferences in childhood reflecting the different foods offered to children because they were known to have been small at birth and needed "feeding up"?

The difficulty distinguishing between these mechanisms demonstrates the limitations of even the best observational cohort studies. Whatever the reason, these differences (especially in fruits and berries and in processed meats) could confound the presumed relationship between low size at birth and later cardiovascular or metabolic outcomes.

These differences in types of food consumed are reflected in the intake of specific nutrients. Elderly subjects whose birth weight or birth ponderal index was higher consumed a larger proportion of their total energy intake as sugars, fructose, sucrose, and fiber and a lower proportion as fat, especially as mono-unsaturated fats.[91]

As discussed earlier, the adverse effects of higher salt intakes on hypertension[46] and the beneficial effects of exercise on type 2 diabetes (Figure 4.9)[47] were only seen in subjects in the Helsinki cohort who had smaller body size at birth, not in those with larger body size at birth.

The Helsinki cohort also identified associations between infantile body size and the amount of leisure time physical activity (LTPA).[92] Among 2003 subjects from the 1934–1944 cohort, LTPA at age 57 to 70 years was significantly higher in subjects who were heavier or longer at birth, or heavier at 2 years of age.[92] These effects persisted even when adult BMI was taken into account.[92] Once again, this could confound the apparent association between lower body size at birth or at age 2 years and later development of CHD or type 2 diabetes.

Physical fitness (as measured by the VO_{2max}) in adulthood was unaffected by body size at birth,[93] but was positively associated with height or weight at 2 years.[93] Adult VO_{2max} was also associated with greater height gains between 0 to 2 years and 2 to 7 years, but not between 7 and 11 years, and greater weight gains between 0 to 2 years but not between 2 to 7 years or 7 to 11 years.

Although birth weight does not seem to affect VO_{2max} in the elderly,[93] it may affect resting metabolic rate.[94] From the 1934–1944 Helsinki cohort, 896 elderly men and women had resting energy expenditure assessed.[94] In the women, the resting metabolic rate adjusted for current age and fat-free mass was negatively correlated with birth weight, that is, those of lighter birth weight had higher adjusted resting energy expenditure. In men, the pattern was different, and a U-shaped relationship between birth weight and adjusted resting energy expenditure was seen. Males with the highest or lowest birth weight had the highest adjusted energy expenditure as adults.[94]

CATCH-UP GROWTH OF PRETERM INFANTS

Postnatal growth of preterm infants is known to be poor between birth and the time of hospital discharge or near term-expected age,[95–100] but after hospital discharge some degree of catch-up growth occurs in most preterm infants.[95,96,98–100] Catch-up is largely complete by 2 to 3 years but may continue to a lesser degree throughout the rest of childhood and adolescence.[95,96,98–100]

For example, in one cohort of very low birth weight infants (VLBW, birth weight < 1.5 kg) 20% were below the third percentile for weight at birth, increasing to 54% at term.[95] Subsequent catch-up growth reduced the number below the third percentile to 33% at 8 months and to 8% at 8 years.[95] Similar changes were seen for length-for-age.[95] Between 8 and 20 years there was no further weight or height catch-up in males, but some catch-up in weight, but not height, in females.[96] Catch-up growth is slower in SGA preterm infants than in AGA preterm infants,[95] and at age 8 years approximately 18 to 20% of SGA VLBW infants are below the third percentile for weight or height, while only 6% of AGA VLBW infants are below the 3rd centile.[95]

Catch-up growth may be less complete, or slower, in infants with major morbidities,[98] SGA infants (especially males),[96] and in more preterm infants.[99, 100] For example, Farooqi et al. examined the growth of 246 very preterm (23 to 25 weeks gestation) infants born in Sweden.[101] In this population, growth continued to worsen between term and 3 months corrected age, with decreases noted in both weight and length Z-score.[101] After this, there was steady catch-up growth in weight and length/height until at least 11 years of age. However, almost no further catch-up in head circumference was seen after 3 months corrected age (Figure 4.16).

Late preterm infants (gestational age 32 weeks to 35 weeks 6 days) may also have ongoing growth deficits. They appear to be smaller than their term-born peers until at least 4 years of age[102] and even over this narrow range of gestational ages, more preterm infants seem to grow more slowly.[103]

In summary, the growth pattern of preterm infants is one of:

- *Ex utero* growth restriction after birth
- A high incidence of small body size at discharge and at term-corrected age (both weight and height below the third percentile)
- Increased rates of growth between birth and 2 to 3 years (early catch-up growth)
- Reduced weight, height, head circumference, and BMI at age 2 to 3 years
- Rates of growth after 2 to 3 years are probably also increased, but less so than before age 2 to 3 years

The growth pattern of preterm infants is very reminiscent of the high-risk pattern of growth seen in term infants.[104] If the *in utero* effects in the fetus are applicable to the *ex utero* events in preterm infants, then small body size at term-expected age should increase the risk for CHD, type 2 diabetes, hypertension (based on retrospective cohort, prospective cohort, and case-control studies), and poorer cognitive outcome. More rapid growth during the first 2 to 3 years after term-expected age would be expected to increase the risk of CHD, type 2 diabetes, hypertension, and obesity, but may improve cognitive outcome (based on prospective cohort studies and case-control cohorts).

The obvious implication for neonatologists is to minimize the amount of *ex utero* growth restriction (EUGR) in preterm infants, as this would reduce the risk of both cognitive deficits and long-term adverse metabolic outcomes.

In later chapters, we will review the evidence that catch-up growth in preterm infants affects cognitive (see Chapter 7) or metabolic outcomes (see Chapter 6). However, putting those questions aside for now, if EUGR does develop in preterm infants, one is left with the classic dilemma;[104] does encouraging catch-up growth improve neurodevelopmental outcomes at the cost of metabolic outcomes, or does avoidance of catch-up growth reduce the risk of adult-onset diabetes, hypertension, and CHD, but at the cost of impaired neurodevelopment?

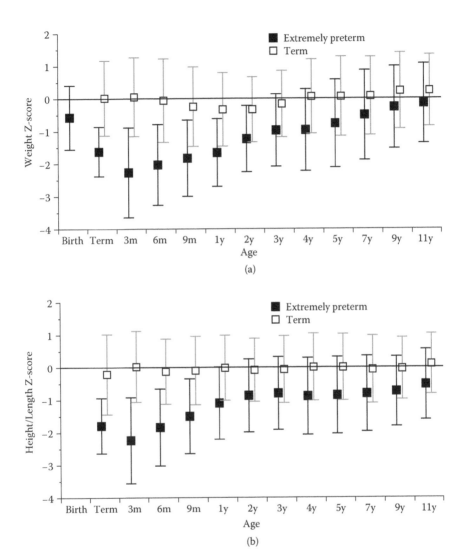

FIGURE 4.16 Comparison between weight Z-score (mean ±1 SD), height/length Z-score, BMI Z-score, and head circumference Z-score in extremely preterm and term infants between birth and 11 years of age. Catch-up growth in weight, length, and BMI occurs between 3 months and 11 years of age, catch-up in head circumference is complete by 8 months of age. (Data from Reference 101.)   *(continued)*

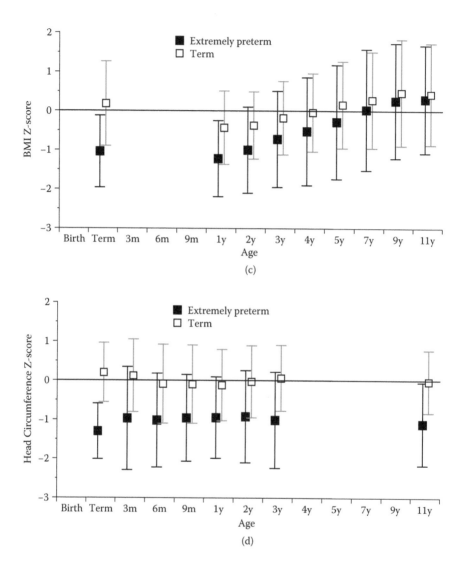

FIGURE 4.16 (CONTINUED)   Comparison between weight Z-score (mean ±1 SD), height/length Z-score, BMI Z-score, and head circumference Z-score in extremely preterm and term infants between birth and 11 years of age. Catch-up growth in weight, length, and BMI occurs between 3 months and 11 years of age, catch-up in head circumference is complete by 8 months of age. (Data from Reference 101.)

THRIFTY PHENOTYPE

The thrifty phenotype hypothesis is a popular explanation for the link between low birth weight or IUGR and later metabolic diseases. It states that the phenotypic development of the fetus is modified by *in utero* exposures including dietary, toxic, and endocrine factors. For example, when a fetus is exposed to malnutrition *in utero*, phenotypic changes occur due to the developmental *plasticity* of the individual at that critical time period. If these changes are adaptive (beneficial) and increase the chance of the fetus surviving to birth, the fetus may be born alive but with low birth weight. After birth, however, the phenotypic changes that developed *in utero* continue (are *programmed*). Postnatally the infant may be exposed to different conditions than existed prenatally, for example nutrient supply may be less limited or even available to excess (i.e., there is *mismatching* between pre- and postnatal conditions). In these new conditions, the previously beneficial adaptations that become programmed *in utero* may become maladaptive and increase the risk of adult diseases such as insulin resistance/diabetes or hypertension. The fetus has therefore traded short-term benefit (survival) for long-term harm (an increased risk of adult-onset diseases).

Animal models support the relationship between nutritional (or other) exposures in critical fetal periods and an effect on long-term postnatal phenotype, and suggest multiple mechanisms that may link the two.[5, 105–109]

As these nutritional insults lead to IUGR, it is an obvious supposition that physical growth of tissues, or of specific cell types, may be partly responsible for the increases in hypertension and diabetes.[105, 106, 108] Decreases in pancreatic beta-cell mass have been reported in animal models of IUGR and could predispose to development of diabetes in later life.[105, 107, 108, 110] Similarly, reductions in nephron number, glomeruli number, or renal size *in utero* are observed in animal models and could predispose to the development of hypertension as animals age.[105, 106, 108, 109] It is also possible that exposure to elevated levels of maternal corticosteroids, which is common in maternal dietary manipulation studies, may either accentuate other effects or be directly response for the change in phenotype.[105, 108]

EPIGENETICS AND FETAL "PROGRAMMING"

Another popular and intensively studied mechanism is *in utero* epigenetic modifications.[111–116] The term *epigenetics* was first used in the 1940s to describe the process by which the environment interacted with the genotype to produce a phenotype.[117, 118] It is now usually defined as "heritable changes in gene expression not attributable to nucleotide sequence variation."[112] There are multiple ways in which the long-term expression of genes can be modified without altering the underlying base sequence. The two most widely studied mechanisms are changes in DNA methylation and histone modifications.[112–114]

DNA Methylation[119]

Cytokine residues within CpG islands in DNA can be enzymatically methylated, which reduces the binding of transcription factors and so reduces expression of the gene.[113] Specific transcription blocking proteins can also bind to the methylated

DNA and further limit gene transcription.[113] In the process of normal development, DNA becomes demethylated in germ cells[112] and methylation patterns become re-established during development, partly in response to *in utero* conditions.[112] DNA methylation patterns are relatively stable during later life, but do diverge in mono-zygotic twins with increasing age and with exposure to different life events.[120] DNA methylation is an attractive and plausible mechanistic explanation for the thrifty phe-notype as it presents the prospect of the fetus as an epigenetic "blank sheet" follow-ing DNA de-methylation, in which *in utero* exposures (including maternal diet) can "write on" during DNA re-methylation, leading to long-lasting, possibly permanent, changes in gene expression.

Histone Modifications[121]

The DNA helix is condensed in nucleosomes where the DNA is wrapped around his-tone proteins. These proteins can be modified by methylation, acetylation, or phos-phorylation. The process is complex and still incompletely understood, but histone modification can either open-up local DNA structure and make genes more assess-able and therefore increase transcription, or decrease gene transcription.[121]

Epigenetically modified genes are typically either imprinted or metastable epial-leles.[112] In imprinted genes, either the maternal or paternal copy of the gene is deacti-vated epigenetically and individuals only express one copy of the gene.[112] For example, genes promoting fetal growth are typically paternal imprinted (the paternal copy is expressed) while those moderating fetal growth are usually maternally imprinted. In metastable epialleles, both copies of the gene are expressed, but one or both haplotypes can be modified epigenetically to alter the level of expression of the gene.[112]

Epigenetic modification has been an active area of research to try to identify mechanisms underlying the thrifty phenotype because of their biological plausibil-ity, the development of high-throughput automated methods of quantifying DNA methylation, and because the agouti mouse provides such a compelling "proof of concept" of the link between *in utero* exposures (including dietary exposures), epi-genetic modifications, and long-term phenotype (including the risk of diabetes).

THE AGOUTI MOUSE

The agouti gene codes for either a black pigment (eumelanin, "a" allele) or a yellow pigment (phaeomelanin, "A" allele) and brief expression of the A allele in hair fol-licles leads to a brown "agouti" coat color in AA or Aa genotypes, rather than the black coat of the aa genotype.[122]

In the agouti viable yellow (Avy/a) mouse, a retrotransposon (IAP) inserted upstream of the agouti promoter leads to ectopic expression of the agouti gene in all tissues, and results in a yellow coat, obesity, adult onset diabetes, and tumor devel-opment.[122] The level of agouti gene expression is affected by methylation of CpG islands in the IAP region. Increased methylation leads to reduced expression of the agouti gene and is seen phenotypically as a darker coat, and reduced rates of obesity and adult onset diabetes. The change in coat color (from yellow to mottled to tan) provides a simple phenotypic marker of the level of DNA methylation (from low to medium to high) and predicts the development of other phenotypic changes such as obesity and diabetes.[122, 123] The agouti gene is therefore an example of a metastable epiallele—epigenetic changes (in this case, DNA methylation) are able to alter the expression of the gene without changes in the nucleotide sequence.[112]

In utero exposures have been shown to affect the agouti phenotype. Maternal BPA treatment decreases agouti gene methylation, increases agouti gene expression, and shifts the phenotypic distribution toward the yellow coat/diabetic end of the spectrum.[123] In contrast, a maternal diet rich in methyl donors (choline, betaine, folate, B_{12}) increases DNA methylation, decreases gene transcription, and pushes the phenotype of offspring toward the brown coat/non-diabetic end of the spectrum.[124] As Avy/a animals pass through multiple generations, the phenotype gradually shifts toward the yellow coat/high-risk phenotype via the maternal line. This trans-generational effect is also prevented by maternal methyl donor supplementation.[125]

Another example of isogenic rodents with obvious changes in phenotype due to a metastable epiallele is the Axin fused mouse. These animals show wide variations in the amounts of tail kinking despite being genetically identical. Once again, the explanation is variable amounts of methylation in a retrotransposon, this time in the $Axin^{fu}$ gene. The degree of tail kinking is inversely correlated with the amount of methylation of the gene.[126] A methyl donor supplemented diet given to the pregnant dams increases DNA methylation of Axin fused gene in the fetuses, reduces gene transcription, and changes the phenotype of the offspring (reducing the amount of tail kinking by 50%).[126]

The agouti mouse provides dramatic "proof of concept" that the epigenome of the offspring is susceptible to modification based on maternal dietary exposures. There is now a large amount of literature on epigenetic modifications and its role in the developmental origin of adult diseases.[115, 116] Intervention shown to lead to epigenetic changes includes maternal or paternal dietary changes (low-protein, low-calorie, or high-fat diets), other exposures during pregnancy (smoke, uterine artery ligation, or toxic exposures), or postnatal dietary restriction or nutritional supplementation (see reviews).[112, 115, 116] Here, we will concentrate on the effect of epigenetic modifications in human cohorts.

EPIGENETIC EFFECTS IN HUMAN COHORTS

The Dutch Famine

The epigenetic effects of exposure to the Dutch famine have been examined in a number of studies.[127–131] Famine exposure has been shown to reduce the methylation of several genes including IGF2[128, 129] (especially at DMR0)[131] and INSIG1 insulin induced gene 1 (INSIG1)[129] and increase the methylation of the leptin gene[129] and the DMR1 region of IGF2.[131] Periconceptional famine exposure may have a larger effect on DNA methylation than exposure in mid- or late pregnancy,[128, 129] but later exposure is also associated with changes in methylation.[129]

Effect on Birth Weight and Later Body Size

Levels of methylation of some genes can affect body size at birth.[132] For example, methylation of LINE-1 and AluYb8 in the placenta is positively associated with birth weight,[133] and decreased methylation of IGF2[134] or increased methylation of leptin DMR[135] increases the incidence of being born SGA.

Methylation levels of exon 1F of the glucocorticoid receptor are similar in SGA and AGA newborns, but are significantly increased in those born LGA.[136] LGA infants may also have increased methylation of a PLAGL1 DMR.[134]

In preterm infants, no differences in methylation of the leptin, INSIG1, or IGF2 genes are seen between those with a birth weight Z-score less than –1 and those with a birth weight Z-score greater than –1.[137]

Lower levels of leptin DMR methylation are associated with higher serum leptin concentrations and increased BMI at 17 months of age,[135] and at 12 months of age, overweight infants have higher levels of H19 methylation, but no differences in IGF2 DMR methylation.[138]

THE THRIFTY GENOTYPE

The thrifty phenotype is not the only possible explanation for the link between low birth weight and insulin resistance in later life. An alternative explanation is that both low birth weight and later development of type 2 diabetes are manifestations of the same insulin-resistant genotype.[139] This has been called the *fetal insulin hypothesis* or the *thrifty genotype*.[139]

Insulin is a potent fetal growth factor and changes in fetal insulin concentration or fetal insulin action are known to affect birth weight.[140] Decreased fetal insulin secretion (e.g., in pancreatic agenesis) or decreased insulin action (e.g., Donohue or Leprechaun syndrome, due to a mutation in the insulin receptor) leads to birth weights well below the fifth percentile for age.[140] Conversely, in the infant of a diabetic mother, maternal hyperglycemia leads to fetal hyperglycemia, fetal hyperinsulinemia, and macrosomia (or large-for-gestational-age).[140] The classic example of a genotype leading both to low birth weight and later diabetes is the glucokinase mutation.

THE GLUCOKINASE MUTATION

Glucokinase is important in glucose sensing and is a rare cause of mono-genic diabetes.[141] Subjects who are heterozygous for the mutation have decreased insulin secretion by about 30%.[140] A father carrying the mutation is at increased risk of development of type 2 diabetes (maturity onset diabetes of the young 2, MODY2) and has a 50% chance of passing the mutation on to his children. A fetus carrying the mutation has decreased insulin secretion *in utero* and as a result is born with a birth weight approximately 500 g less than otherwise expected, and is also at increased risk of later insulin resistance.[141] In twins discordant for the mutation, the affected twin is approximately 500 g lighter than the non-affected twin.[141] Thus, the same mutation causes both low birth weight and later insulin resistance.

If the mother is a carrier of the glucokinase mutation, maternal hyperglycemia (secondary to maternal insulin resistance) occurs.[141] This leads to fetal hyperglycemia and fetal hyperinsulinemia with the result that birth weight is *increased* by 600 g.[141] If both parents carry the mutation, the opposing effects of fetal hyperglycemia and decreased fetal insulin secretion cancel each other out and birth weight is similar to cases where neither parent carries the mutation.[141]

The glucokinase mutation is rare, but data from the Pima Indians (who have a very high rate of diabetes) suggest that this model may have wider applicability.[142] In the Gila River Indian community, paternal diabetes is associated with a small but significant decrease in birth weight (by 78 g).[142] This suggests that the fathers may have some genetic predisposition to lower insulin secretion or action, which increases their risk of diabetes and impairs insulin-stimulated growth in their offspring.[142]

For genetic factors to explain the relationship between birth size and later insulin resistance, one would expect that heritable genetic traits are responsible for both variations in birth size and variations in the incidence of type 2 diabetes, and that some genetic traits are responsible for both such effects.

HERITABILITY OF PHENOTYPIC TRAITS

The heritability of a trait is an estimate of how much of the variation in the trait is explained by heritable genetic factors. It can be estimated by comparing parents and offspring, siblings, or, most classically, twins. For example, if the heights of pairs of monozygotic twins were more closely correlated than height for pairs of dizygotic twins, this would suggest that common genetic factors (which are shared by monozygotic twins) were responsible for some of the variation in height. The greater the difference between pairs of monozygotic twins and pairs of dizygotic twins, the greater the role of genetic factors and the less the role of environmental factors (which are shared to a similar degree by monozygotic and dizygotic twins).

Many measures of body size in adults and children, including weight, height, and BMI, are moderately or highly heritable.[143–145] Heritability of birth weight is low to moderate,[146–148] but heritability of body weight increases considerably within the first 6 to 12 months of life[147–149] and beyond.[145, 146] Heritability of fetal weight in the second trimester is lower than during the third trimester, and lower than the heritability birth weight.[150] It is also lower in preterm than in term infants.[149]

Postnatal growth rates are highly heritable in both term infants between 1 and 6 months, 6 and 12 months, and during childhood,[144, 151] and in preterm infants,[152] but much less heritable for term infants in the first month of life.[151]

There is a much higher than expected concordance rate for the diagnosis of type 2 diabetes in monozygotic twins than expected by chance.[153] If a monozygotic twin had a diagnosis of type 2 diabetes at age 52 to 65 years, 58% of the co-twins also had diabetes, compared to 17% of dizygotic, and 10% expected by chance.[153] However, at earlier ages (42 to 55 years) the concordance rate is similar for mono- and dizygotic twins.[153] Despite this, estimates for the heritability of fasting glucose or fasting insulin levels are variable.[143, 144] The heritability of systolic blood pressure in adults is also moderately high.[143, 154, 155]

POTENTIAL CONFOUNDING GENETIC FACTORS

The glucokinase gene mutation is the best-known potential genetic cause for both lower birth weight and increased risk of insulin resistance, and is an important "proof of concept" for the fetal insulin hypothesis.[140–142] Although there is not clear evidence that such "thrifty genes" are the frequent cause of such an association, several candidate gene mutations and polymorphisms have been described.

INS VNTR

Difference in repeat number in the variable nucleotide tandem repeat region (VNTR) of the insulin (INS) gene have been associated with the development of higher BMI and insulin resistance,[156–158] although this may only occur when transmitted via the paternal line.[157] Polymorphisms within INS-VNTR may also significantly affect birth weight, length, and head circumference,[159, 160] particularly if paternally transmitted.[160]

ACE I/D POLYMORPHISMS

The insertion/deletion (I/D) polymorphism in intron 16 of the angiotensin-converting enzyme (ACE) gene affects adult disease risk. The D allele is associated with an increased risk of diabetes and with increased cardiovascular mortality in subjects with type 2 diabetes from genotype II to ID to DD.[161] In adults, the low-risk I allele is associated with higher birth weight and birth length Z-scores.[162] The high-risk D-allele of the ACE I/D polymorphism may, therefore, present phenotypically as both smaller size at birth and as increased risk of type 2 diabetes.

The same polymorphism may also modify the relationship between small size at birth and later insulin resistance. The low-risk I allele has been shown to improve insulin response and reduce serum glucose during an oral glucose challenge, but only in subjects who were small at birth.[162, 163] The relationship between low birth weight and later glucose intolerance may therefore be reduced by the presence of the D allele.

PPAR-GAMMA

A polymorphism in the PPAR-gamma gene affects the risk of type 2 diabetes. The Pro12Pro variant has increased transcription activity and is associated with poorer insulin sensitivity and a higher risk of type 2 diabetes than the low-risk Pro12Ala allele.[164]

The Pro12Pro mutation has not been directly correlated with birth weight,[165] but higher placental expression of PPAR-gamma (which would be expected in Pro12Pro individuals) is seen in AGA and LGA subjects compared to SGA subjects[166] and PPAR-gamma gene expression does correlate with birth weight.[166]

The main effect of Pro12Pro appears to be permissive. In the presence of the high-risk Pro12Pro mutation, low birth weight is a risk factor for the development of type 2 diabetes.[165] In subjects with the lower risk Pro12Ala variant, birth weight does not affect the risk of type 2 diabetes.[165] The polymorphism may act in a similar way to the ACE I/D polymorphism by modifying the relationship between low birth weight and later insulin resistance.

GLYCOPROTEIN PC-1

Polymorphisms in the PC-1 gene also appear to have a modifying or permissive effect on the relationship between low birth weight and type 2 diabetes.[164]

In subjects from the 1923–1933 Helsinki birth cohort, the 121Q variant (which has greater inhibitory effect on the insulin receptor) is associated with an increased risk of type 2 diabetes or hypertension, but only in those with birth lengths less than 49 cm.[167] In those with birth length greater than 49 cm, the presence or absence of the 121Q variant had no effect on the risk of type 2 diabetes.[167] In the presence of the 121Q variant, insulin resistance is inversely related to birth length. In those without the 121Q variant, birth length had such no effect.[167]

GLUCOCORTICOID RECEPTOR HAPLOTYPES

Several other genetic markers, including the glucocorticoid receptor haplotype 3,[168] may plan a permissive role in the fetal origins of adult disease. In the Helsinki 1924–1933 birth cohort, lower length at birth was associated with impaired glucose tolerance or diabetes, but only if glucocorticoid receptor haplotype 3 was present.[168] Haplotype 3 was associated with significantly higher cortisol levels (375 nmol/L in non-carriers, 392 nmol/L in heterozygotes, and 431 nmol/L in subjects homozygous for haplotype 3, p for trend = 0.05).[168] Carriers of haplotype 3 also had an inverse relationship between length at birth, and adult cortisol levels and free cortisol index (lower birth weight subjects having higher adult cortisol levels and free cortisol index). In subjects who did not carry the type 3 haplotype, length at birth had no effect on cortisol levels or free cortisol index.[168] The same was also seen for impaired glucose tolerance. In carriers of haplotype 3, the incidence of impaired glucose tolerance decreased with increasing birth length from 60% in the lowest length tertile, to 42% in the middle length tertile, to 37% in the highest length tertile (p for trend = 0.0007). In subjects without the type 3 haplotype, the incidence of impaired glucose tolerance was similar in all three birth length tertiles (47%, 55%, and 50%; p for trend = 0.9).[168]

MITOCHONDRIAL BP16189

A polymorphism (T->C) at bp 16189 of mitochondrial DNA has been associated with higher fasting insulin levels in men, even accounting for age and BMI,[169] and it may be expressed phenotypically as both low body size at birth and increase risk of type 2 diabetes.[170]

In subjects with rapid postnatal growth, the bp16189 mutation was associated with lower ponderal index at birth and significantly increased risk of adult type 2 diabetes (OR 5.1 [95% confidence interval 1.2–21.8]).[170] However, in subjects that did not have rapid postnatal growth, the mutation had no effect on either ponderal index at birth or the risk of developing type 2 diabetes.[170]

IGF2/H19

The IGF2/H19 complex is an example of the difficulty in distinguishing genetic and epigenetic effects on gene transcription and fetal programming. The IGF2 and H19 loci are closely related imprinted genes on human chromosome 11 (11p15.5).[171] The IGF2 gene is paternally imprinted, meaning that the maternal copy has been epigenetically silenced and only the paternal copy is transcribed.[172] The H19 gene is maternally imprinted and only the allele inherited from the mother is expressed.[172]

H19 appears to regulate the transcription of IGF2. For example, in mice over-expression of H19 down-regulates IGF2 transcription and leads to reduced birth size.[173] Conversely, under-expression of H19 increases IGF2 transcription and increases size at birth.[173] A similar situation is seen in humans. Beckwith-Wiedermann syndrome is a genetic disorder leading to marked overgrowth of the fetus, large body size at birth, and increased risk of tumor formation. One cause of Beckwith-Wiedermann syndrome is increased methylation of H19 DMR,[171] which leads to decreased H19 transcription and increased IGF2 transcription. The opposite defect, a loss of methylation of H19, leads to fetal growth failure and to Russell-Silver Dwarfism.[171]

In the Avon ALSPAC cohort, a common single nucleotide polymorphism (2992C>T) in the H19 gene of the mother or the offspring was associated with a significant increase in birth weight.[174] The presence of the same SNP in the father had no effect on birth weight,[172, 174] presumably because the paternal inherited allele is silenced in the fetus. The presence of the 2992T allele in the mother was associated with higher cord IGF2 levels and with an increased birth weight even if not transmitted to the offspring.[174] Postnatal growth between birth and 3 years of age was slower in those with the 2992T allele, so that by 3 years of age weight, height, and head circumference were similar in the CC, CT, and TT genotypes,[174] suggesting that this slower postnatal growth rate is to compensate for higher *in utero* growth rates.

Other studies have confirmed that maternally transmitted SNPs in H19 or IGF2 may affect fetal growth[175–177] and this is not due to changes in blood glucose levels in the pregnant women.[176] There is intriguing preliminary evidence that paternally transmitted SNPs may, however, worsen maternal glucose tolerance.[178]

In recent years, the effect of methylation of DMRs in the IGF2 and H19 loci has been the subject of many studies. Decreased IGF2 methylation is associated with increased cord IGF-II.[179] Increased levels of IGF-II in cord blood, in turn, are associated with higher birth weight.[179] Decreased IGF2 methylation also appears to decrease the risk of LBW or SGA birth.[134]

IGF2 methylation appears to be responsive to maternal nutritional status. Subjects exposed to the Dutch Famine have decreased IGF2 methylation at the DMR0 loci, but increased DMR1 methylation.[131] H19 methylation, in contrast, does not affect IGF-II levels[179] or the risk of being overweight at 1 year,[138] and is not affected by exposure to the Dutch Famine.[131] Increased average methylation across IGF2 and H19 combined has no effect on birth weight but is associated with increased subcutaneous adiposity at 17 years, but not with total or visceral adiposity or with BMI.[180]

Indeed, it is probably simplistic to consider DNA methylation as a purely epigenetic event (independent from the underlying DNA base sequence). As DNA methylation occurs at cytosine bases in CpG islands, a polymorphism replacing a C with a T would obviously affect methylation, as it is impossible to methylate a C base that is no longer present .[181] In subjects exposed to the Dutch Famine, several SNPs modify the effect of the famine on DNA methylation.[131] More broadly, it seems that local and distant genetic factors modify DNA methylation throughout the genome.[182–184] These interactions are complex and are an active area of research.

OTHER MUTATIONS

The bp192 mutation of the IGF1 promoter is known to increase circulating IGF-I levels, and affect the risk of CHD, and type 2 diabetes and stroke in adults.[185, 186] It is also associated with increased blood pressure in children.[187] It leads to higher IGF-I levels, and may increase birth weight in subjects either homozygous or heterozygous for the mutation,[185] although data are contradictory,[188] but is associated with reduced postnatal growth rates.[185, 188]

The TNF-alpha 308A/G polymorphism may affect both body size in early life, and the risk of later disease. The GG genotype is associated with lower birth weight and lower birth length.[189] In AGA (but not SGA) subjects, the GG genotype is also associated with higher blood pressure and increased insulin resistance.[189]

Pulizzi et al.[30] examined the effect of nine genes (TCF7L2, HHEX, PPARG, KCNJ11, SLC30A8, IGF2BP2, CDKAL1, CDKN2A/2B, and JAZF1) known to be associated with an increased risk of developing type 2 diabetes. None of the alleles associated with increased risk of diabetes was associated with lower birth weight (and one was associated with higher birth weight).[30] However, the high-risk variants of HHEX, CDKN2A/2B, and JAZF1 (and all nine genes pooled) showed a significant interaction with birth weight; that is, the effect of the genes on the risk of type 2 diabetes depended on the subjects' birth weight.[30] In each case, the high-risk allele had more of an effect on the long-term risk of type 2 diabetes in low birth weight individuals, and less effect on those born at higher birth weight.[30]

GENOTYPE OR PHENOTYPE?

It seems clear that low body size at birth and more rapid postnatal weight gain are risk factors for later insulin resistance, coronary artery disease, and hypertension. Genetic factors are also important, but even in genetically identical individuals, *in utero* growth modifies the risk of later metabolic diseases. For example, in an isogenic rodent model (where all individuals are genetically identical) naturally occurring differences in birth weight (reflecting differences in *in utero* growth) modify the risk of insulin resistance with the highest risk seen in pups of lower birth weight.[190] The same is seen in monozygotic twins (who are also genetically identical).[191] When twins are discordant for a diagnosis of type 2 diabetes, the diabetic twin is more likely to have been born at a lower birth weight than the non-diabetic twin.[191] This is seen also in dizygotic twins.[191]

Just as first suggested by Hattersley,[139] genotypic changes do not appear to be an alternative to that *thrifty phenotype* hypothesis; instead, they appear to be complimentary to it.

We are therefore left with a model (Figure 4.17, A, upper panel) that combines both phenotypic and genetic factors. In response to fetal under-nutrition, a series of phenotypic changes occur (either through epigenetic mechanisms, alterations in tissue size and growth, or by some other mechanism). This phenotype leads to survival at lower birth weight, but at the cost of an increased risk of insulin resistance and adult onset diseases. At the same time, genotypic factors may be at play. They may act to increase the risk of both low birth weight birth and of later insulin resistance. Potential genetic mechanisms that act in this way could include the glucokinase gene mutation, INS VNTR polymorphisms, and the ACE I/D polymorphism. Other genetic factors (e.g., PPAR-gamma Pro12Pro mutation, PC-1 mutation, and glucocorticoid receptor haplotype 3) may modify relationship between low birth weight and final adult phenotype (e.g., type 2 diabetes).

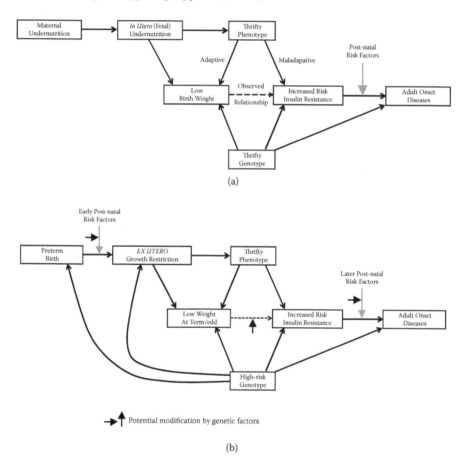

FIGURE 4.17   Conceptual model of the interaction between phenotype and genotype of the relationship between low birth weight, insulin resistance, and adult onset diseases in subjects exposed to *in utero* malnutrition (a, upper panel), and the interaction between phenotype and genotype on the relationship between preterm birth, *ex utero* growth restriction, insulin resistance, and adult onset diseases in subjects exposed to *in utero* malnutrition (b, lower panel).

A similar but more complex mechanism could be at play in preterm infants (Figure 4.17, B, lower panel). Preterm birth leads to *ex utero* growth restriction, the risk of which is modified by a range of early postnatal actors (including nutrition intake, co-morbidities, etc.; see Chapter 3). *Ex utero* growth restriction leads directly to small body size at term-expected age, and may also lead to development of a thrifty phenotype (through changes in tissue growth, epigenetic modifications, or some other mechanism). The thrifty phenotype leads to both reduced body size at term and to an increased risk of insulin resistance in later life. This in turn leads to adult onset diseases (such as type 2 diabetes) although the likelihood of progression may be modified by postnatal factors (such as diet, exercise, and social factors). Genotypic factors may interact with this model at multiple steps. Genetic factors may increase the risk of preterm birth, or reduce postnatal growth rates in infants born preterm; they may affect body size at birth or the risk of insulin resistance (e.g., the glucokinase mutation, or the INS VNTR and ACE I/D polymorphisms). Alternatively, genetic factors may modify the link between body size at birth and the subsequent development of insulin resistance and adult onset diseases (possible examples include the Pro12Pro allele, the 121Q variant of the PC-1 gene, the ACE I/D polymorphisms, and high-risk alleles of HHEX, CDKN2A/B, and JAFK1). Finally, genetic factors may modify the effect of postnatal/environmental exposures on the relationship between preterm birth and *ex utero* growth restriction in preterm infants, or the effect of postnatal factors on risk of developing adult onset diseases due to differences in insulin resistance.

SUMMARY AND CONCLUSIONS

It seems very likely that in term infants, small size at birth is associated with an increase risk of some adult diseases (for example, insulin resistance and type 2 diabetes) and possibly poorer cognitive outcomes. More rapid growth in the first 2 to 3 years of life may also be associated with an increased risk of insulin resistance and type 2 diabetes, but may be associated with improved cognitive outcomes.

The mechanisms linking early growth and long-term outcomes are still unclear, and an active source of investigation. However, it seems likely that *in utero* changes in tissue growth and structure, epigenetic modification of disease-associated genetic loci, and underlying genetic susceptibilities to poor fetal growth, rapid postnatal growth, and long-term insulin resistance, act in combination to result in the high-risk phenotype.

REFERENCES

1. Barker DJP, Ed. *Fetal and Infant Origins of Adult Disease*. London: BMJ Publishing Group; 1992.
2. Barker DJ, Osmond C, Golding J, Kuh D, Wadsworth ME. Growth in utero, blood pressure in childhood and adult life, and mortality from cardiovascular disease. *BMJ* 1989;298:564–567.
3. Barker DJ. Fetal programming of coronary heart disease. *Trends Endocrinol Metab* 2002;13:364–368.

4. Gram IT, Jacobsen BK, Straume B, Arnesen E, Lochen ML, Lund E. Early origin of coronary heart disease. Earlier published work supports the "Barker hypothesis." *BMJ* 1995;310:1468.

5. Calkins K, Devaskar SU. Fetal origins of adult disease. *Curr Probl Pediatr Adolesc Health Care* 2011;41:158–176.

6. Barker DJ, Winter PD, Osmond C, Margetts B, Simmonds SJ. Weight in infancy and death from ischaemic heart disease. *Lancet* 1989;2:577–580.

7. Osmond C, Barker DJ, Winter PD, Fall CH, Simmonds SJ. Early growth and death from cardiovascular disease in women. *BMJ* 1993;307:1519–1524.

8. Hales CN, Barker DJ, Clark PM, et al. Fetal and infant growth and impaired glucose tolerance at age 64. *BMJ* 1991;303:1019–1022.

9. Barker DJ, Bull AR, Osmond C, Simmonds SJ. Fetal and placental size and risk of hypertension in adult life. *BMJ* 1990;301:259–262.

10. Ravelli GP, Stein ZA, Susser MW. Obesity in young men after famine exposure in utero and early infancy. *N Engl J Med* 1976;295:349–353.

11. Eriksson JG, Forsen TJ. Childhood growth and coronary heart disease in later life. *Ann Med* 2002;34:157–161.

12. Eriksson JG. Early growth and adult health outcomes: lessons learned from the Helsinki Birth Cohort Study. *Matern Child Nutr* 2005;1:149–154.

13. Golding J. The Avon Longitudinal Study of Parents and Children (ALSPAC): study design and collaborative opportunities. *Eur J Endocrinol* 2004;151 Suppl 3:U119–123.

14. Golding J, Pembrey M, Jones R. ALSPAC: the Avon Longitudinal Study of Parents and Children. I. Study methodology. *Paediatr Perinat Epidemiol* 2001;15:74–87.

15. Lumey LH, Stein AD, Susser E. Prenatal famine and adult health. *Annu Rev Public Health* 2011;32:237–262.

16. Susser M, Stein Z. Timing in prenatal nutrition: a reprise of the Dutch Famine Study. *Nutr Rev* 1994;52:84–94.

17. Eriksson JG, Forsen T, Tuomilehto J, Winter PD, Osmond C, Barker DJ. Catch-up growth in childhood and death from coronary heart disease: longitudinal study. *BMJ* 1999;318:427–431.

18. Forsen T, Eriksson JG, Tuomilehto J, Osmond C, Barker DJ. Growth in utero and during childhood among women who develop coronary heart disease: longitudinal study. *BMJ* 1999;319:1403–1407.

19. Eriksson JG, Forsen T, Tuomilehto J, Osmond C, Barker DJ. Early growth and coronary heart disease in later life: longitudinal study. *BMJ* 2001;322:949–953.

20. Barker DJ, Forsen T, Eriksson JG, Osmond C. Growth and living conditions in childhood and hypertension in adult life: a longitudinal study. *J Hypertens* 2002;20:1951–1956.

21. Barker DJ, Osmond C, Forsen TJ, Kajantie E, Eriksson JG. Trajectories of growth among children who have coronary events as adults. *N Engl J Med* 2005;353:1802–1809.

22. Forsen T, Osmond C, Eriksson JG, Barker DJ. Growth of girls who later develop coronary heart disease. *Heart* 2004;90:20–24.

23. Forsen TJ, Eriksson JG, Osmond C, Barker DJ. The infant growth of boys who later develop coronary heart disease. *Ann Med* 2004;36:389–392.

24. Barker DJ, Eriksson JG, Forsen T, Osmond C. Fetal origins of adult disease: strength of effects and biological basis. *Int J Epidemiol* 2002;31:1235–1239.

25. Eriksson JG. Early growth and coronary heart disease and type 2 diabetes: findings from the Helsinki Birth Cohort Study (HBCS). *Am J Clin Nutr* 2011;94:1799S–1802S.

26. Eriksson J, Forsen T, Tuomilehto J, Osmond C, Barker D. Size at birth, childhood growth and obesity in adult life. *Int J Obes Relat Metab Disord* 2001;25:735–740.

27. Eriksson J, Forsen T, Osmond C, Barker D. Obesity from cradle to grave. *Int J Obes Relat Metab Disord* 2003;27:722–727.

28. Yliharsila H, Kajantie E, Osmond C, Forsen T, Barker DJ, Eriksson JG. Birth size, adult body composition and muscle strength in later life. *Int J Obes (Lond)* 2007;31:1392–1399.

29. Forsen T, Eriksson J, Tuomilehto J, Reunanen A, Osmond C, Barker D. The fetal and childhood growth of persons who develop type 2 diabetes. *Ann Intern Med* 2000;133:176–182.

30. Pulizzi N, Lyssenko V, Jonsson A, et al. Interaction between prenatal growth and high-risk genotypes in the development of type 2 diabetes. *Diabetologia* 2009;52:825–829.

31. Lithell HO, McKeigue PM, Berglund L, Mohsen R, Lithell UB, Leon DA. Relation of size at birth to non-insulin dependent diabetes and insulin concentrations in men aged 50–60 years. *BMJ* 1996;312:406–410.

32. Eriksson JG, Osmond C, Kajantie E, Forsen TJ, Barker DJ. Patterns of growth among children who later develop type 2 diabetes or its risk factors. *Diabetologia* 2006;49:2853–2858.

33. Eriksson JG, Forsen T, Tuomilehto J, Osmond C, Barker DJ. Early adiposity rebound in childhood and risk of Type 2 diabetes in adult life. *Diabetologia* 2003;46:190–194.

34. Eriksson J, Forsen T, Tuomilehto J, Osmond C, Barker D. Fetal and childhood growth and hypertension in adult life. *Hypertension* 2000;36:790–794.

35. Kajantie E, Osmond C, Barker DJ, Forsen T, Phillips DI, Eriksson JG. Size at birth as a predictor of mortality in adulthood: a follow-up of 350,000 person-years. *Int J Epidemiol* 2005;34:655–663.

36. Barker DJ, Osmond C, Kajantie E, Eriksson JG. Growth and chronic disease: findings in the Helsinki Birth Cohort. *Ann Hum Biol* 2009;36:445–458.

37. Raikkonen K, Forsen T, Henriksson M, et al. Growth trajectories and intellectual abilities in young adulthood: the Helsinki Birth Cohort Study. *Am J Epidemiol* 2009;170:447–455.

38. Raikkonen K, Kajantie E, Pesonen AK, et al. Early life origins cognitive decline: findings in elderly men in the Helsinki Birth Cohort Study. *PLoS One* 2013;8:e54707.

39. Kajantie E, Barker DJ, Osmond C, Forsen T, Eriksson JG. Growth before 2 years of age and serum lipids 60 years later: the Helsinki Birth Cohort Study. *Int J Epidemiol* 2008;37:280–289.

40. Eriksson JG, Forsen T, Tuomilehto J, Osmond C, Barker DJ. Early growth, adult income, and risk of stroke. *Stroke* 2000;31:869–874.

41. von Bonsdorff MB, Rantanen T, Sipila S, et al. Birth size and childhood growth as determinants of physical functioning in older age: the Helsinki Birth Cohort Study. *Am J Epidemiol* 2011;174:1336–1344.

42. Osmond C, Kajantie E, Forsen TJ, Eriksson JG, Barker DJ. Infant growth and stroke in adult life: the Helsinki Birth Cohort Study. *Stroke* 2007;38:264–270.

43. Barker DJ, Forsen T, Uutela A, Osmond C, Eriksson JG. Size at birth and resilience to effects of poor living conditions in adult life: longitudinal study. *BMJ* 2001;323:1273–1276.

44. Phillips DI, Handelsman DJ, Eriksson JG, Forsen T, Osmond C, Barker DJ. Prenatal growth and subsequent marital status: longitudinal study. *BMJ* 2001;322:771.

45. Kajantie E, Raikkonen K, Henriksson M, et al. Childhood socioeconomic status modifies the association between intellectual abilities at age 20 and mortality in later life. *J Epidemiol Community Health* 2010;64:963–969.

46. Perala MM, Moltchanova E, Kaartinen NE, et al. The association between salt intake and adult systolic blood pressure is modified by birth weight. *Am J Clin Nutr* 2011;93:422–426.

47. Eriksson JG, Yliharsila H, Forsen T, Osmond C, Barker DJ. Exercise protects against glucose intolerance in individuals with a small body size at birth. *Prev Med* 2004;39:164–167.

48. Golding J. Children of the nineties. A longitudinal study of pregnancy and childhood based on the population of Avon (ALSPAC). *West Engl Med J* 1990;105:80–82.

49. Ong KK, Ahmed ML, Emmett PM, Preece MA, Dunger DB. Association between postnatal catch-up growth and obesity in childhood: prospective cohort study. *BMJ* 2000;320:967–971.

50. Ong KK, Dunger DB. Birth weight, infant growth and insulin resistance. *Eur J Endocrinol* 2004;151 Suppl 3:U131–139.

51. Karaolis-Danckert N, Buyken AE, Bolzenius K, Perim de Faria C, Lentze MJ, Kroke A. Rapid growth among term children whose birth weight was appropriate for gestational age has a longer lasting effect on body fat percentage than on body mass index. *Am J Clin Nutr* 2006;84:1449–1455.

52. Stettler N, Kumanyika SK, Katz SH, Zemel BS, Stallings VA. Rapid weight gain during infancy and obesity in young adulthood in a cohort of African Americans. *Am J Clin Nutr* 2003;77:1374–1378.

53. Stettler N, Bovet P, Shamlaye H, Zemel BS, Stallings VA, Paccaud F. Prevalence and risk factors for overweight and obesity in children from Seychelles, a country in rapid transition: the importance of early growth. *Int J Obes Relat Metab Disord* 2002;26:214–219.

54. Ong KK, Loos RJ. Rapid infancy weight gain and subsequent obesity: systematic reviews and hopeful suggestions. *Acta Paediatr* 2006;95:904–908.

55. Ong KK, Petry CJ, Emmett PM, et al. Insulin sensitivity and secretion in normal children related to size at birth, postnatal growth, and plasma insulin-like growth factor-I levels. *Diabetologia* 2004;47:1064–1070.

56. Bhargava SK, Sachdev HS, Fall CH, et al. Relation of serial changes in childhood body-mass index to impaired glucose tolerance in young adulthood. *N Engl J Med* 2004;350:865–875.

57. Whincup PH, Bredow M, Payne F, Sadler S, Golding J. Size at birth and blood pressure at 3 years of age. The Avon Longitudinal Study of Pregnancy and Childhood (ALSPAC). *Am J Epidemiol* 1999;149:730–739.

58. Jones A, Charakida M, Falaschetti E, et al. Adipose and height growth through childhood and blood pressure status in a large prospective cohort study. *Hypertension* 2012;59:919–925.

59. Gale CR, O'Callaghan FJ, Bredow M, Martyn CN. The influence of head growth in fetal life, infancy, and childhood on intelligence at the ages of 4 and 8 years. *Pediatrics* 2006;118:1486–1492.

60. Emond AM, Blair PS, Emmett PM, Drewett RF. Weight faltering in infancy and IQ levels at 8 years in the Avon Longitudinal Study of Parents and Children. *Pediatrics* 2007;120:e1051–1058.

61. Heinonen K, Raikkonen K, Pesonen AK, et al. Prenatal and postnatal growth and cognitive abilities at 56 months of age: a longitudinal study of infants born at term. *Pediatrics* 2008;121:e1325–1333.

62. Ekelund U, Ong K, Linne Y, et al. Upward weight percentile crossing in infancy and early childhood independently predicts fat mass in young adults: the Stockholm Weight Development Study (SWEDES). *Am J Clin Nutr* 2006;83:324–330.

63. Ekelund U, Ong KK, Linne Y, et al. Association of weight gain in infancy and early childhood with metabolic risk in young adults. *J Clin Endocrinol Metab* 2007;92:98–103.

64. Lawlor DA, Cooper AR, Bain C, et al. Associations of birth size and duration of breast feeding with cardiorespiratory fitness in childhood: findings from the Avon Longitudinal Study of Parents and Children (ALSPAC). *Eur J Epidemiol* 2008;23:411–422.

65. Tapp RJ, Williams C, Witt N, et al. Impact of size at birth on the microvasculature: the Avon Longitudinal Study of Parents and Children. *Pediatrics* 2007;120:e1225–1228.

66. Ibanez L, Ong K, Dunger DB, de Zegher F. Early development of adiposity and insulin resistance after catch-up weight gain in small-for-gestational-age children. *J Clin Endocrinol Metab* 2006;91:2153–2158.

67. Ibanez L, Suarez L, Lopez-Bermejo A, Diaz M, Valls C, de Zegher F. Early development of visceral fat excess after spontaneous catch-up growth in children with low birth weight. *J Clin Endocrinol Metab* 2008;93:925–928.
68. Ibanez L, Lopez-Bermejo A, Suarez L, Marcos MV, Diaz M, de Zegher F. Visceral adiposity without overweight in children born small for gestational age. *J Clin Endocrinol Metab* 2008;93:2079–2083.
69. Ibanez L, Lopez-Bermejo A, Diaz M, Suarez L, de Zegher F. Low-birth weight children develop lower sex hormone binding globulin and higher dehydroepiandrosterone sulfate levels and aggravate their visceral adiposity and hypoadiponectinemia between six and eight years of age. *J Clin Endocrinol Metab* 2009;94:3696–3699.
70. Soto N, Bazaes RA, Pena V, et al. Insulin sensitivity and secretion are related to catch-up growth in small-for-gestational-age infants at age 1 year: results from a prospective cohort. *J Clin Endocrinol Metab* 2003;88:3645–3650.
71. Mericq V, Ong KK, Bazaes R, et al. Longitudinal changes in insulin sensitivity and secretion from birth to age three years in small- and appropriate-for-gestational-age children. *Diabetologia* 2005;48:2609–2614.
72. Ibanez L, Lopez-Bermejo A, Diaz M, Marcos MV, Casano P, de Zegher F. Abdominal fat partitioning and high-molecular-weight adiponectin in short children born small for gestational age. *J Clin Endocrinol Metab* 2009;94:1049–1052.
73. Deng HZ, Li YH, Su Z, et al. Association between height and weight catch-up growth with insulin resistance in pre-pubertal Chinese children born small for gestational age at two different ages. *Eur J Pediatr* 2011;170:75–80.
74. Leunissen RW, Oosterbeek P, Hol LK, Hellingman AA, Stijnen T, Hokken-Koelega AC. Fat mass accumulation during childhood determines insulin sensitivity in early adulthood. *J Clin Endocrinol Metab* 2008;93:445–451.
75. Ravelli AC, van Der Meulen JH, Osmond C, Barker DJ, Bleker OP. Obesity at the age of 50 y in men and women exposed to famine prenatally. *Am J Clin Nutr* 1999;70:811–816.
76. Roseboom TJ, van der Meulen JH, Osmond C, Barker DJ, Ravelli AC, Bleker OP. Adult survival after prenatal exposure to the Dutch famine 1944–45. *Paediatr Perinat Epidemiol* 2001;15:220–225.
77. Painter RC, Roseboom TJ, Bossuyt PM, Osmond C, Barker DJ, Bleker OP. Adult mortality at age 57 after prenatal exposure to the Dutch famine. *Eur J Epidemiol* 2005;20:673–676.
78. van Abeelen AF, Veenendaal MV, Painter RC, et al. Survival effects of prenatal famine exposure. *Am J Clin Nutr* 2012;95:179–183.
79. Painter RC, De Rooij SR, Bossuyt PM, et al. A possible link between prenatal exposure to famine and breast cancer: a preliminary study. *Am J Hum Biol* 2006;18:853–856.
80. Roseboom TJ, van der Meulen JH, Ravelli AC, Osmond C, Barker DJ, Bleker OP. Effects of prenatal exposure to the Dutch famine on adult disease in later life: an overview. *Twin Res* 2001;4:293–298.
81. Kyle UG, Pichard C. The Dutch Famine of 1944-1945: a pathophysiological model of long-term consequences of wasting disease. *Curr Opin Clin Nutr Metab Care* 2006;9:388–394.
82. Ravelli AC, van der Meulen JH, Michels RP, et al. Glucose tolerance in adults after prenatal exposure to famine. *Lancet* 1998;351:173–177.
83. Antonov AN. Children born during the siege of Leningrad in 1942. *J Pediatr* 1947;30:250–259.
84. Stanner SA, Bulmer K, Andres C, et al. Does malnutrition in utero determine diabetes and coronary heart disease in adulthood? Results from the Leningrad siege study, a cross sectional study. *BMJ* 1997;315:1342–1348.
85. Koupil I, Shestov DB, Sparen P, Plavinskaja S, Parfenova N, Vagero D. Blood pressure, hypertension and mortality from circulatory disease in men and women who survived the siege of Leningrad. *Eur J Epidemiol* 2007;22:223–234.

86. Larciprete G, Valensise H, Di Pierro G, et al. Intrauterine growth restriction and fetal body composition. *Ultrasound Obstet Gynecol* 2005;26:258–262.

87. Padoan A, Rigano S, Ferrazzi E, Beaty BL, Battaglia FC, Galan HL. Differences in fat and lean mass proportions in normal and growth-restricted fetuses. *Am J Obstet Gynecol* 2004;191:1459–1464.

88. Hemachandra AH, Klebanoff MA. Use of serial ultrasound to identify periods of fetal growth restriction in relation to neonatal anthropometry. *Am J Hum Biol* 2006;18:791–797.

89. Ay L, Van Houten VA, Steegers EA, et al. Fetal and postnatal growth and body composition at 6 months of age. *J Clin Endocrinol Metab* 2009;94:2023–2030.

90. Beltrand J, Nicolescu R, Kaguelidou F, et al. Catch-up growth following fetal growth restriction promotes rapid restoration of fat mass but without metabolic consequences at one year of age. *PLoS One* 2009;4:e5343.

91. Perala MM, Mannisto S, Kaartinen NE, et al. Body size at birth is associated with food and nutrient intake in adulthood. *PLoS One* 2012;7:e46139.

92. Salonen MK, Kajantie E, Osmond C, et al. Prenatal and childhood growth and leisure time physical activity in adult life. *Eur J Public Health* 2011;21:719–724.

93. Salonen MK, Kajantie E, Osmond C, et al. Developmental origins of physical fitness: the Helsinki Birth Cohort Study. *PLoS One* 2011;6:e22302.

94. Sandboge S, Moltchanova E, Blomstedt PA, et al. Birth-weight and resting metabolic rate in adulthood: sex-specific differences. *Ann Med* 2012;44:296–303.

95. Hack M, Weissman B, Borawski-Clark E. Catch-up growth during childhood among very low-birth-weight children. *Arch Pediatr Adolesc Med* 1996;150:1122–1129.

96. Hack M, Schluchter M, Cartar L, Rahman M, Cuttler L, Borawski E. Growth of very low birth weight infants to age 20 years. *Pediatrics* 2003;112:e30–38.

97. Ehrenkranz RA, Younes N, Lemons JA, et al. Longitudinal growth of hospitalized very low birth weight infants. *Pediatrics* 1999;104:280–289.

98. Bertino E, Milani S, Boni L, et al. Evaluation of postnatal weight growth in very low birth weight infants. *J Pediatr Gastroenterol Nutr* 2007;45 Suppl 3:S155–158.

99. Gibson A, Carney S, Wales JK. Growth and the premature baby. *Horm Res* 2006;65 Suppl 3:75–81.

100. Gibson AT, Carney S, Cavazzoni E, Wales JK. Neonatal and post-natal growth. *Horm Res* 2000;53:42–49.

101. Farooqi A, Hagglof B, Sedin G, Gothefors L, Serenius F. Growth in 10- to 12-year-old children born at 23 to 25 weeks' gestation in the 1990s: a Swedish national prospective follow-up study. *Pediatrics* 2006;118:e1452–1465.

102. Bocca-Tjeertes IF, Kerstjens JM, Reijneveld SA, de Winter AF, Bos AF. Growth and predictors of growth restraint in moderately preterm children aged 0 to 4 years. *Pediatrics* 2011;128:e1187–1194.

103. Bocca-Tjeertes IF, van Buuren S, Bos AF, Kerstjens JM, Ten Vergert EM, Reijneveld SA. Growth of preterm and full-term children aged 0-4 years: integrating median growth and variability in growth charts. *J Pediatr* 2012;161:460–465 e1.

104. Thureen PJ. The neonatologist's dilemma: catch-up growth or beneficial undernutrition in very low birth weight infants: What are optimal growth rates? *J Pediatr Gastroenterol Nutr* 2007;45 Suppl 3:S152–154.

105. Xita N, Tsatsoulis A. Fetal origins of the metabolic syndrome. *Ann N Y Acad Sci* 2010;1205:148–155.

106. Van Abeelen AF, Veenendaal MV, Painter RC, et al. The fetal origins of hypertension: a systematic review and meta-analysis of the evidence from animal experiments of maternal undernutrition. *J Hypertens* 2012;30:2255–2267.

107. Portha B, Chavey A, Movassat J. Early-life origins of type 2 diabetes: fetal programming of the beta-cell mass. *Exp Diabetes Res* 2011;2011:105076.

108. McMullen S, Mostyn A. Animal models for the study of the developmental origins of health and disease. *Proc Nutr Soc* 2009;68:306–320.

109. Vuguin PM. Animal models for small for gestational age and fetal programming of adult disease. *Horm Res* 2007;68:113–123.

110. Garofano A, Czernichow P, Breant B. In utero undernutrition impairs rat beta-cell development. *Diabetologia* 1997;40:1231–1234.

111. Murrell A, Rakyan VK, Beck S. From genome to epigenome. *Hum Mol Genet* 2005;14 Spec No 1:R3–R10.

112. Wadhwa PD, Buss C, Entringer S, Swanson JM. Developmental origins of health and disease: brief history of the approach and current focus on epigenetic mechanisms. *Semin Reprod Med* 2009;27:358–368.

113. Gluckman PD, Hanson MA, Beedle AS. Non-genomic transgenerational inheritance of disease risk. *Bioessays* 2007;29:145–154.

114. Waterland RA, Michels KB. Epigenetic epidemiology of the developmental origins hypothesis. *Annu Rev Nutr* 2007;27:363–388.

115. Bocock PN, Aagaard-Tillery KM. Animal models of epigenetic inheritance. *Semin Reprod Med* 2009;27:369–379.

116. Seki Y, Williams L, Vuguin PM, Charron MJ. Minireview: Epigenetic programming of diabetes and obesity: animal models. *Endocrinology* 2012;153:1031–1038.

117. Waddington CH. The epigenotype. 1942. *Int J Epidemiol* 2012;41:10–13.

118. Waddington CH. The epigenotype. *Endeavour* 1942;1.

119. Bergman Y, Cedar H. DNA methylation dynamics in health and disease. *Nat Struct Mol Biol* 2013;20:274–281.

120. Fraga MF, Ballestar E, Paz MF, et al. Epigenetic differences arise during the lifetime of monozygotic twins. *Proc Natl Acad Sci USA* 2005;102:10604–10609.

121. Bannister AJ, Kouzarides T. Regulation of chromatin by histone modifications. *Cell Res* 2011;21:381–395.

122. Dolinoy DC. The agouti mouse model: an epigenetic biosensor for nutritional and environmental alterations on the fetal epigenome. *Nutr Rev* 2008;66 Suppl 1:S7–11.

123. Wolff GL, Kodell RL, Moore SR, Cooney CA. Maternal epigenetics and methyl supplements affect agouti gene expression in Avy/a mice. *FASEB J* 1998;12:949–957.

124. Cooney CA, Dave AA, Wolff GL. Maternal methyl supplements in mice affect epigenetic variation and DNA methylation of offspring. *J Nutr* 2002;132:2393S–2400S.

125. Waterland RA, Travisano M, Tahiliani KG, Rached MT, Mirza S. Methyl donor supplementation prevents transgenerational amplification of obesity. *Int J Obes (Lond)* 2008;32:1373–1379.

126. Waterland RA, Dolinoy DC, Lin JR, Smith CA, Shi X, Tahiliani KG. Maternal methyl supplements increase offspring DNA methylation at Axin Fused. *Genesis* 2006;44:401–406.

127. Heijmans BT, Tobi EW, Lumey LH, Slagboom PE. The epigenome: archive of the prenatal environment. *Epigenetics* 2009;4:526–531.

128. Heijmans BT, Tobi EW, Stein AD, et al. Persistent epigenetic differences associated with prenatal exposure to famine in humans. *Proc Natl Acad Sci USA* 2008;105:17046–17049.

129. Tobi EW, Lumey LH, Talens RP, et al. DNA methylation differences after exposure to prenatal famine are common and timing- and sex-specific. *Hum Mol Genet* 2009;18:4046–4053.

130. de Rooij SR, Costello PM, Veenendaal MV, et al. Associations between DNA methylation of a glucocorticoid receptor promoter and acute stress responses in a large healthy adult population are largely explained by lifestyle and educational differences. *Psychoneuroendocrinology* 2012;37:782–788.

131. Tobi EW, Slagboom PE, van Dongen J, et al. Prenatal famine and genetic variation are independently and additively associated with DNA methylation at regulatory loci within IGF2/H19. *PLoS One* 2012;7:e37933.

132. Banister CE, Koestler DC, Maccani MA, Padbury JF, Houseman EA, Marsit CJ. Infant growth restriction is associated with distinct patterns of DNA methylation in human placentas. *Epigenetics* 2011;6:920–927.

133. Wilhelm-Benartzi CS, Houseman EA, Maccani MA, et al. In utero exposures, infant growth, and DNA methylation of repetitive elements and developmentally related genes in human placenta. *Environ Health Perspect* 2012;120:296–302.

134. Liu Y, Murphy SK, Murtha AP, et al. Depression in pregnancy, infant birth weight and DNA methylation of imprint regulatory elements. *Epigenetics* 2012;7:735–746.

135. Obermann-Borst SA, Eilers PH, Tobi EW, et al. Duration of breastfeeding and gender are associated with methylation of the LEPTIN gene in very young children. *Pediatr Res* 2013;74:344–349.

136. Filiberto AC, Maccani MA, Koestler D, et al. Birthweight is associated with DNA promoter methylation of the glucocorticoid receptor in human placenta. *Epigenetics* 2011;6:566–572.

137. Tobi EW, Heijmans BT, Kremer D, et al. DNA methylation of IGF2, GNASAS, INSIGF and LEP and being born small for gestational age. *Epigenetics* 2011;6:171–176.

138. Perkins E, Murphy SK, Murtha AP, et al. Insulin-like growth factor 2/H19 methylation at birth and risk of overweight and obesity in children. *J Pediatr* 2012;161:31–39.

139. Hattersley AT, Tooke JE. The fetal insulin hypothesis: an alternative explanation of the association of low birthweight with diabetes and vascular disease. *Lancet* 1999;353:1789–1792.

140. Frayling TM, Hattersley AT. The role of genetic susceptibility in the association of low birth weight with type 2 diabetes. *Br Med Bull* 2001;60:89–101.

141. Hattersley AT, Beards F, Ballantyne E, Appleton M, Harvey R, Ellard S. Mutations in the glucokinase gene of the fetus result in reduced birth weight. *Nat Genet* 1998;19:268–270.

142. Lindsay RS, Dabelea D, Roumain J, Hanson RL, Bennett PH, Knowler WC. Type 2 diabetes and low birth weight: the role of paternal inheritance in the association of low birth weight and diabetes. *Diabetes* 2000;49:445–459.

143. Vattikuti S, Guo J, Chow CC. Heritability and genetic correlations explained by common SNPs for metabolic syndrome traits. *PLoS Genet* 2012;8:e1002637.

144. Beardsall K, Ong KK, Murphy N, et al. Heritability of childhood weight gain from birth and risk markers for adult metabolic disease in prepubertal twins. *J Clin Endocrinol Metab* 2009;94:3708–3713.

145. Poveda A, Jelenkovic A, Salces I, Ibanez ME, Rebato E. Heritability variations of body linearity and obesity indicators during growth. *Homo* 2012;63:301–310.

146. Dubois L, Ohm Kyvik K, Girard M, et al. Genetic and environmental contributions to weight, height, and BMI from birth to 19 years of age: an international study of over 12,000 twin pairs. *PLoS One* 2012;7:e30153.

147. Johnson L, Llewellyn CH, van Jaarsveld CH, Cole TJ, Wardle J. Genetic and environmental influences on infant growth: prospective analysis of the Gemini twin birth cohort. *PLoS One* 2011;6:e19918.

148. van Dommelen P, de Gunst MC, van der Vaart AW, Boomsma DI. Genetic study of the height and weight process during infancy. *Twin Res* 2004;7:607–616.

149. Gielen M, Lindsey PJ, Derom C, et al. Modeling genetic and environmental factors to increase heritability and ease the identification of candidate genes for birth weight: a twin study. *Behav Genet* 2008;38:44–54.

150. Mook-Kanamori DO, van Beijsterveldt CE, Steegers EA, et al. Heritability estimates of body size in fetal life and early childhood. *PLoS One* 2012;7:e39901.

151. Touwslager RN, Gielen M, Mulder AL, et al. Changes in genetic and environmental effects on growth during infancy. *Am J Clin Nutr* 2011;94:1568–1574.
152. Brescianini S, Giampietro S, Cotichini R, Lucchini R, De Curtis M. Genetic and environmental components of neonatal weight gain in preterm infants. *Pediatrics* 2012;129:e455–459.
153. Newman B, Selby JV, King MC, Slemenda C, Fabsitz R, Friedman GD. Concordance for type 2 (non-insulin-dependent) diabetes mellitus in male twins. *Diabetologia* 1987;30:763–768.
154. Fagard RH, Loos RJ, Beunen G, Derom C, Vlietinck R. Influence of chorionicity on the heritability estimates of blood pressure: a study in twins. *J Hypertens* 2003;21:1313–1318.
155. Almgren P, Lehtovirta M, Isomaa B, et al. Heritability and familiality of type 2 diabetes and related quantitative traits in the Botnia Study. *Diabetologia* 2011;54:2811–2819.
156. Waterworth DM, Bennett ST, Gharani N, et al. Linkage and association of insulin gene VNTR regulatory polymorphism with polycystic ovary syndrome. *Lancet* 1997;349:986–990.
157. Huxtable SJ, Saker PJ, Haddad L, et al. Analysis of parent-offspring trios provides evidence for linkage and association between the insulin gene and type 2 diabetes mediated exclusively through paternally transmitted class III variable number tandem repeat alleles. *Diabetes* 2000;49:126–130.
158. Mitchell SM, Hattersley AT, Knight B, et al. Lack of support for a role of the insulin gene variable number of tandem repeats minisatellite (INS-VNTR) locus in fetal growth or type 2 diabetes-related intermediate traits in United Kingdom populations. *J Clin Endocrinol Metab* 2004;89:310–317.
159. Lindsay RS, Hanson RL, Wiedrich C, Knowler WC, Bennett PH, Baier LJ. The insulin gene variable number tandem repeat class I/III polymorphism is in linkage disequilibrium with birth weight but not Type 2 diabetes in the Pima population. *Diabetes* 2003;52:187–193.
160. Dunger DB, Ong KK, Huxtable SJ, et al. Association of the INS VNTR with size at birth. ALSPAC Study Team. Avon Longitudinal Study of Pregnancy and Childhood. *Nat Genet* 1998;19:98–100.
161. Ruiz J, Blanche H, Cohen N, et al. Insertion/deletion polymorphism of the angiotensin-converting enzyme gene is strongly associated with coronary heart disease in non-insulin-dependent diabetes mellitus. *Proc Natl Acad Sci USA* 1994;91:3662–3665.
162. Kajantie E, Rautanen A, Kere J, et al. The effects of the ACE gene insertion/deletion polymorphism on glucose tolerance and insulin secretion in elderly people are modified by birth weight. *J Clin Endocrinol Metab* 2004;89:5738–5741.
163. Cambien F, Leger J, Mallet C, Levy-Marchal C, Collin D, Czernichow P. Angiotensin I-converting enzyme gene polymorphism modulates the consequences of in utero growth retardation on plasma insulin in young adults. *Diabetes* 1998;47:470–475.
164. Eriksson JG. Gene polymorphisms, size at birth, and the development of hypertension and type 2 diabetes. *J Nutr* 2007;137:1063–1065.
165. Eriksson JG, Lindi V, Uusitupa M, et al. The effects of the Pro12Ala polymorphism of the peroxisome proliferator-activated receptor-gamma2 gene on insulin sensitivity and insulin metabolism interact with size at birth. *Diabetes* 2002;51:2321–2324.
166. Diaz M, Bassols J, Lopez-Bermejo A, Gomez-Roig MD, de Zegher F, Ibanez L. Placental expression of peroxisome proliferator-activated receptor gamma (PPARgamma): relation to placental and fetal growth. *J Clin Endocrinol Metab* 2012;97:E1468–1472.
167. Kubaszek A, Markkanen A, Eriksson JG, et al. The association of the K121Q polymorphism of the plasma cell glycoprotein-1 gene with type 2 diabetes and hypertension depends on size at birth. *J Clin Endocrinol Metab* 2004;89:2044–2047.

168. Rautanen A, Eriksson JG, Kere J, et al. Associations of body size at birth with late-life cortisol concentrations and glucose tolerance are modified by haplotypes of the gluco-corticoid receptor gene. *J Clin Endocrinol Metab* 2006;91:4544–4551.

169. Poulton J, Brown MS, Cooper A, Marchington DR, Phillips DI. A common mitochondrial DNA variant is associated with insulin resistance in adult life. *Diabetologia* 1998;41:54–58.

170. Casteels K, Ong K, Phillips D, Bendall H, Pembrey M. Mitochondrial 16189 variant, thinness at birth, and type-2 diabetes. ALSPAC study team. Avon Longitudinal Study of Pregnancy and Childhood. *Lancet* 1999;353:1499–1500.

171. Soejima H, Higashimoto K. Epigenetic and genetic alterations of the imprinting disorder Beckwith-Wiedemann syndrome and related disorders. *J Hum Genet* 2013;58:402–409.

172. Vambergue A, Fajardy I, Dufour P, et al. No loss of genomic imprinting of IGF-II and H19 in placentas of diabetic pregnancies with fetal macrosomia. *Growth Horm IGF Res* 2007;17:130–136.

173. Gabory A, Ripoche MA, Le Digarcher A, et al. H19 acts as a trans regulator of the imprinted gene network controlling growth in mice. *Development* 2009;136:3413–3421.

174. Petry CJ, Ong KK, Barratt BJ, et al. Common polymorphism in H19 associated with birthweight and cord blood IGF-II levels in humans. *BMC Genet* 2005;6:22.

175. Adkins RM, Somes G, Morrison JC, et al. Association of birth weight with polymor-phisms in the IGF2, H19, and IGF2R genes. *Pediatr Res* 2010;68:429–434.

176. Petry CJ, Seear RV, Wingate DL, et al. Maternally transmitted foetal H19 variants and associations with birth weight. *Hum Genet* 2011;130:663–670.

177. Narayanan RP, Fu B, Payton A, et al. IGF2 gene polymorphisms and IGF-II concen-tration are determinants of longitudinal weight trends in type 2 diabetes. *Exp Clin Endocrinol Diabetes* 2013;121:361–367.

178. Petry CJ, Seear RV, Wingate DL, et al. Associations between paternally transmitted fetal IGF2 variants and maternal circulating glucose concentrations in pregnancy. *Diabetes* 2011;60:3090–3096.

179. Hoyo C, Fortner K, Murtha AP, et al. Association of cord blood methylation fractions at imprinted insulin-like growth factor 2 (IGF2), plasma IGF2, and birth weight. *Cancer Causes Control* 2012;23:635–645.

180. Huang RC, Galati JC, Burrows S, et al. DNA methylation of the IGF2/H19 imprinting control region and adiposity distribution in young adults. *Clin Epigenetics* 2012;4:21.

181. Burris HH, Braun JM, Byun HM, et al. Association between birth weight and DNA methylation of IGF2, glucocorticoid receptor and repetitive elements LINE-1 and Alu. *Epigenomics* 2013;5:271–281.

182. Bell JT, Pai AA, Pickrell JK, et al. DNA methylation patterns associate with genetic and gene expression variation in HapMap cell lines. *Genome Biol* 2011;12:R10.

183. Gertz J, Varley KE, Reddy TE, et al. Analysis of DNA methylation in a three-gen-eration family reveals widespread genetic influence on epigenetic regulation. *PLoS Genet* 2011;7:e1002228.

184. Meaburn EL, Schalkwyk LC, Mill J. Allele-specific methylation in the human genome: implications for genetic studies of complex disease. *Epigenetics* 2010;5:578–582.

185. Vaessen N, Janssen JA, Heutink P, et al. Association between genetic variation in the gene for insulin-like growth factor-I and low birthweight. *Lancet* 2002;359:1036–1037.

186. van Rijn MJ, Slooter AJ, Bos MJ, et al. Insulin-like growth factor I promoter polymor-phism, risk of stroke, and survival after stroke: the Rotterdam study. *J Neurol Neurosurg Psychiatry* 2006;77:24–27.

187. van Houten VA, Mook-Kanamori DO, van Osch-Gevers L, et al. A variant of the IGF-I gene is associated with blood pressure but not with left heart dimensions at the age of 2 years: the Generation R Study. *Eur J Endocrinol* 2008;159:209–216.

188. Landmann E, Geller F, Schilling J, Rudloff S, Foeller-Gaudier E, Gortner L. Absence of the wild-type allele (192 base pairs) of a polymorphism in the promoter region of the IGF-I gene but not a polymorphism in the insulin gene variable number of tandem repeat locus is associated with accelerated weight gain in infancy. *Pediatrics* 2006;118:2374–2379.
189. Casano-Sancho P, Lopez-Bermejo A, Fernandez-Real JM, et al. The tumour necrosis factor (TNF)-alpha-308GA promoter polymorphism is related to prenatal growth and postnatal insulin resistance. *Clin Endocrinol (Oxf)* 2006;64:129–135.
190. Roghair RD, Aldape G. Naturally occurring perinatal growth restriction in mice programs cardiovascular and endocrine function in a sex- and strain-dependent manner. *Pediatr Res* 2007;62:399–404.
191. Poulsen P, Vaag AA, Kyvik KO, Moller Jensen D, Beck-Nielsen H. Low birth weight is associated with NIDDM in discordant monozygotic and dizygotic twin pairs. *Diabetologia* 1997;40:439–446.

5 Effect of Postnatal Growth in the Large-for-Gestational-Age Infants

Rae-Chi Huang and Elizabeth A. Davis

INTRODUCTION

Large-for-gestational-age (LGA) neonates are defined as babies born weighing greater than the 90th percentile for their gestational age as compared to their relevant population and ethnic background. LGA is becoming increasingly prevalent mostly due to increasing maternal obesity and to a lesser extent due to decreasing maternal smoking.[1] This was illustrated by a Swedish study where the prevalence of LGA births increased 23% between 1992 and 2001.[1] There are many immediate problems related to LGA deliveries such as prolonged vaginal delivery, shoulder dystocia, brachial plexus injury, neonatal hypoglycemia, and respiratory distress. However, there are also longer-term sequelae of LGA, in particular an increased risk of the metabolic syndrome.

"Fetal programming" was first suggested by David Barker and his colleagues when he observed that low birth weight babies in Hertfordshire in the United Kingdom were at increased risk of subsequent coronary vascular disease,[2] type 2 diabetes,[3] and the metabolic syndrome.[4] As low birth weight is a surrogate measure of suboptimal *in utero* environment/growth, the term "fetal programming" (or the developmental origins of health and disease) was used to refer to the lifelong effects on metabolism and other non-communicable diseases that result from *in utero* events.

In contemporary populations, it has been observed that both low and high birth weight babies have a greater risk of the metabolic syndrome, as first observed in a study of over 1000 Pima Indians followed up at 20 to 39 years of age with an oral glucose tolerance test. In a contemporary Western population, a similar U-shaped relationship was demonstrated, where both the highest and the lowest quintiles of birth weight were associated with greater metabolic risk (Figure 5.1).[5,6,7]

The medical issue of high birth weight babies is increasing in both prevalence and importance due to the escalation of maternal and childhood obesity. There is evidence that high birth weight babies are at risk of subsequent development of the

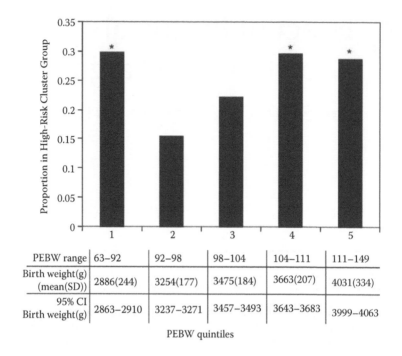

PEBW range	63–92	92–98	98–104	104–111	111–149
Birth weight(g) (mean(SD))	2886(244)	3254(177)	3475(184)	3663(207)	4031(334)
95% CI Birth weight(g)	2863–2910	3237–3271	3457–3493	3643–3683	3999–4063

PEBW quintiles

FIGURE 5.1   Proportion of subjects in the high metabolic risk cluster, by quintile percentage of expected birth weight (PEBW; * indicates a significant difference from the lowest quintile, quintile 2.). (From Reference 5 with permission of the authors.)

metabolic syndrome.[8] The increased risk observed in high birth weight babies can be exacerbated by early infant and childhood postnatal growth patterns.[9] This chapter outlines the effects of pregnancy environment, large birth size, and early life growth patterns on subsequent risk of the metabolic syndrome.

FETAL PROGRAMMING

Although "fetal programming" describes a phenomenon whereby the fetal environment affects risk of outcomes of offspring, including the metabolic syndrome, two further concepts have emerged.

1. The long-term effects of a suboptimal antenatal environment are exacerbated by a suboptimal postnatal environment. There is evidence that the full phenotypic manifestation of "fetal programming" may be contingent on the additional exposure to a suboptimal postnatal environment. A suboptimal postnatal environment includes a poor diet, lack of physical activity, and environmental exposures that impact postnatal growth trajectories in infancy and childhood.

2. Animal studies show that *in utero* over-nutrition is also associated with an increased risk of the offspring developing subsequent obesity and related disease. The animal data relating to this includes work that shows that high-fat maternal and paternal diets are associated with increased risk of adult obesity,[10] taste preference in the offspring for "junk" food,[11] hypothalamic leptin resistance,[12] and altered hypothalamic[10] and liver[13] gene expression.

METABOLIC SYNDROME IN CHILDREN

The obstetrician, neonatologist, pediatrician, and public health physician have increasing roles in managing and preventing the metabolic syndrome in children. The importance lies in the increasing prevalence of the disease, its early development, and persistent tracking from childhood into adult life.

INCREASING LEVELS OF CHILDHOOD OBESITY AND THE METABOLIC SYNDROME

There is a global epidemic of obesity that is projected to cause increases in adult heart disease, diabetes, and a range of co-morbidities. Childhood obesity and overweight have increased two- to threefold in recent decades. With each of the National Health and Nutrition Examination Survey (NHANES) follow-up studies, there have been progressive increases in overweight. For example, among 12- to 19-year-olds, 5.0% were overweight in 1976 to 1980, 10.5% in 1988 to 1994, and 15.5% in 1995 to 2000.[14] Similar increases were seen in 6- to 11-year-olds as well, increasing from 6.5% to 11.3% to 15.3% over the three surveys.[14]

The increases in childhood obesity are paralleled by increases in the metabolic syndrome in children. Weiss and colleagues have shown that the prevalence of the metabolic syndrome increased as the severity of obesity increased in childhood. With each 0.5 Z-score increase in BMI, there is an increase in the risk of the metabolic syndrome quantified by an odds ratio of 1.55 (95% confidence interval, 1.16 to 2.08) among overweight and obese children.[15]

METABOLIC SYNDROME IN CHILDREN

Defining the metabolic syndrome in children has been challenging and there is no current consensus. In adults, the metabolic syndrome describes a cluster of abnormalities comprising four major components:

1. Central obesity
2. Insulin resistance
3. Hypertension
4. Dyslipidemia[16]

Adult definitions of the metabolic syndrome differ. For example, the World Health Organization (WHO) criteria include evidence of insulin resistance and two of the following criteria: obesity, increased waist-to-hip ratio, elevated HDL cholesterol, elevated triglycerides, hypertension, or proteinuria. In the metabolic syndrome, these individual risk factors impart synergistic effects for cardiovascular risk. Different definitions have different criteria for the individual components of the metabolic syndrome. For example, the cut-offs for fasting glucose levels vary for the different consensus definitions: the International Diabetes Federation (IDF) criteria and the National Cholesterol Education Program (NCEP) criteria are for a fasting glucose ≥5.6 mM, the WHO criteria are for a fasting glucose ≥6.1 mM or a 2-h glucose of ≥7.6 mM.[17–19] The presence of a clinical diagnosis of diabetes mellitus would satisfy all three groups.

There are numerous modifications of metabolic syndrome definitions for children.[20] Therefore, obtaining prevalence figures for the metabolic syndrome in children is difficult. In the NHANES III cohort (1988–1994) (using an NCEP-related definition), nearly 10% of adolescents aged 12 years or older met diagnostic criteria for the metabolic syndrome. [21]

TRACKING OF THE METABOLIC SYNDROME FROM CHILDHOOD INTO ADULT LIFE

Type 2 diabetes, insulin resistance, and the metabolic syndrome are increasing in prevalence in childhood and are increasingly the purview of the pediatrician. The metabolic syndrome[22] and its components (hypertension,[22] dyslipidemia, obesity,[23] and insulin resistance[24]) have been shown to track from childhood into adulthood. Bao and colleagues investigated the large longitudinal Bogalusa Study cohort and found that among subjects initially in the highest quintile of a multiple cardiovascular risk index, 61% remained there 8 years later. In adult life, these cardiovascular risk factors translate into increased risk for atherosclerotic diseases.[25]

RISK FACTORS FOR LARGE-FOR-GESTATIONAL-AGE BIRTH

The causes of LGA are multifactorial. Significant risk factors include:

1. Gestational diabetes
2. Pregestational diabetes
3. Maternal obesity
4. Gestational weight gain
5. Genetic predisposition
6. Multiparity
7. Male gender
8. Ethnicity

GESTATIONAL AND PREGESTATIONAL DIABETES

The most well recognized cause of LGA babies is gestational diabetes. Maternal diabetes is associated with double to triple the risk of an LGA delivery. In a large study of 12,950 deliveries, diet- treated gestational diabetes was associated with an increased prevalence of LGA (29%) compared to those born to mothers without diabetes (11%).[26] Pregestational diabetes was also associated with increased prevalence of LGA (38% compared to 12%). With each 1 mmol/L (18 mg/dL) increase in maternal plasma glucose at 28 weeks, the baby was on average 48 g heavier at birth.[27]

MATERNAL OBESITY

Maternal obesity is an increasing global problem. It is associated with more than double the risk of stillbirth and perinatal deaths, as well as fetal birth defects such as neural tube defects, abdominal wall defects, heart defects, and multiple congenital anomalies. It is also associated with macrosomia and LGA. Because of these problems, babies born to obese mothers are 3.5 times more likely to be admitted to the intensive care unit than their appropriate for gestational age peers.[28, 29] Obesity is increasing in many Western populations, including among men and women of reproductive age.[30] Combined with the decreases in maternal smoking during pregnancy, observations of increased rates of LGA are being made.[1]

EXCESSIVE GESTATIONAL WEIGHT GAIN

Gestational weight gain is strongly associated with having an LGA neonate. It is also associated with other adverse neonatal outcomes. Gestational weight gain of more than 18 kg is associated with need for assisted ventilation, seizures, hypoglycemia, polycythemia, and meconium aspiration syndrome as well as LGA.[31] The Institute of Medicine issued guidelines in 1990 for recommended weight gain during pregnancy depending on pregravid BMI and other maternal factors.[32]

Recommended weight gain during pregnancy depends on the pre-pregnancy BMI (Table 5.1). Additionally, adolescents and African-Americans should gain weight at the upper end of the recommended range, and short women (<157 cm) should gain weight at the lower end of the recommended range. Weight gains above these recommendations are consistently associated with greater risk for LGA and macrosomia, irrespective of whether the mother is underweight, normal or overweight, or

TABLE 5.1
Recommended Pregnancy Weight Gains in Underweight, Normal Weight, and Overweight Mothers[134]

Prepregnancy Maternal Weight Category	Prepregnancy Body Mass Index	Recommended Weight Gain
Underweight	<18.5 kg/m²	28–40 lb (12.7–18.1 kg)
Normal weight	18.5–24.9 kg/m²	25–35 lb (11.3–15.9 kg)
Overweight	>25.0–29.9 kg/m²	15–25 lb (6.8–11.3 kg)
Obese	>30 kg/m²	11–20 lb (5.0–9.7 kg)

her degree of obesity. In contrast, weight gains below the recommendations did not necessarily protect against LGA.[32]

GENETIC FACTORS

Some genetic polymorphisms have been shown to modify the risk of LGA. The 737.738 polymorphism of insulin-like growth factor 1 (IGF-1) comprises a variable number of microsatellite repeats of the cystosine-adenine (CA) in the promoter region of IGF-1. Homozygosity for variant type alleles was associated with a significantly increased risk of being born LGA compared to appropriate for gestational age (AGA), compared to the heterozygous state or homozygous wild type.[33] The -11391G>A polymorphism of the adiponectin gene has also been associated with LGA and subsequent plasma adiponectin levels at 23 to 25 years of age.[34]

OTHER RISK FACTORS

Multiparity and male gender are further factors associated with a greater risk of LGA.[26] African Americans have a lower rate of LGA than other American populations.[26]

LONG-TERM SEQUELAE OF LGA

RELATIONSHIP BETWEEN SIZE AT BIRTH AND SIZE IN LATER LIFE

Overall, increasing birth weight, adjusted for sex and gestational age, weakly predicts larger childhood and adult body size and body mass index. In a meta-analysis, which included 643,902 people from 66 studies, high birth weight (>4000 g) was associated with increased risk of overweight (OR = 1.66; 95% CI 1.55–1.77).[35] In the East Flanders Prospective Twin study, a 1 kg increase in birth weight is associated with a 4.2 kg increase in adult weight, a 3.3 cm increase in height, and 0.49 kg/m² increase in BMI.[36] These findings may reflect, in part, the U-shaped association between birth weight and obesity-related disease that has been described (Figure 5.1).

A more consistent relationship has been seen between LGA and subsequent obesity. LGA babies are at greater risk of obesity and probably more prone to fat development in infancy compared to neonates of appropriate birth weight for their gestational age.[37] They develop greater childhood length, weight, BMI, skin fold thickness, and head circumference.[38] Greater skin folds have been identified in LGA babies by 3 years of age.[38] These differences in skin fold thickness are present well before overt onset of the metabolic manifestations. For example, those children who will subsequently develop metabolic risk have greater skin fold thicknesses in young childhood (by 3 years old) than those of lower risk.[39]

Extremes of birth weight also affect body composition (fat percentage and distribution). Lower birth weight is clearly associated with greater adiposity, greater fat percentage, and greater central fat distribution in childhood and adulthood compared to appropriately sized newborns (see Chapter 4). LGA is also associated with increased adipose tissue development. This may already be developing *in utero*. A study investigating newborns with dual X-ray absorptiometry (DEXA) within days of their delivery show that LGA infants have higher total body fat mass and bone mineral content, and lower lean body mass expressed as an absolute amount and as a percentage of total body weight.[37]

RELATIONSHIP BETWEEN LGA AND METABOLIC SYNDROME

LGA is associated with greater body size through the neonatal period, infancy, and early childhood and possibly with increased fat percentage. Therefore, Boney and colleagues investigated the association between LGA and risk for the metabolic syndrome in childhood.[8] In this longitudinal cohort study of children aged 6 to 11 years, they identified four groups of children:

1. LGA with control mothers
2. LGA with mother with gestational diabetes mellitus (LGA/GDM)
3. Appropriately grown neonates for gestational age (AGA) of control mothers
4. AGA with mothers with gestational diabetes

LGA status and maternal obesity increased the risk of metabolic syndrome approximately twofold, with hazard ratios of 2.19 (95% CI 1.25–3.82) and 1.81 (95% CI 1.03–3.19), respectively. Gestational diabetes mellitus was not independently associated with the risk of offspring metabolic syndrome. The interaction term between LGA and GDM was significantly associated with insulin resistance between 9 and 11 years, but not with the metabolic syndrome. The prevalence of the metabolic syndrome was highest in the LGA/GDM infants, who had a 50% prevalence of metabolic syndrome. LGA in the absence of GDM was associated with a lower prevalence of the metabolic syndrome at 29%. The other two groups had a prevalence of 18 and 21%.

Obese mothers without clinical diagnosis of GDM had infants at higher risk of the metabolic syndrome. This suggests that obese mothers without a diagnosis of GDM already experience a level of maternal glucose dysregulation that is associated with fetal hyperinsulinism and insulin resistance. This concurs with other studies that show that even in the absence of overt gestational diabetes in the mother, LGA infants have greater insulin resistance compared to those born to AGA.[40] In another study, *in utero* exposure to gestational diabetes increased insulin secretion and lowered HDL-C by 5 to 10 years of age, independent of the child's current weight status.[41] The exposure also resulted in greater central adiposity even for children within a normal weight range. Further work is required to dissect out the relative causative roles of LGA, GDM, pre-gestational diabetes mellitus, and maternal obesity upon offspring risk of the metabolic syndrome.

GENDER DIFFERENCES IN THE RELATIONSHIP BETWEEN LGA WITH THE METABOLIC SYNDROME

Boney et al. did not show a gender difference in the relationship between LGA and the metabolic syndrome.[8] However, our understanding is still incomplete; many animal and human studies on "fetal programming" suggest a strong effect of gender of the offspring. It has also been observed that female fetuses are more likely to develop

LGA due to excessive maternal weight gain in pregnancy than are male fetuses.[42] Huang et al. showed that females who developed metabolic syndrome risk in adolescence were more likely to have been LGA compared to males, and to have increased adiposity in infancy (apparent at 3 years old).[39]

RELATIONSHIP BETWEEN EARLY GROWTH AND ADULT HEALTH

Evidence over the last half century indicates that early nutrition and growth affect long-term cardiovascular health. Early growth acceleration promotes abnormal vascular biology[43] with early atherosclerosis.[44] Some studies show that rapid postnatal growth is associated with increased risk of obesity-related disease.[45, 46] Infant obesity is also associated with childhood and adult obesity.[23]

The definition of rapid postnatal growth is variable in the literature; however, the most frequent definition is a Z-score change greater than 0.67 in weight for age between two different ages in childhood.[47] This has mostly focused on the concept of "catch-up" growth related to rapid postnatal growth after a period of growth restriction *in utero* (i.e., in IUGR or SGA infants). However, the detrimental effect of rapid postnatal growth also holds for babies who are not growth retarded at birth and are AGA at birth.[46]

There is a suggestion that LGA babies are independently at increased risk of the metabolic syndrome. It is not as well established whether these individuals experience particular detrimental effects with continuation of postnatal weight gain. There is, however, accumulating evidence that this is likely to be the case.[8] There is also an emerging suggestion that "catch down" growth early in life in these babies may be beneficial for reducing their long-term adverse metabolic profiles.

Longitudinal Statistical Models of Postnatal Growth

Life course adiposity trajectories have been defined using longitudinal statistical techniques, which are data driven. Different patterns of growth can be identified using such techniques. Obesity trajectories have been identified with growth mixture modeling techniques;[7, 8] for example, Li et al. demonstrated an "early-onset overweight" trajectory,[48] and Ventura et al.[49] used growth mixture modeling using continuous BMI and identified four distinct BMI trajectories including an upward percentile group, which was associated with more metabolic risk factors.

In an Australian study with longitudinal data from over 1000 children, seven distinct growth trajectories during childhood were identified (Figure 5.2). Based on body adiposity at seven time points between birth and 14 years, distinct growth trajectories were identified using semi-parametric mixture modeling (Table 5.2).[50]

Trajectory 1 corresponds to babies that are above average size at 2 years and remain so through childhood. Trajectory 3 starts with a similar high adiposity to Trajectory 1 but decreases throughout childhood years to reach a similar level of adiposity to the "reference/normal" population by 14 years old.[50]

While strictly speaking not all Trajectory 1 and 3 children are LGA, it does demonstrate that postnatal growth plays a role in cardiovascular risk outside of the subsets of SGA, AGA, and preterm babies. Comparisons of Trajectories 1 and 3 give some

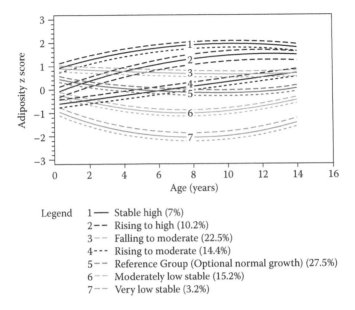

Legend
1 —— Stable high (7%)
2 – – Rising to high (10.2%)
3 – – Falling to moderate (22.5%)
4 - - - Rising to moderate (14.4%)
5 – – Reference Group (Optional normal growth) (27.5%)
6 – – Moderately low stable (15.2%)
7 – – Very low stable (3.2%)

FIGURE 5.2   Seven growth trajectories between birth and 14 years. (Figure is copyright the authors, and is reproduced from Reference 50. With permission of the authors.)

TABLE 5.2
Seven Distinct Growth Trajectories during Childhood Based on Data from Over 1000 Australian Children

Trajectory	Percentage of Cohort (%)	Adiposity Z-score Birth	Childhood Course in Adiposity	Adiposity Z-score at Age 14 Years
1, "stable high"	7.0	High	Stable	High
2, "rising to high"	10.2	Average	Increasing	High
3, "falling to moderate"	22.5	High	Decreasing	Average
4, "rising to moderate"	14.4	Low	Increasing	Average
5, "reference/normal"	27.5	Average	Stable	Average
6, "stable low"	15.2	Low average	Stable	Low
7, "stable very low"	3.2	Very low	Stable	Very low

Note: See Reference 50 and Figure 5.2.

insight into the associations of childhood growth with metabolic risk in larger infants. As we will discuss later, catch-down growth (Trajectory 3) is associated with improved metabolic outcomes such as lower blood pressure and reduced insulin resistance.

These longitudinal models also suggest that babies who have grown at greater rates *in utero* and born at greater than average weight also have greater weight gain postnatally and develop risk for the metabolic syndrome (Trajectory 1 in Figure 5.2).[50] These observational studies to date, however, cannot establish causation or direction of effects.

EFFECT OF POSTNATAL GROWTH ON THE COMPONENTS OF THE METABOLIC SYNDROME

Body Composition

Early life growth patterns affect subsequent body composition. Rapid postnatal growth is associated with increased risk of later life obesity, central adiposity, and increased fat percentage. Most of the literature has focused on the SGA neonate with "catch-up" growth (see Chapter 4). For example, Ong and colleagues showed that among 848 full-term singleton infants from the Avon Longitudinal (ALSPAC) cohort, children who showed catch-up growth between birth and 2 years old had greater total and central fat at 5 years old than other children.[46] Of interest in the ALSPAC cohort, almost a third of participants with rapid growth between 0 and 2 years were not initially growth restricted. Of those with rapid growth, the mean birth weight and length measures were –0.53 and –0.23 Z scores, respectively. Therefore, in a contemporary well-nourished cohort, average sized babies with rapid postnatal growth were at increased risk of obesity.[46] These studies show that catch-up growth or postnatal growth is associated with a future risk of cardiovascular disease even in normal sized newborns and that the effect is not restricted to SGA or preterm babies. There is less direct evidence of the effect of postnatal growth on LGA babies. A recent case-control study (n = 515) investigated LGA and AGA subjects at ages 9 to 10 years old and again at 23 to 25 years old. In comparison to those without catch-down growth, LGA subjects with at least 0.67 SD catch-down growth in childhood had lower BMI (23.5 ± 4.4 vs. 24.9 ± 4.1 kg/m^2, $p < 0.05$) and waist circumference (80.4 ± 11.9 vs. 84.4 ± 13.1 cm, $p < 0.05$) at 23 to 25 years of age.[33]

Insulin Resistance

As for the other cardiovascular outcomes, insulin resistance has also been associated with rapid weight gain in early life. Similar to the other risk factors, the focus of most studies has been on SGA babies.[51]

Evidence in AGA and LGA Infants

The effect of accelerated postnatal growth on insulin resistance is also applicable to AGA babies. Weight gain from birth to 3 months is significantly associated with raised serum insulin levels and increased homeostatic model assessment of insulin resistance (HOMA-IR) score in adolescents aged 17 years who were born SGA and AGA.[52]

Other supportive evidence for this comes from the Australian longitudinal prospective cohort previously described (Figure 5.2, Table 5.2). Trajectories 1 and 3 both showed high size at birth (3.53 kg) but Trajectory 3 had a lower BMI by age 14 years old (26.4 vs. 29.4 kg/m^2). Trajectory 1, which continued to show a rising adiposity to middle childhood, was associated with increased homeostasis model of insulin resistance (HOMA-IR) at age 14 years, compared to children who grew following the optimal adiposity trajectory. However, Trajectory 3, which showed "catch-down" growth, did not show elevated insulin resistance (Table 5.3).[50]

Trajectories 1 and 3 are characterized by a mean birth size of approximately 1 SD greater than the mean, so not all infants in these groups are LGA. However, they may provide some insight into whether postnatal growth affects metabolic risk in LGA

TABLE 5.3

Trajectories 1 and 3 Demonstrate Different Levels of Insulin Resistance

	Males		Females	
	Trajectory 1	Trajectory 3	Trajectory 1	Trajectory 3
Fasting Insulin	16.4	10.8	18.2	11.3
	(13.8–19.0)	(9.5–12.1)	(15.2–21.2)	(10.5–12.2)
HOMA-IR	3.6	2.4	3.9	2.3
	(3.0–4.2)	(2.1–2.8)	(3.2–4.5)	(2.2–2.5)

infants. It is not possible to ascertain if the pattern of downward growth velocity is protective against insulin resistance or if this growth pattern occurs independently in those with a lower inherent risk of insulin resistance. This will only be untangled with intervention studies.

Blood Pressure

Evidence in SGA and AGA Infants

Several studies demonstrate an association between early catch-up in weight (in infants born SGA or AGA) and later-life blood pressure.[52–55] Rapid weight gain from birth to 1 year of age (adjusted for gestational age) was associated with increased systolic blood pressure in young adult life.[54] Excessive weight gain between birth and 3 months of age was associated with increased systolic blood pressure in adolescents who were born at full term.[52] Yet another study of adult men and women who developed hypertension showed they were lighter and shorter at birth but became heavier and taller between 7 and 15 years of age compared to those with normotension.[55]

Evidence in LGA Infants

Studies of the effect of weight gain in infancy and the effect on later-life blood pressure have rarely looked at LGA neonates. One study showed that babies who are LGA and do not cross down percentiles in early childhood are likely to develop higher blood pressure. In this study, LGA subjects with at least 0.67 SD catch-down growth in childhood had lower diastolic (77 ± 7 vs. 72 ± 11 mm Hg, $p < 0.05$) blood pressure at 23 to 25 years of age, compared to those without catch-down growth.[33] In another study comparing Trajectories 1 and 3 from the seven previously described trajectories (Figure 5.2, Table 5.2), it has been shown that catch-down growth (Trajectory 3) was associated with lower blood pressure than in those who remained larger (Trajectory 1).[50] These larger infants therefore show metabolic benefits in catch-down growth with lower blood pressure and lower insulin resistance, even though not all the infants were strictly LGA.

Serum Lipid Levels

The evidence for an association between early weight gain and subsequent lipid profiles is less robust than for body size, body composition, fasting insulin, or blood pressure. Some studies show that rapid weight gain in the first 3 months of life is associated with a more adverse lipid profile in adolescents and early adulthood.[5] A Japanese study showed that rapid weight gain between both the periods of 0 to 18 months and 18 months to 3 years was associated with an adverse lipid profile and elevated BMI. However, the association with an adverse lipid profile disappeared after adjustment for BMI.[56] In contrast, weight gain in the first 20 months of life had no effect on serum lipid levels in a group of >2000 males aged 18 years.[57] Therefore, the association between early weight gain and later serum lipid levels remains controversial.

To date, no studies have focused on LGA babies.

Coronary Artery Disease

Barker et al. investigated a cohort born at Helsinki University Central Hospital from 1934 to 1944 that had an average of 11 measurements of height and weight from birth to 2 years and 6 measurements from 2 to 11 years. Males who developed coronary heart disease as adults were born thin, and females who developed coronary artery disease were thin by 6 months of age. On average, those who developed subsequent coronary artery disease had a birth weight approximately 0.2 SD below the mean. After 2 years of age, the BMI of subjects with coronary artery disease rose progressively compared with other children. By 11 years old, their BMI exceeded the average BMI of 11-year-olds. The increase in BMI after 2 years of age predicted later coronary events more strongly than did BMI attained at a particular age.[45]

This is supported by animal studies that show that postnatal overfeeding of Wistar rats in early life can induce persistent changes in the hypothalamus, which promotes the subsequent development of the metabolic syndrome and obesity-related disease.[58]

PATTERNS OF INFANT AND CHILDHOOD GROWTH IN LGA INFANTS

SHORT- AND MEDIUM-TERM CHANGES IN WEIGHT

Babies born to mothers with gestational diabetes are at greatly increased risk of LGA. The majority of studies show that in the first few months after birth, there is slower growth in terms of weight and height, resulting in differences in weight and height being lost by 12 months of age.[59–61] Some studies show that the initial differences in weight are no longer present by 3 months of age.[61] Furthermore, higher levels of maternal glucose are correlated with greater initial catch-down growth in the first few months immediately after birth.[27] However, this *early* normalization of body weight was not maintained beyond infancy. By 5 years of age, weight increased and by 8 years of age, more than half of the offspring from mothers with gestational diabetes had a weight above the 90th percentile.[59]

In a study that excluded preterm babies,[62] 38% of LGA babies born to mothers with gestational diabetes were above the 90th percentile for BMI between 4 and 7 years old. There appears to be a dose effect with higher maternal glucose levels during pregnancy being associated with higher subsequent body size at 7 years of age. A small study (n = 27) showed that higher 1-hour post-prandial glucose level of an oral glucose tolerance test at 24 to 28 weeks gestation was associated with greater lean and fat mass at 5 to 10 years of age.[63] At 4 years old, female offspring of diabetic mothers had larger subscapular and triceps skin fold thickness, higher 30- and

120-minute insulin levels, and clustering of cardiovascular risk factors compared to control children.[64, 65]

CATCH-DOWN GROWTH

A study showed that LGA without catch-down growth by 5 to 8 years was associated with greater BMI, central adiposity, and diastolic BP than in LGA subjects with catch-down growth.[33] Huang and colleagues also showed two growth trajectories with birth size that was 1 SD greater than the mean birth size (#1 and #3 in Figure 5.4). Trajectory 1, which did not show catch-down growth, was associated with higher levels of metabolic risk. However, Trajectory 3, which did show catch-down growth, showed no evidence of elevated metabolic risk.[50] Therefore, currently there is evidence that LGA is associated with increased subsequent metabolic risk coupled with some early evidence that catch-down growth is associated with a decreased risk. Direct evidence that inducing the catch-down growth will ameliorate risk is currently lacking. Nevertheless, it seems likely that an intervention that induces catch-down growth by lifestyle changes is likely to induce metabolic benefits. Therefore, the results of well-designed intervention studies will allow recommendations to be made.

TIMING OF WEIGHT CHANGE

The timing of the critical period, or periods, of postnatal weight gain continues to be debated. The current literature is mostly concerned with SGA infants, rather than LGA infants, and has considered variable ages and variable intervals for the calculation of growth rates. The majority of studies have examined the period between birth and 2 years of age, but results are very heterogeneous. Some studies suggest that the period between birth and 6 months is critical.[66, 67] Other studies favor the first few months of life.[68, 69] In some studies, later weight gain is a major determinant of childhood obesity. For example, Law et al. showed in a systematic review that weight gain before 12 months of age had no effect on blood pressure at 22 years, but rapid weight gain between 1 and 5 years was associated with higher adult blood pressure.[70] Still others have investigated rapid growth up to adolescence and beyond. Ong et al. showed that "catch-up" growth between the ages of birth to 2 years old was associated with greater BMI, percentage body fat, and waist circumference at 5 years.[46] Barker et al. showed that those who went on to develop coronary heart disease were still thin at 2 years and gained weight rapidly between 2 and 11 years of age.[45] Despite the variable time periods, the majority of studies have reported a strong positive relationship between rapid weight gain in earlier life (age < 5 years) and obesity-related disease.[47]

It is likely that there are multiple periods of critical weight gain or upward percentile crossing and that there are likely to be multiple opportunities for intervention to prevent future cardiovascular risk. Upward percentile crossing in infancy and childhood may be different processes and amenable to separate opportunities for obesity prevention.[71] Ekelund showed that increasing weight gain during two separate time periods (infancy and childhood) were both independently associated with larger body mass index, fat mass, relative fat mass, fat-free mass, and waist circumference at 17 years old.[71]

Therefore, there is still debate about whether infant or childhood weight gain has greater effect on long-term outcomes of metabolic risk. The majority of the data relating to timing of weight change is from observational studies, which cannot demonstrate direction of causation.

Concerning LGA babies, the first question that needs to be focused on in future studies is whether inducing catch-down growth can ameliorate metabolic risk. If so, the timing and rapidity of this to maintain normal neurological development and reduce metabolic syndrome risk will be an important question to investigate. The initial work in this field suggests the need to focus on obesity intervention during the early preschool years.[72]

AMOUNT OR RATE OF WEIGHT GAIN

There is no consensus on the amount of weight gain, or on the rapidity of weight gain, that is required to have an effect on subsequent obesity-related metabolic disease. However, in general, an increase in 0.67 SD has been considered to have significant clinical effect and corresponds to an upward crossing of percentiles on growth charts.[9]

WHAT ABOUT ADIPOSITY REBOUND?

Adiposity rebound has been defined as a period of increasing BMI that occurs after an early childhood nadir. It marks the start of the second rise in BMI that usually occurs between 3 and 7 years of age.[73] At higher BMI percentiles, the age of adiposity rebound tends to occur earlier (Figure 5.3). Both an upward crossing of percentiles of BMI and a higher overall BMI percentile are associated with an early adiposity rebound. It predicts future adiposity. However, upward BMI percentile crossing rather than the early timing of the adiposity rebound is a more direct indicator of future obesity.

MODIFIERS OF EARLY POSTNATAL GROWTH

BIRTH WEIGHT

Lower birth weight is associated with greater postnatal growth. However, it is likely that postnatal growth from any birth size is associated independently with greater metabolic risk. In Figure 5.2, Trajectories 1, 2, and 4 are all associated with greater adolescent fasting insulin, homeostasis model of insulin resistance (HOMA-IR), and blood pressure. These trajectories begin from different starting points: low, middle, and high birth weights. They all share the characteristic of accelerated infant weight gain. This suggests that accelerated weight gain across the whole spectrum of birth weight occurs and is associated with increased metabolic risk.

BREAST-FEEDING

Disentangling potential confounding variables from the effect of breast-feeding per se is difficult, but overall the evidence suggests that artificial feeding stimulates a

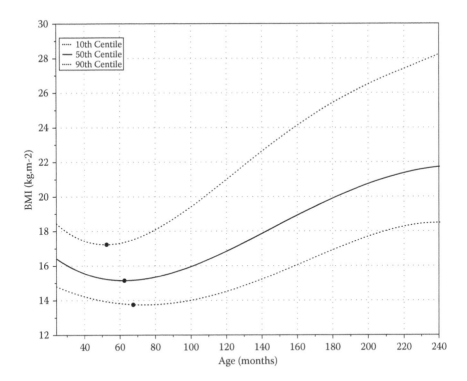

FIGURE 5.3   Age at adiposity rebound (black dots) for subjects with BMI on the 10th, 50th, and 90th percentile for age.

higher postnatal growth velocity with the adiposity rebound occurring earlier, whereas breastfeeding has been shown to promote slower growth.[74]

Breast-feeding is also associated with reduced metabolic risk later in life. Systematic reviews suggest that breast-feeding is linked to a modest reduction in the risk of later overweight and obesity. A recent meta-analysis investigated the effect of infant feeding type on body composition in healthy, term infants.[75] Fifteen studies were included in the systematic review. At 12 months of age, fat mass was higher in formula-fed infants compared to breast-fed infants. Interestingly, before 12 months, the reverse was true and fat mass was lower in formula-fed infants compared to breast-fed infants.

Furthermore, multiple meta-analyses have investigated the effect of the exclusivity and duration of breast-feeding on overweight and obesity later in life. Arenz et al. showed that breast-feeding has a small but consistent protective effect on subsequent overweight/obesity with adjusted OR 0.78 (95% CI 0.71 to 0.85).[76] In 4 out of 8 of the studies, a dose effect relationship was seen, with longer duration of breast-feeding being more protective.[76] Harder et al. showed that duration of breast-feeding was inversely associated with risk of overweight with a 4% decrease in risk per additional month of breast-feeding.[77] Horta et al. showed a pooled estimate of the risk of overweight or obese of OR = 0.78 (95% CI 0.72 to 0.84) with breast-feeding.

Despite the consistent findings of these meta-analyses, some publication and selection bias is probable. Smaller studies show greater protective effects than larger studies,[78] and the magnitude of the protective effect of breast-feeding is diminished in studies that have more variables.[79]

There are many potential mechanisms for the differences between breast-feeding and artificial feeding. The main difference in composition between breast milk and infant formulas is that breast milk has lower protein concentration as well as the presence of growth factors and hormones. The early protein hypothesis proposes that higher infant protein intake results in increased growth rate and adiposity.[80] Increased protein intake in infants stimulates the release of insulin and IGF-1, which stimulates growth.[81] Infant formulas can contain up to 70% higher protein content than breast milk. This effect could be especially important for preterm infants as their protein requirements are much higher and there is an ongoing trend to further increase protein intakes.

There may also be behavioral differences between breast- and bottle-fed babies. Bottle-feeding is controlled by the parent and as a consequence the baby may develop less self-regulation and internalization of satiety mechanisms, resulting in different caloric intakes. A breast-fed infant is more likely to regulate his or her energy intake based upon satiety cues.[74]

TIMING OF INTRODUCTION OF SOLIDS

Currently some studies show no evidence that earlier introduction of solids to infants increases subsequent obesity risk,[82] while others show an increased risk of obesity at 3 years of age with introduction of solids before the age of 4 months.[83] Other than timing, the quality and quantity of foods may be a consideration.

PHYSICAL ACTIVITY AND SEDENTARY BEHAVIORS IN CHILDHOOD

With increasing childhood obesity, there has been a public health focus on increasing regular physical activity in children and minimizing the time children spend in sedentary pursuits such as television and computer viewing. From the National Health and Nutritional Examination Survey 2003–2004, 42% of 6- to 11-year-olds in the United States performed the recommended level of 1 hour of physical activity per day and this fell to less than 8% among older children.[84] Children also spend large amounts of time in sedentary activities. For example, from the earlier NHANES III survey (1988–1994) over a quarter of 6- to 18-year-olds watched more than 4 hours of television per day and two thirds watched more than 2 hours per day.[85]

Nevertheless, it is currently not possible to provide an evidence-based answer to whether regular exercise is necessary for normal childhood growth and body composition, but exercise has no effect on rate of height increase in childhood or on adult stature. It does increase bone mineral density, muscle mass, volume, and cardiorespiratory fitness during childhood and adolescence.[86, 87]

MATERNAL SMOKING DURING PREGNANCY

Maternal smoking during pregnancy is associated with low birth weight, in the order of 150 g less than babies of non-smoking mothers.[88] However, LGA infants born to mothers who smoked during pregnancy have increased metabolic risk compared to LGA infants whose mothers did not smoke. In an Australian study, it was shown that babies who were in the upper quintile of birth size and also had mothers who smoked in pregnancy had an OR of 14.0 (95% CI 3.8 to 51.1) for high metabolic risk at 8 years old compared to babies in quintile 2 of birth size born to mothers who did not smoke.[5]

A similar effect can be seen across the entire birth weight range. One meta-analysis showed maternal prenatal smoking had an adjusted OR 1.50 (95% CI 1.36–1.65) for overweight at ages 3 to 33 years, compared with children whose mothers were non-smokers during pregnancy.[89]

Animal studies support the relationship between *in utero* exposure to cigarette smoke and metabolic risk. Prenatal nicotine exposure in rats has been shown to affect the development of pancreatic islet cells and adipose tissue.[90] Specifically, it led to a reduction in pancreatic islet size and number. It was also associated with an increase in regional white adipose tissue and adipose cell size. These and related gene expression alterations could lead to future metabolic disturbance, increased risk of obesity, and diabetes.

SOCIOECONOMIC STATUS

Postnatal growth patterns have been shown to be influenced by socioeconomic status. Socioeconomic variables explained 21.4% of the variation in maximum gain in weight-for-age Z-score achieved from birth to 12 months of age.[91] In a British study, lower socioeconomic status was associated with greater weight gain in infancy.[92]

GENDER

Gender differences have been observed in animals and humans. In an Australian population study, the importance of accelerated adiposity gain was seen only in males when the analysis was done separately for boys and girls.[50] This needs to be studied further to see if gender differences in fetal programming persist when the subjects become adults.

MECHANISMS FOR "FETAL PROGRAMMING" OF METABOLIC RISK

EPIGENETICS

A potential molecular mechanism for the relationship between LGA and subsequent offspring development of the metabolic syndrome is epigenetics. Epigenetics is defined as the study of inherited changes in gene expression caused by mechanisms other than changes in the underlying DNA sequence, such as DNA methylation and histone acetylation. Epigenetics appears to be the key molecular mechanism for fetal programming.

An early life (*in utero*) environmental challenge can cause epigenetic changes in the offspring.[93] Such epigenetic changes can lead to long-term changes in gene expression and metabolism, ultimately affecting long-term disease risk. Lillycrop and colleagues showed that *in utero* protein restriction was associated with persistent, gene-specific epigenetic changes that induced persistent changes in gene expression and the metabolic processes that the genes controlled. They showed that peroxisome proliferator-activated receptor alpha (PPAR-α) and glucocorticoid receptor (Nr3c1) gene methylation in the liver was lower, and PPAR-α and Nr3c1 expression higher, in rodents exposed to a low protein *in utero* environment compared with control pups. This was associated with a reduction in expression of a primary enzyme involved in DNA methylation, DNA methyltransferase.[93] Notably, the genes affected were related to obesity and cardio-metabolic pathways. Other early life environments (including maternal high-fat diet[94] and maternal perinatal care[95]) have now been associated with epigenetic changes in animal studies.

Similar findings have been seen in humans. For example, childhood stress[96] and maternal anxiety/depression during pregnancy[97] are associated with epigenetic changes in offspring.[98]

DNA methylation of specific CpGs within the promoter of retinoid X receptor alpha (RXR-alpha) gene in umbilical cord at birth is associated with childhood fat mass at 6 and 9 years in two independent cohorts.[98] Greater methylation of RXR-alpha was additionally associated with lower maternal carbohydrate intake in early pregnancy, which had previously been linked with greater neonatal adiposity.

Role of Adipokines, Ghrelin, and Other Hormones on Postnatal Growth

Ghrelin

Ghrelin is a peptide hormone that that has an effect on growth hormone secretion and energy balance, and is likely to have a role in pre- and postnatal growth. Its serum levels have been considered to have prognostic value for postnatal catch-up growth. Higher ghrelin levels were associated with more weight gain over the first 12 weeks of life.[99] In addition, LGA-born, non-obese, prepubertal children have lower ghrelin levels when compared with age and BMI matched AGA children.[100] Experimentally, ghrelin infusion has been associated with increased weight and adiposity in mice.[101]

Adiponectin

Adiponectin is one of the main adipokines. It is produced by the adipose tissue and has insulin sensitizing and antiatherogenic properties. Those with accelerated infant growth have lowered levels of adiponectin.[102] A fall in adiponectin levels in the first two years of life is associated with greater weight gain in SGA infants.[103]

LGA infants develop greater insulin resistance and lower adiponectin levels compared to AGA infants despite similar BMI at a mean age of 4.8 ± 0.3 years old.[104]

Leptin

Leptin is associated with fat mass in adults. It appears that this is also true in neonates and infants. LGA neonates have greater concentrations of leptin in the cord blood.[105] The usual weight loss that occurs in breast-fed babies in the first 4 days after delivery is associated with a 26% decrease in plasma leptin levels.

Vickers and colleagues demonstrated that neonatal leptin treatment in rats from postnatal day 3 to 13 slowed postnatal weight gain and normalized long-term caloric intake, body weight, and fasting glucose and insulin levels.[106] The leptin administration reversed the effects of maternal under-nutrition. The equivalent study to show if leptin administration reverses the programming effects of maternal over-nutrition has not been done. In humans, cases of rare monogenic obesity clearly show that genetic factors in the leptin signaling pathways affect infant appetite and therefore postnatal growth.[107]

FTO Gene

The FTO (fat mass and obesity associated) gene was identified by several genome-wide association studies to be associated with obesity. FTO encodes a protein with a novel C-terminal alpha-helical domain and an N-terminal double-strand beta-helix domain, which is conserved in Fe(II) and 2-oxoglutarate-dependent oxygenase family. Mice with a deletion of FTO show postnatal growth retardation and reduced IGF-1 levels.[108] In humans, the rs9939609 SNP in FTO is not associated with birth weight but is associated with weight, ponderal index, and total, truncal, and abdominal fat mass by two weeks.[109]

FETAL PROGRAMMING ACROSS GENERATIONS AND THE OBESITY EPIDEMIC

Obesity in a mother around the time of pregnancy is associated with having an overweight child at risk of type 2 diabetes and the metabolic syndrome.[8] Consequently, there is a propensity for increasing obesity and the emergence of complications at increasingly younger ages with each progressive generation. Transgenerational fetal programming is therefore relevant to the obesity epidemic. Maternal obesity, before and during pregnancy, can cause developmental changes in offspring, which lead to obesity. Evidence for this includes observations that maternal weight gain and development of type 2 diabetes mellitus between two pregnancies is associated with increased body weight in the second child.[110] Further, children born after maternal weight loss from bariatric surgery are less prone to obesity compared to siblings born before surgery.[111]

In a human population, there are persistent obesogenic influences over successive generations due to shared lifestyle within a family and a community. Two scenarios have been identified in animals. The first is an amplification of an epigenotype and phenotype associated with increased disease risk with each successive generation.[112, 113] Waterland et al.[113] used three generations of mice with the environmentally labile agouti viable yellow genetic variant. The genetic tendency for obesity in these mice was progressively exacerbated when passed through successive generations of obese females. In this animal model, the transgenerational amplification of body weight was prevented by a methyl-supplemented diet.[113]

The second is a progressive metabolic and epigenetic adjustment, akin to natural selection.[114] The epigenetic consequences of sustained energy intake over many generations has been explored in rats.[115] When rats were exposed to increased energy intake in F0 and the challenge was continued until F3, the offspring in each generation exhibited progressive metabolic adjustment via changes in the epigenetic regulation of transcription. Work is still required to ascertain which scenario occurs in humans to help predict the consequences of the obesity epidemic into the future.

CLINICAL AND PUBLIC HEALTH IMPLICATIONS

LGA babies have a baseline risk of future metabolic risk and this increased risk is exacerbated by sustained accelerated postnatal growth. The clinical implications of this are that childhood obesity prevention needs to start very early.

Clinicians should recommend that LGA infants be breast-fed whenever possible, as indeed should all infants, irrespective of birth weight. The benefits of catch-down growth should be investigated. The optimum degree and timing for this catch-down growth, however, is unclear. Further guidelines regarding how or, when to safely intervene to avoid weight gain in the first few months of life are still pending. The World Health Organization global strategy for infant and young child feeding recommends exclusive breast-feeding for the first 6 months of life. A recent study shows that LGA infants who were breast-fed for at least 12 months achieved a similar BMI at 4 years of age as AGA infants.[116]

The lack of understanding, and absence of clear guidance on catch-down growth, presents both parents and health-care professionals with problems. In many cultures, larger "chubbier" babies are perceived to be healthier, and weight gain is highly desirable (usually "the more the better"). Clear evidence of benefit and best practice for catch-down growth is currently missing. This evidence is required before advocating changing this highly engrained behavior.

CHILDHOOD AND INFANT WEIGHT MANAGEMENT

Pediatric obesity interventions are required to combat the childhood obesity epidemic. It is likely that earlier focus is required in the earlier preschool period.[72] This will entail careful monitoring of early childhood growth and family history of metabolic risk by maternal health nurses, pediatricians, and general practitioners, particularly after deliveries complicated by LGA, gestational diabetes, and maternal obesity. There is also a need to address the parental underestimation of childhood overweight. This is an issue highlighted by Baughcum et al., who showed that nearly 80% of mothers did not perceive their overweight preschool child as overweight.[117] It is likely that early referral to childhood weight management programs will be beneficial for ameliorating metabolic complications.[118–120]

INTERPREGNANCY INTERVENTION

Avoidance of maternal weight gain between pregnancies should also be advocated. Villamour et al. showed that those women who gained more than 3 BMI points between pregnancies increased their risk increased their risk of having an LGA baby (Odds Ratio 1.87 (95% CI 1.72–2.04)). The implications are that women of normal BMI should be advised to maintain a healthy BMI prior to pregnancy. More controversial is when and how much weight loss should be advocated for women who are overweight or obese prior to pregnancy.[110] The controversy exists because there is some evidence that weight loss or suboptimal nutrition at critical time periods during the periconceptional period results in increased risk of fetal programming of metabolic risk. Therefore, firm advice at this stage regarding timing of weight loss is pending future intervention studies.

PREGNANCY INTERVENTIONS

Lifestyle counseling has been shown to be effective in preventing gestational diabetes and reducing LGA.[121] Several further studies are in the process of being completed and results are pending to assess how effective pregnancy intervention can be in reducing LGA. Randomized controlled trials are currently pending, investigating dietary and lifestyle advice for women with borderline gestational diabetes[122] and limiting weight gain in overweight and obese women during pregnancy.[123] Follow-up of these and other trials will be required to ascertain if there is also a long-term benefit on metabolic syndrome risk in the offspring.

PREVENTION AND TREATMENT OF GESTATIONAL DIABETES

Prevention and treatment of gestational diabetes has also been shown to reduce LGA births.[124] Strategies such as the use of continuous glucose monitoring through pregnancy[125] and postprandial rather than fasting glucose levels should be recommended. A randomized controlled trial that investigated continuous glucose monitoring with standard antenatal care demonstrated a reduced risk of macrosomia (OR = 0.36, 95% CI of 0.13 to 0.98).[125] Oral hypoglycemic agents, such as metformin, are also increasingly being used as first line medical management of gestational diabetes mellitus.[126]

MANAGEMENT OF MATERNAL OBESITY DURING PREGNANCY

Advice about optimal weight gain for obese mothers during pregnancy is not clear. It is suggested that ideal pregnancy weight gain depends on the degree of obesity. For example, gains of 9.1 to 13.5 kg for obesity class 1, 5.0 to 9 kg for obesity class 2, 2.2 to <5.0 kg for obesity class 3 white women, and <2.2 kg for obesity class 3 black women are appropriate.[127] Some studies suggest that 25 lb or 11.4 kg should be recommended as the maximum amount of pregnancy weight gain in morbidly obese women (defined as a BMI >35) to prevent LGA in their offspring.[128]

A systematic review examining antenatal interventions for overweight and obese pregnant mothers did not show any differences in LGA outcomes.[129] However, at that point there were only three studies included with 366 women.

EXERCISE IN PREGNANCY

Leading professional bodies such as the American College of Obstetricians and Gynecologists and Royal College of Obstetricians and Gynecologists recommend 30 minutes of daily moderate intensity physical activity for pregnant women. Despite this, only a small proportion of healthy pregnant women meet these targets.[130] Furthermore, many women who previously exercised cease or curtail their exercise when they become pregnant.[131] The benefits of moderate exercise in pregnancy include reducing the risk of LGA.[132] This is aside from the significant benefits which accrue to the mother in terms of reduction in preeclampsia, gestational diabetes, and elevation in mood. From the work of Boney et al. it is clear that both LGA and maternal obesity were associated with increased risk of offspring metabolic syndrome,[8] both of which are reduced with exercise.

MATERNAL DIETARY INTERVENTIONS DURING PREGNANCY

Dietary interventions in pregnancy are currently being investigated. For example, a randomized controlled trial of a low-glycemic-index diet in pregnancy demonstrated a reduction in gestational weight gain and glucose intolerance in the mothers. However, it did not show a reduction in LGA neonates.[133]

CONCLUSIONS/SUMMARY

In summary, LGA infants are at increased risk of the metabolic syndrome in later life. This will almost inevitably become an increasing public health concern due to the escalating prevalence of childhood and maternal obesity. Some amelioration of this risk is possible by addressing factors affecting postnatal growth. Evidence to date, mostly based on observational studies, shows that catch-down growth may reduce baseline risk to levels comparable to AGA babies. Intervention studies are currently underway and more such studies will be required to guide recommendations regarding the optimum amount and timing of catch-down growth to advocate, as well as optimum methods to achieve this safely.

REFERENCES

1. Surkan PJ, Hsieh CC, Johansson ALV, Dickman PW, Cnattingius S. Reasons for increasing trends in large for gestational age births. *Obstet Gynecol.* 2004; **104**(4): 720–6.
2. Barker DJP, Gluckman PD, Godfrey KM, Harding JE, Owens JA, Robinson JS. Fetal nutrition and cardiovascular disease in adult life. *Lancet.* 1993; **341**(8850): 938–41.
3. Hales CN, Barker DJP, Clark PMS, Cox LJ, Fall C, Osmond C, et al. Fetal and infant growth and impaired glucose-tolerance at age 64. *Br Med J.* 1991; **303**(6809): 1019–22.
4. Barker DJP, Hales CN, Fall CHD, Osmond C, Phipps K, Clark PMS. Type 2 (non-insulin-dependent) diabetes-mellitus, hypertension and hyperlipidemia (Syndrome-X): relation to reduced fetal growth. *Diabetologia.* 1993; **36**(1): 62–7.
5. Huang RC, Burke V, Newnham JP, Stanley FJ, Kendall GE, Landau LI, et al. Perinatal and childhood origins of cardiovascular disease. *Int J Obes* (Lond). 2007; **31**(2): 236–44.

6. McCance DR, Pettitt DJ, Hanson RL, Jacobsson LTH, Knowler WC, Bennett PH. Birthweight and non-insulin-dependent diabetes: thrifty genotype, thrifty phenotype, or surviving small baby genotype. *Br Med J.* 1994; **308**(6934): 942–5.

7. Wei JN, Sung FC, Li CY, Chang CH, Lin RS, Lin CC, et al. Low birth weight and high birth infants are both at an increased risk to have type 2 diabetes among schoolchildren in Taiwan. *Diabetes Care.* 2003; **26**(2): 343–8.

8. Boney CM, Verma A, Tucker R, Vohr BR. Metabolic syndrome in childhood: Association with birth weight, maternal obesity, and gestational diabetes mellitus. Pediatrics. 2005; **115**(3): E290–E6.

9. Kerkhof GF, Hokken-Koelega ACS. Rate of neonatal weight gain and effects on adult metabolic health. *Nat Rev Endocrinol.* 2012; **8**(11): 689–92.

10. Chang GQ, Gaysinskaya V, Karatayev O, Leibowitz SF. Maternal high-fat diet and fetal programming: increased proliferation of hypothalamic peptide-producing neurons that increase risk for overeating and obesity. *J Neurosci.* 2008; **28**(46): 12107–19.

11. Bayol SA, Farrington SJ, Stickland NC. A maternal 'junk food' diet in pregnancy and lactation promotes an exacerbated taste for 'junk food' and a greater propensity for obesity in rat offspring. *Br J Nutr.* 2007; **98**(4): 843–51.

12. Ferezou-Viala J, Roy AF, Serougne C, Gripois D, Parquet M, Bailleux V, et al. Long-term consequences of maternal high-fat feeding on hypothalamic leptin sensitivity and diet-induced obesity in the offspring. *Am J Physiol-Regul Integr Comp Physiol.* 2007; **293**(3): R1056–R62.

13. Strakovsky RS, Zhang XY, Zhou D, Pan YX. Gestational high fat diet programs hepatic phosphoenolpyruvate carboxykinase gene expression and histone modification in neonatal offspring rats. *J Physiol-London.* 2011; **589**(11): 2707–17.

14. Ogden CL, Kuczmarski RJ, Flegal KM, Mei Z, Guo S, Wei R, et al. Centers for Disease Control and Prevention 2000 growth charts for the United States: Improvements to the 1977 National Center for Health Statistics version. *Pediatrics.* 2002; **109**(1): 45–60.

15. Weiss R, Dziura J, Burgert TS, Tamborlane WV, Taksali SE, Yeckel CW, et al. Obesity and the metabolic syndrome in children and adolescents. *NEJM.* 2004; **350**(23): 2362–74.

16. Reaven G. Metabolic syndrome: Pathophysiology and implications for management of cardiovascular disease. *Circulation.* 2002; **106**(3): 286–8.

17. Alberti KG, Zimmet P, Shaw J. Metabolic syndrome: a new world-wide definition. A consensus statement from the International Diabetes Federation. *Diabetic Med.* 2006; **23**(5): 469–80.

18. Zimmet P, George K, Alberti MM, Kaufman F, Tajima N, Silink M, et al. The metabolic syndrome in children and adolescents: an IDF consensus report. *Pediatr Diabetes.* 2007; **8**(5): 299–306.

19. Cleeman JI, Grundy SM, Becker D, Clark LT, Cooper RS, Denke MA, et al. Executive summary of the Third Report of the National Cholesterol Education Program (NCEP) expert panel on detection, evaluation, and treatment of high blood cholesterol in adults (Adult Treatment Panel III). *JAMA.* 2001; **285**(19): 2486–97.

20. Ford ES, Li C. Defining the metabolic syndrome in children and adolescents: will the real definition please stand up? *J Pediatr.* 2008; **152**(2): 160–4.

21. de Ferranti SD, Gauvreau K, Ludwig DS, Neufeld EJ, Newburger JW, Rifai N. Prevalence of the metabolic syndrome in American adolescents: findings from the Third National Health and Nutrition Examination Survey. *Circulation.* 2004; **110**(16): 2494–7.

22. Bao WH, Threefoot SA, Srinivasan SR, Berenson GS. Essential hypertension predicted by tracking of elevated blood-pressure from childhood to adulthood: the Bogalusa Heart Study. *Am J Hypertens.* 1995; **8**(7): 657–65.

23. Baird J, Fisher D, Lucas P, Kleijnen J, Roberts H, Law C. Being big or growing fast: systematic review of size and growth in infancy and later obesity. *Br Med J.* 20.

24. Burke GL, Webber LS, Srinivasan SR, Radhakrishnamurthy B, Freedman DS, Berenson GS. Fasting plasma glucose and insulin levels and their relationship to cardiovascular risk factors in children: Bogalusa Heart Study. *Metabol Clinical Experiment* 1986; **35**(5): 441–6.

25. Berenson GS, Srinivasan SR, Bao WH, Newman WP, Tracy RE, Wattigney WA, et al. Association between multiple cardiovascular risk factors and atherosclerosis in children and young adults. *NEJM*. 1998; **338**(23): 1650–6.

26. Ehrenberg HM, Mercer BM, Catalano PM. The influence of obesity and diabetes on the prevalence of macrosomia. *Am J Obstet Gynecol*. 2004; **191**(3): 964–8.

27. Stenhouse E, Wright DE, Hattersley AT, Millward BA. Maternal glucose levels influence birthweight and 'catch-up' and 'catch-down' growth in a large contemporary cohort. *Diabetic Med*. 2006; **23**(11): 1207–12.

28. Galtier-Dereure F, Boegner C, Bringer J. Obesity and pregnancy: complications and cost. *Am J Clin Nutr*. 2000; **71**(5): 1242S–8S.

29. Guelinckx I, Devlieger R, Beckers K, Vansant G. Maternal obesity: pregnancy complications, gestational weight gain and nutrition. *Obes Rev*. 2008; **9**(2): 140–50.

30. Kim SY, Dietz PM, England L, Morrow B, Callaghan WM. Trends in pre-pregnancy obesity in nine states, 1993–2003. *Obesity*. 2007; **15**(4): 986–93.

31. Stotland NE, Cheng YW, Hopkins LM, Caughey AB. Gestational weight gain and adverse neonatal outcome among term infants. *Obstet Gynecol*. 2006; **108**(3): 635–43.

32. Siega-Riz AM, Viswanathan M, Moos MK, Deierlein A, Mumford S, Knaack J, et al. A systematic review of outcomes of maternal weight gain according to the Institute of Medicine recommendations: birthweight, fetal growth, and postpartum weight retention. *Am J Obstet Gynecol*. 2009; **201**(4): e1–14.

33. Espineira AR, Fernandes-Rosa FL, Bueno AC, de Souza RM, Moreira AC, de Castro M, et al. Postnatal growth and cardiometabolic profile in young adults born large for gestational age. *Clin Endocrinol*. 2011; **75**(3): 335–41.

34. Bueno AC, Espineira AR, Fernandes-Rosa FL, de Souza RM, de Castro M, Moreira AC, et al. Adiponectin: serum levels, promoter polymorphism, and associations with birth size and cardiometabolic outcome in young adults born large for gestational age. *Eur J Endocrinol*. 2010; **162**(1): 53–60.

35. Schellong K, Schulz S, Harder T, Plagemann A. Birth weight and long-term overweight risk: systematic review and a meta-analysis including 643,902 persons from 66 studies and 26 countries globally. *Plos One*. 2012; **7**(10).

36. Loos RJF, Beunen G, Fagard R, Derom C, Vlietinck R. Birth weight and body composition in young adult men: a prospective twin study. *Int J Obes*. 2001; **25**(10): 1537–45.

37. Hammami M, Walters JC, Hockman EM, Koo WWK. Disproportionate alterations in body composition of large for gestational age neonates. *J Pediatr*. 2001; **138**(6): 817–21.

38. Hediger ML, Overpeck MD, Kuczmarski RJ, McGlynn A, Maurer KR, Davis WW. Muscularity and fatness of infants and young children born small- or large-for-gestational-age. *Pediatrics*. 1998; **102**(5): e60.

39. Huang R-C, Mori TA, Burrows S, Ha CL, Oddy WH, Herbison C, et al. Sex dimorphism in the relation between early adiposity and cardiometabolic risk in adolescents. *J Clin Endocrinol Metab*. 2012; **97**(6): E1014–E22.

40. Evagelidou EN, Kiortsis DN, Bairaktari ET, Giapros VI, Cholevas VK, Tzallas CS, et al. Lipid profile, glucose homeostasis, blood pressure, and obesity-anthropometric markers in macrosomic offspring of nondiabetic mothers. *Diabetes Care*. 2006; **29**(6): 1197–201.

41. Chandler-Laney PC, Bush NC, Granger WM, Rouse DJ, Mancuso MS, Gower BA. Overweight status and intrauterine exposure to gestational diabetes are associated with children's metabolic health. *Pediatric Obesity*. 2012; **7**(1): 44–52.

42. Sojo L, Garcia-Patterson A, Maria MA, Martin E, Ubeda J, Adelantado JM, et al. Are birth weight predictors in diabetic pregnancy the same in boys and girls? *Eur J Obstet Gynecol Reprod Biol.* 2010; **153**(1): 32–7.

43. Singhal A, Cole TJ, Fewtrell M, Deanfield J, A. L. Is slower early growth beneficial for long-term cardiovascular health? *Circulation.* 2004; **109**(9): 1008–13.

44. Singhal A. Early Growth and later atherosclerosis. In: Shamir RTD, Phillip M, Eds. *Nutrition and Growth*: Karger; 2013.

45. Barker DJP, Osmond C, Forsen TJ, Kajantie E, Eriksson JG. Trajectories of growth among children who have coronary events as adults. *NEJM.* 2005; **353**(17): 1802–9.

46. Ong KKL, Ahmed ML, Emmett PM, Preece MA, Dunger DB. Avon Longitudinal Study P. Association between postnatal catch-up growth and obesity in childhood: prospective cohort study. *Br Med J.* 2000; **320**(7240): 967–71.

47. Monteiro POA, Victora CG. Rapid growth in infancy and childhood and obesity in later life: a systematic review. *Obes Rev.* 2005; **6**(2): 143–54.

48. Li CY, Goran MI, Kaur H, Nollen N, Ahluwalia JS. Developmental trajectories of overweight during childhood: Role of early life factors. *Obesity.* 2007; **15**(3): 760–71.

49. Ventura AK, Loken E, Birch LL. Developmental trajectories of girls' BMI across childhood and adolescence. *Obesity.* 2009; **17**(11): 2067–74.

50. Huang RC, de Klerk NH, Smith A, Kendall GE, Landau LI, Mori TA, et al. Lifecourse childhood adiposity trajectories associated with adolescent insulin resistance. *Diabetes Care.* 2011; **34**(4): 1019–25.

51. Leunissen RWJ, Kerkhof GF, Stijnen T, Hokken-Koelega A. Timing and tempo of first-year rapid growth in relation to cardiovascular and metabolic risk profile in early adulthood. *JAMA.* 2009; **301**(21): 2234–42.

52. Fabricius-Bjerre S, Jensen RB, Faerch K, Larsen T, Molgaard C, Michaelsen KF, et al. Impact of birth weight and early infant weight gain on insulin resistance and associated cardiovascular risk factors in adolescence. *Plos One.* 2011; **6**(6): e20595.

53. Huxley RR, Shiell AW, Law CM. The role of size at birth and postnatal catch-up growth in determining systolic blood pressure: a systematic review of the literature. *J Hypertension.* 2000; **18**(7): 815–31.

54. Jarvelin MR, Sovio U, King V, Lauren L, Xu BZ, McCarthy MI, et al. Early life factors and blood pressure at age 31 years in the 1966 northern Finland birth cohort. *Hypertension.* 2004; **44**(6): 838–46.

55. Eriksson J, Forsen T, Tuomilehto J, Osmond C, Barker D. Fetal and childhood growth and hypertension in adult life. *Hypertension.* 2000; **36**(5): 790–4.

56. Fujita Y, Kouda K, Nakamura H, Iki M. Association of rapid weight gain during early childhood with cardiovascular risk factors in Japanese adolescents. *J Epidemiol.* 2013; **23**(2): 103–8.

57. Horta BL, Victora CG, Lima RC, Post P. Weight gain in childhood and blood lipids in adolescence. *Acta Paediatr.* 2009; **98**(6): 1024–8.

58. Plagemann A, Harder T, Rake A, Voits M, Fink H, Rohde W, et al. Perinatal elevation of hypothalamic insulin, acquired malformation of hypothalamic galaninergic neurons, and syndrome X-like alterations in adulthood of neonatally overfed rats. *Brain Res.* 1999; **836**(1–2): 146–55.

59. Silverman BL, Rizzo T, Green OC, Cho NH, Winter RJ, Ogata ES, et al. Long-term prospective evaluation of offspring of diabetic mothers. *Diabetes.* 1991; **40**: 121–5.

60. Rizzo TA, Dooley SL, Metzger BE, Cho NH, Ogata ES, Silverman BL. Prenatal and perinatal influences on long-term psychomotor development in offspring of diabetic mothers. *Am J Obstet Gynecol.* 1995; **173**(6): 1753–8.

61. Dode M, Santos IS, Gonzalez DA. Anthropometry from birth to 24 months among offspring of women with gestational diabetes: 2004 Pelotas Birth Cohort. *J Dev Orig Health Dis.* 2011; **2**(3): 144–51.

62. Vohr BR, McGarvey ST, Tucker R. Effects of maternal gestational diabetes on offspring adiposity at 4–7 years of age. *Diabetes Care.* 1999; **22**(8): 1284–91.

63. Chandler-Laney PC, Bush NC, Rouse DJ, Mancuso MS, Gower BA. Maternal glucose concentration during pregnancy predicts fat and lean mass of prepubertal offspring. *Diabetes Care.* 2011; **34**(3): 741–5.

64. Krishnaveni GV, Hill JC, Leary SD, Venna SR, Saperia J, Saroja A, et al. Antheopometry, glucose tolerance, and insulin concentrations in Indian children: Relationships to maternal glucose and insulin concentrations during pregnancy. *Diabetes Care.* 2005; **28**(12): 2919–25.

65. Krishnaveni GV, Veena SR, Hill JC, Kehoe S, Karat SC, Fall CHD. Intrauterine exposure to maternal diabetes is associated with higher adiposity and insulin resistance and clustering of cardiovascular risk markers in Indian children. *Diabetes Care.* 2010; **33**(2): 402–4.

66. Dennison BA, Edmunds LS, Stratton HH, Pruzek RM. Rapid infant weight gain predicts childhood over-weight. *Obesity.* 2006; **14**(3): 491–9.

67. Dubois L, Girard M. Early determinants of overweight at 4.5 years in a population-based longitudinal study. *Int J Obes.* 2006; **30**(4): 610–7.

68. Stettler N, Stallings VA, Troxel AB, Zhao J, Schinnar R, Nelson SE, et al. Weight gain in the first week of life and overweight in adulthood—A cohort study of European American subjects fed infant formula. *Circulation.* 2005; **111**(15): 1897–903.

69. Stettler N, Zemel BS, Kumanyika S, Stallings VA. Infant weight gain and childhood overweight status in a multicenter, cohort study. *Pediatrics.* 2002; **109**(2): 194–9.

70. Law CM, Shiell AW, Newsome CA, Syddall HE, Shinebourne EA, Fayers PM, et al. Fetal, infant, and childhood growth and adult blood pressure: a longitudinal study from birth to 22 years of age. *Circulation.* 2002; **105**(9): 1088–92.

71. Ekelund U, Ong K, Linne Y, Neovius M, Brage S, Dunger DB, et al. Upward weight percentile crossing in infancy and early childhood independently predicts fat mass in young adults: the Stockholm Weight Development Study (SWEDES). *Am J Clin Nutr.* 2006; **83**(2): 324–30.

72. Lee JM, Lim S, Zoellner J, Burt BA, Sandretto AM, Sohn W, et al. Don't children grow out of their obesity? Weight transitions in early childhood. *Clin Pediatr.* 2010; **49**(5): 466–9.

73. Cole TJ. Children grow and horses race: is the adiposity rebound a critical period for later obesity? *BMC Pediatr.* 2004; **4**: 6.

74. Oddy WH. Infant feeding and obesity risk in the child. *Breastfeed Rev.* 2012; **20**(2): 7–12.

75. Gale C, Logan KM, Santhakumaran S, Parkinson JRC, Hyde MJ, Modi N. Effect of breastfeeding compared with formula feeding on infant body composition: a systematic review and meta-analysis. *Am J Clin Nutr.* 2012; **95**(3): 656–69.

76. Arenz S, Ruckerl R, Koletzko B, von Kries R. Breast-feeding and childhood obesity: a systematic review. *Int J Obesity.* 2004; **28**(10): 1247–56.

77. Harder T, Bergmann R, Kallischnigg G, Plagemann A. Duration of breastfeeding and risk of overweight: a meta-analysis. *Am J Epidemiol.* 2005; **162**(5): 397–403.

78. Owen CG, Martin RM, Whincup PH, Smith GD, Cook DG. Does breastfeeding influence risk of type 2 diabetes in later life? A quantitative analysis of published evidence. *Am J Clin Nutr.* 2006; **84**(5): 1043–54.

79. Ip S, Chung M, Raman G, Chew P, Magula N, DeVine D, et al. Breastfeeding and maternal and infant health outcomes in developed countries. *Evidence Report/Technology Assessment.* 2007; (153): 1–186.

80. Koletzko B, von Kries R, Closa Monasterolo R, Escribano Subias J, Scaglioni S, Giovannini M, et al. Can infant feeding choices modulate later obesity risk? *Am J Clin Nutr.* 2009; **89**(5): S1502–S8.

81. Koletzko B, Broekaert I, Demmelmair H, Franke J, Hannibal I, Oberle D. Protein intake in the first year of life: A risk factor for later obesity? The EU Childhood Obesity project. In: Koletzko B, Dodds P, Akerblom H, Ashwell M, Eds. *Early Nutrition and Its Later Consequences: New Opportunities: Perinatal Programming of Adult Health.* Berlin: Springer-Verlag; 2005, 69–79.

82. Gillman MW, Rifas-Shiman SL, Camargo CA, Berkey CS, Frazier AL, Rockett HRH, et al. Risk of overweight among adolescents who were breastfed as infants. *JAMA.* 2001; **285**(19): 2461–7.

83. Huh SY, Rifas-Shiman SL, Taveras EM, Oken E, Gillman MW. Timing of solid food introduction and risk of obesity in preschool-aged children. *Pediatrics.* 2011; **127**(3): E544–E51.

84. Troiano RP, Berrigan D, Dodd KW, Masse LC, Tilert T, McDowell M. Physical activity in the United States measured by accelerometer. *Med Sci Sports Exercise.* 2008; **40**(1): 181–8.

85. Andersen RE, Crespo CJ, Bartlett SJ, Cheskin LJ, Pratt M. Relationship of physical activity and television watching with body weight and level of fatness among children: results from the Third National Health and Nutrition Examination Survey. *JAMA.* 1998; **279**(12): 938–42.

86. Beunen GP, Malina RM, Renson R, Simons J, Ostyn M, Lefevre J. Physical activity and growth, maturation and preformance: a longitudinal study. *Med Sci Sports Exercise.* 1992; **24**(5): 576–85.

87. Morris FL, Naughton GA, Gibbs JL, Carlson JS, Wark JD. Prospective ten-month exercise intervention in premenarcheal girls: positive effects on bone and lean mass. *J Bone Min Res.* 1997; **12**(9): 1453–62.

88. Kramer MS. Dterminants of low birth-weight: methodological assessments and meta-analysis. *Bull World Health Organ.* 1987; **65**(5): 663–737.

89. Oken E, Levitan EB, Gillman MW. Maternal smoking during pregnancy and child overweight: systematic review and meta-analysis. *Int J Obes.* 2008; **32**(2): 201–10.

90. Somm E, Schwitzgebel VM, Vauthay DM, Camm EJ, Chen CY, Giacobino JP, et al. Prenatal nicotine exposure alters early pancreatic islet and adipose tissue development with consequences on the control of body weight and glucose metabolism later in life. *Endocrinology.* 2008; **149**(12): 6289–99.

91. Ashworth A, Morris SS, Lira PIC. Postnatal growth patterns of full-term low birth weight infants in Northeast Brazil are related to socioeconomic status. *J Nutr.* 1997; **127**(10): 1950–6.

92. Wijlaars L, Johnson L, van Jaarsveld CHM, J. W. Socioeconomic status and weight gain in early infancy. *Int J Obes.* 2011; **35**(7): 963–70.

93. Lillycrop KA, Slater-Jefferies JL, Hanson MA, Godfrey KM, Jackson AA, Burdge GC. Induction of altered epigenetic regulation of the hepatic glucocorticoid receptor in the offspring of rats fed a protein-restricted diet during pregnancy suggests that reduced DNA methyltransferase-1 expression is involved in impaired DNA methylation and changes in histone modifications. *Br J Nutr.* 2007; **97**(6): 1064–73.

94. Dudley KJ, Sloboda DM, Connor KL, Beltrand J, Vickers MH. Offspring of mothers fed a high fat diet display hepatic cell cycle inhibition and associated changes in gene expression and DNA methylation. *Plos One.* 2011; **6**(7): e21662.

95. Weaver ICG, Cervoni N, Champagne FA, D'Alessio AC, Sharma S, Seckl, Jr., et al. Epigenetic programming by maternal behavior. *Nature Neurosci.* 2004; **7**(8): 847–54.

96. McGowan PO, Sasaki A, D'Alessio AC, Dymov S, Labonte B, Szyf M, et al. Epigenetic regulation of the glucocorticoid receptor in human brain associates with childhood abuse. *Nature Neurosci.* 2009; **12**(3): 342–8.

97. Oberlander TF, Weinberg J, Papsdorf M, Grunau R, Misri S, Devlin AM. Prenatal exposure to maternal depression, neonatal methylation of human glucocorticoid receptor gene (NR3C1) and infant cortisol stress responses. *Epigenetics.* 2008; **3**(2): 97–106.

98. Godfrey KM, Sheppard A, Gluckman PD, Lillycrop KA, Burdge GC, McLean C, et al. Epigenetic gene promoter methylation at birth is associated with child's later adiposity. *Diabetes.* 2011; **60**(5): 1528–34.

99. Fidanci K, Meral C, Suleymanoglu S, Pirgon O, Karademir F, Aydinoz S, et al. Ghrelin levels and postnatal growth in healthy infants 0–3 months of age. *J Clin Res Pediatr Endocrinol.* 2010; **2**(1): 34–8.

100. Darendeliler F, Poyrazoglu S, Bas F, Sancakli O, Gokcay G. Ghrelin levels are decreased in non-obese prepubertal children born large for gestational age. *Eur J Endocrinol.* 2009; **160**(6): 951–6.

101. Tschop M, Smiley DL, Heiman ML. Ghrelin induces adiposity in rodents. *Nature.* 2000; **407**(6806): 908–13.

102. Cianfarani S, Martinez C, Maiorana A, Scire G, Spadoni GL, Boemi S. Adiponectin levels are reduced in children born small for gestational age and are inversely related to postnatal catch-up growth. *J Clin Endocrinol Metab.* 2004; **89**(3): 1346–51.

103. Iniguez G, Soto N, Avila A, Salazar T, Ong K, Dunger D, et al. Adiponectin levels in the first two years of life in a prospective cohort: relations with weight gain, leptin levels and insulin sensitivity. *J Clin Endocrinol Metab.* 2004; **89**(11): 5500–3.

104. Darendeliler F, Poyrazoglu S, Sancakli O, Bas F, Gokcay G, Aki S, et al. Adiponectin is an indicator of insulin resistance in non-obese prepubertal children born large for gestational age (LGA) and is affected by birth weight. *Clin Endocrinol.* 2009; **70**(5): 710–6.

105. Marchini G, Fried G, Ostlund E, Hagenas L. Plasma leptin in infants: relations to birth weight and weight loss. *Pediatrics.* 1998; **101**(3): 429–32.

106. Vickers MH, Gluckman PD, Coveny AH, Hofman PL, Cutfield WS, Gertler A, et al. Neonatal leptin treatment reverses developmental programming. *Endocrinology.* 2005; **146**(10): 4211–6.

107. Farooqi IS, O'Rahilly S. Monogenic obesity in humans. Ann Rev Med; 2005. pp. 443–457.

108. Gao X, Shin YH, Li M, Wang F, Tong QA, Zhang PM. The fat mass and obesity associated gene FTO functions in the brain to regulate postnatal growth in mice. *Plos One.* 2010; **5**(11): e14005.

109. Lopez-Bermejo A, Petry CJ, Diaz M, Sebastiani G, de Zegher F, Dunger DB, et al. The association between the FTO gene and fat mass in humans develops by the postnatal age of two weeks. *J Clin Endocrinol Metab.* 2008; **93**(4): 1501–5.

110. Villamor E, Cnattingius S. Interpregnancy weight change and risk of adverse pregnancy outcomes: a population-based study. *Lancet.* 2006; **368**(9542): 1164–70.

111. Kral JG, Biron S, Simard S, Hould F-S, Lebel S, Marceau S, et al. Large maternal weight loss from obesity surgery prevents transmission of obesity to children who were followed for 2 to 18 years. *Pediatrics.* 2006; **118**(6): E1644–E9.

112. Cropley JE, Dang THY, Martin DIK, Suter CM. The penetrance of an epigenetic trait in mice is progressively yet reversibly increased by selection and environment. *Proc R Soc B-Biol Sci.* 2012; **279**(1737): 2347–53.

113. Waterland RA, Travisano M, Tahiliani KG, Rached MT, Mirza S. Methyl donor supplementation prevents transgenerational amplification of obesity. *Int J Obes.* 2008; **32**(9): 1373–9.

114. Hoile SP, Lillycrop KA, Thomas NA, Hanson MA, Burdge GC. Dietary protein restriction during f-0 pregnancy in rats induces transgenerational changes in the hepatic transcriptome in female offspring. *Plos One.* 2011; **6**(7).

115. Hoile SP, Irvine NA, Kelsall CK, Feunteun A, Lillycrop KA, Torrens C, et al. Fat content of maternal diet alters female offspring fatty acid status through epigenetic regulation of Fads2. *J Dev Orig Health Dis.* 2011; **2**: S21.

116. Camurdan MO, Camurdan AD, Polat S, Beyazova U. Growth patterns of large, small, and appropriate for gestational age infants: impacts of long-term breastfeeding: a retrospective cohort study. *J Pediatr Endocrinol Metabol.* 2011; **24**(7-8): 463–8.
117. Baughcum AE, Chamberlin LA, Deeks CM, Powers SW, Whitaker RC. Maternal perceptions of overweight preschool children. *Pediatrics.* 2000; **106**(6): 1380–6.
118. Sabin MA, Ford A, Hunt L, Jamal R, Crowne EC, Shield JPH. Which factors are associated with a successful outcome in a weight management programme for obese children? *J Eval Clin Pract.* 2007; **13**(3): 364–8.
119. Davis K, Christoffel KK. Obesity in preschool and school-age children: treatment early and often may be best. *Arch Pediatr Adolesc Med.* 1994; **148**(12): 1257061.
120. Savoye M, Shaw M, Dziura J, Tamborlane WV, Rose P, Guandalini C. Effects of a weight management program on body composition and metabolic parameters in overweight children: a randomized controlled trial. *JAMA.* 2007; **297**(24): 2697–704.
121. Luoto R, Kinnunen TI, Aittasalo M, Kolu P, Raitanen J, Ojala K, et al. Primary prevention of gestational diabetes mellitus and large-for-gestational-age newborns by lifestyle counseling: a cluster-randomized controlled trial. *Plos Medicine.* 2011; **8**(5): e1001036.
122. Crowther CA, Hague WM, Middleton PF, Baghurst PA, McPhee AJ, Tran TS, et al. The IDEAL study: investigation of dietary advice and lifestyle for women with borderline gestational diabetes: a randomised controlled trial–study protocol. *BMC Preg Child.* 2012; **12.**05; **331**(7522): 929–31.
123. Dodd JM, Turnbull DA, McPhee AJ, Wittert G, Crowther CA, Robinson JS. Limiting weight gain in overweight and obese women during pregnancy to improve health outcomes: the LIMIT randomised controlled trial. *BMC Preg Child.* 2011; **11**: 79.
124. Walsh JM, McAuliffe FM. Prediction and prevention of the macrosomic fetus. *Eur J Obstet Gynecol Reprod Biol.* 2012; **162**(2): 125–30.
125. Murphy HR, Rayman G, Lewis K, Kelly S, Johal B, Duffield K, et al. Effectiveness of continuous glucose monitoring in pregnant women with diabetes: randomised clinical trial. *Br Med J.* 2008; **337**(7675): a1680.
126. Rowan JA, Hague WM, Gao WZ, Battin MR, Moore MP, Mi GTI. Metformin versus insulin for the treatment of gestational diabetes. *NEJM.* 2008; **358**(19): 2003–15.
127. Bodnar LM, Siega-Riz AM, Simhan HN, Himes KP, Abrams B. Severe obesity, gestational weight gain, and adverse birth outcomes. *Am J Clin Nutr.* 2010; **91**(6): 1642–8.
128. Bianco AT, Smilen TW, Davis Y, Lopez S, Lapinski R, Lockwood CJ. Pregnancy outcome and weight gain recommendations for the morbidly obese woman. *Obstet Gynecol.* 1998; **91**(1): 97–102.
129. Dodd JM, Grivell RM, Crowther CA, Robinson JS. Antenatal interventions for overweight or obese pregnant women: a systematic review of randomised trials. *Bjog.* 2010; **117**(11): 1316–26.
130. Walsh JM, McGowan C, Byrne J, McAuliffe FM. Prevalence of physical activity among healthy pregnant women in Ireland. *Int J Gynecol Obstetr.* 2011; **114**(2): 154–5.
131. Macera CA, Ham SA, Yore MM, Jones DA, Ainsworth BE, Kimsey CD, et al. Prevalence of physical activity in the United States: Behavioral Risk Factor Surveillance System, 2001. *Prev Chronic Dis.* 2005; **2**(2): A17.
132. Owe KM, Nystad W, Bo K. Association between regular exercise and excessive newborn birth weight. *Obstet Gynecol.* 2009; **114**(4): 770–6.
133. Walsh JM, McGowan CA, Mahony R, Foley ME, McAuliffe FM. Low glycaemic index diet in pregnancy to prevent macrosomia (ROLO study): randomised control trial. *Br Med J.* 2012; **345**: e5605.
134. Rasmussen KM, Yaktine AL, Eds. Weight Gain During Pregnancy: Reexamining the Guidelines. National Academic Press, Washington DC, 2009.

6 Postnatal Growth Failure in Preterm Infants
Metabolic Outcomes

Richard J. Cooke and Ian J. Griffin

INTRODUCTION

Postnatal growth failure (*ex utero* growth restriction, or EUGR) is almost inevitable in preterm infants; the smaller and more immature the infant, the greater the degree of growth failure[1,2] (see Chapter 3). Poor somatic growth reflects poor organ growth and is associated with alterations in organ structure and function.

Postnatal growth is directly related to alterations in brain growth and structure, and slower growth is associated with poorer neurodevelopmental outcome in term and preterm infants.[3] On the other hand, catch-up growth is paralleled by improved function, particularly neurodevelopment, both in term and preterm infants (see Chapter 7).

However, concern exists about catch-up growth and the development of metabolic syndrome.[4–6] In this chapter, the relationship between preterm birth, *ex utero* growth restriction, catch-up growth, and subsequent development of metabolic syndrome will be explored.

EX UTERO GROWTH RESTRICTION

Several factors contribute to the development of EUGR in very low birth weight (VLBW) infants (see Chapter 3). It takes time to establish adequate dietary intakes in the sick, unstable infant[2] and what is "adequate" is not well established. Moreover, sensitive, valid, and robust measures of outcome are not readily available.

The extent to which inadequate intake contributes to EUGR was quantified by Embleton et al.,[2] who prospectively followed nutrient intakes and growth in a group of infants admitted to a neonatal intensive care unit. Actual intake was subtracted from recommended intake to calculate the nutritional deficit, and the cumulative deficit over time was calculated. This was examined in relationship to EUGR, expressed as change in Z-score between birth and a given time point.

The results are presented in Figure 6.1. It took time to establish adequate protein and energy intakes and nutrient deficits accrued in all infants; the smaller and more immature the infant, the greater the deficit. Inadequate intakes were directly

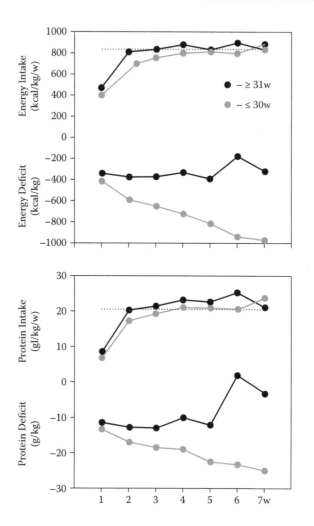

FIGURE 6.1   Weekly energy and protein intakes, and cumulative energy and protein deficits in preterm infants ≥31 w or <32 w. (Data from Reference 2. With permission.)

paralleled by EUGR; the smaller and more immature the infant, the greater the EUGR, with variations in dietary intake accounting for ≈ 50% of variation in EUGR.[2]

These data indicate inadequate intakes of protein and energy are important contributing factors to EUGR. Nevertheless, an important question remains unanswered. After a period of "faltering," should growth parallel that *in utero* or should infants be catching-back to original birth weight percentile? If so, dietary intake must not only meet needs of maintenance and normal growth but also catch-up growth during this critical epoch of growth and development.

MALNUTRITION AND NEURODEVELOPMENTAL OUTCOMES

Malnutrition during infancy is associated with poor growth and altered cognitive function.[3,7] Yet, the inter-relationship is not always so clear-cut as might first appear.[8] Studies are commonly confounded by the effects of socio-economic deprivation and inter-current illness, which not only affect educational processes but also alter nutritional requirements.[8] A vicious cycle is created among malnutrition, altered organ structure/function, development of disease, increased needs, and further malnutrition.

These considerations are magnified in preterm VLBW infant, in whom inter-current illnesses such as sepsis, respiratory distress syndrome, etc. are more common and more severe. At the same time, neurologic insults, peri-/intra-ventricular hemorrhage and periventricular leukomalacia are also more common, further confounding the interpretation of studies examining the relationship between nutrition, growth, and development in these high-risk infants.

An additional confounder is maternal choice. Morley et al. have shown that a mother's choice of feeding may account for an 8-point advantage in Bayley mental development index at 18 months corrected age.[9] Development outcome at 18 months corrected age, while extremely important, therefore, is not a very sensitive or, indeed, timely measure of adequacy/inadequacy of intake in the VLBW infant.

While poor growth in the first few months of life is paralleled by poor development, recovery or catch-up is associated with improved development in preterm infants[10–12] (see Chapter 7).

To examine this issue, Dharmaraj et al. prospectively followed growth between birth and 18 months corrected age and developmental outcome at 18 months corrected age.[13] It was hypothesized that the greater the degree of early growth failure (birth to 28 d), the poorer the development at 18 months corrected age (mca). Infants were, therefore, stratified at 28 d into those with mild (fall in weight Z-score ≤ −1.0; MGF) and severe (fall in weight Z-score > 1.0; SGF to those with mild growth failure (MGF; fall in weight Z-score ≤ −1.0) and those with severe growth failure (SGF; fall in weight Z-score > 1.0) growth failure. This process was repeated at 18 months corrected age. Growth of these infants is presented in Figure 6.2. Between birth and 28 d, Z-scores for weight decreased and then recovered to some degree in all groups. After 28 d, growth continued to improve in infants with MGF at 28 d and 18 mca (MGF-MGF) and SGF at 28 d but mild growth failure (SGF-MGF) at 18 mca. However, growth faltered in the other groups; that is, MGF-SGF and SGF-SGF. The developmental outcome data are presented in Table 6.1. SGF-SGF infants had a reduced mental development index (MDI) and psychomotor development index (PDI) compared to MGF-MGF infants, supporting the idea that poor growth between birth and 28 d is a marker for poor development at 18 mca. However, infants who recovered after 28 d (SGF-MGF) had better MDI and PDI scores than those who did not (SGF-SGF), indicating that catch-up growth between 28 d and 18 mca is paralleled by improved development.

While poor fetal growth is paralleled by altered organ growth, structure, and function,[14] not all organ systems are affected equally. In small-for-gestational-age monkeys, a 30% reduction in body weight was associated with an 8% reduction in brain weight but a greater than 35% reduction in lung, liver, pancreatic, and spleen weights when compared to their appropriately grown counterparts.[15] Thus, the brain

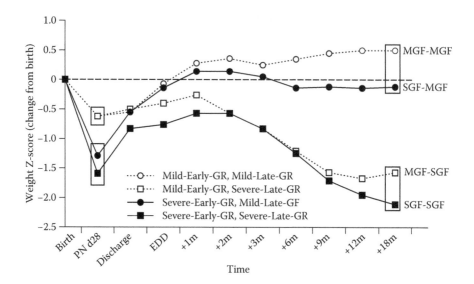

FIGURE 6.2 Growth of VLBW infants from Reference 13 categorized based on their growth at 28 d of life and at 18 m corrected age based on their degree of growth failure (GF), into SGF-SGF (severe GF at 28 d, severe GF at 18 m), SGF-MGF (severe GF at 28 d, mild GF at 18 m), MGF-MGF (mild GF at 28 d, mild GF at 18 m), and MGF-SGF (mild GF at 28 d, severe GF at 18 m). (From Reference 13. With permission.)

TABLE 6.1
Bayley's Mental (MDI) and Psychomotor (PDI) Development Scores

	SGF-SGF	SGF-MGF	MGF-MGF	MGF-SGF
All Infants				
Cerebral Palsy n (%)	5 (31%)	2 (2%)	3 (8%)	4 (17%)
MDI[a]	77 ± 19[a]	95 ± 11[a]	93 ± 18[a]	91 ± 18[a]
PDI[b]	77 ± 22[b]	87 ± 19	90 ± 17[b]	83 ± 19
Infants without Cerebral Palsy				
MDI[c]	88 ± 11[c]	98 ± 16[c]	96 ± 15[c]	93 ± 20
PDI	89 ± 16	91 ± 14	94 ± 13	89 ± 15

[a] Group SGF-SGF < SGF-MGF, MGF-MGF (p = 0.003), MGF-SGF (p = 0.01)

[b] Group SGF-SGF < MGF-MGF (p <.01)

[c] Group SGF-SGF < SGF-MGF (p <.05), MGF-MGF (p <.10)

Note: Infants from Reference 13. VLBW infants were categorized based on their growth at 28 d of life and at 18 m corrected age based on their degree of growth failure (GF), into SGF-SGF (severe GF at 28 d, severe GF at 18 m), SGF-MGF (severe GF at 28 d, mild GF at 18 m), MGF-MGF (mild GF at 28 d, mild GF at 18 m), and MGF-SGF (mild GF at 28 d, severe GF at 18 m).

growth is spared at the expense of other organ systems. This "brain sparing," however, might amplify the effects of under-nutrition on the other systems. Indeed, it may partly contribute to some co-morbidities noted in preterm infants; that is, alterations in immune function and the development infection, alterations in alveolar growth and the development of chronic lung disease, etc.[1] Irrespective, while of utmost importance, development is neither a sensitive nor, indeed, a timely measure of adequacy/inadequacy of intake in these high-risk infants.

THE FETAL ORIGINS OF ADULT DISEASES

OVERVIEW

Despite there being a clear relationship between poor growth and poor development, as well as better growth and better development, concern has been expressed about catch-up growth and the development of insulin resistance[16,17] and metabolic syndrome[4] in VLBW infants. These concerns emanate from the seminal work of Barker et al. who noted that intra-uterine/fetal malnutrition was paralleled by an increased risk for the development of insulin resistance, visceral adiposity, and cardiovascular disease in later life.[18]

Barker speculated that adverse ante-natal or early postnatal influences had permanent effects on body structure, physiology, and metabolism.[18] Depending upon timing, the effect varied. Insults during early gestation permanently reduced body size whereas those during late gestation affected cell structure and function without necessarily altering body size.[19] After delivery, released from *in utero* constraints and fed a normal diet, catch-up growth is paralleled by the development of insulin resistance, visceral adiposity, and other components of the metabolic syndrome.[19]

How this occurs is not fully understood. Inadequate nutrient delivery during a critical epoch of development is thought to alter tissue growth; that is, cell proliferation and differentiation. This, in turn, is associated with changes in organ size, structure, and function, notably the liver, pancreas, and kidney.[18] The relative contributions of different organ systems to the development of insulin resistance are not fully elucidated, but alterations in hepatic metabolism may be key.[20]

Obesity and increased adipose mass are core components of metabolic syndrome. Increased adipose mass is paralleled by an increased free fatty acid (FFA) flux and pro-inflammatory cytokine production. These, in turn, blunt the effects of insulin on liver, muscle, and adipose tissue (Figure 6.3). Hepatic output of glucose and VLDL lipoprotein increase, but HDL output decreases. Hepatic triglyceride synthesis/storage increases. Eventually, ectopic fat accumulation ensues, a result of concomitant oxidative stress, lipid peroxidation, and cytokine production.[21]

Adipose and muscle tissue sensitivity are also important in the development of insulin resistance. Normally, insulin inhibits adipose lipolysis and increases glucose transport into skeletal muscle. With insulin resistance, lipolysis continues, FFA levels increase, and the vicious cycle is perpetuated.[21–23] Macrophage infiltration has also been noted,[24,25] and is associated with adipocyte hypertrophy, thus increasing cytokine release,[26] further antagonizing insulin action. With increased FFA levels, glucose transport into skeletal muscle is also inhibited.[27–29]

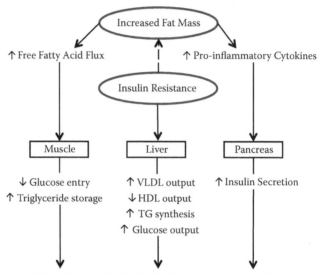

FIGURE 6.3 Schematic representation of inter-relationships between components of the metabolic syndrome.

The relative roles of genetic, intra-uterine, and environmental factors in the pathogenesis of insulin resistance are not clear, but diet also plays a key role.[21] A high-energy, that is, glycemic or fat, content increases insulin needs, fat synthesis, storage, etc. Diets high in trans-fats, branched chained amino acids, ethanol, and fructose content have also been related to increased lipogenesis, and therefore the development of metabolic syndrome.[20] However, whether a "normal" infant diet is likely to do so in VLBW infant with significant fetal or EUGR is unclear.

ANIMAL MODELS

Several animal models are used to study this issue. These include global dietary restriction, protein restriction, or hormonal intervention in rats. Global dietary restriction is associated with short-term and long-term effects on fetal physiology. The effects vary but alterations in blood pressure and vaso-reactivity,[30] glucose homeostasis,[31] pancreatic development,[31] and hypothalamic-pituitary adrenal axis[32] have been shown.

Rat pups born to dams fed a low-protein diet are underweight and short at delivery.[33–35] Pups then fed an unrestricted diet catch-up in weight but not length,[34] and permanent disruption to organ structure and function result.[34]

Diet shortly after birth may amplify the risk of obesity and metabolic disease in later life.[36] However, differences exist in endocrine and metabolic status between fetal growth failure and dietary-induced alterations. With fetal growth failure, fasting plasma insulin and C-peptide levels are increased and there is no reduction in insulin sensitivity.[37] At the same time, hepatic fatty acid synthesis and fat storage in peripheral fat sites is increased.[37]

With diet-induced obesity, insulin levels are not elevated but insulin sensitivity is reduced.[37,38] At the same time, fatty acid synthesis is also decreased and there is increased fat storage in non-adipose tissues.[39,40] Whatever the differential effects of fetal growth failure and dietary induced obesity are on endocrine/metabolic status, both increase the likelihood of development of metabolic syndrome.

Hormonal interventions have also been used to study this issue. Fetal gluco-corticoid exposure in rats is associated with fetal growth failure,[40,41] elevated blood pressure, enhanced hypothalamic-pituitary-adrenal (HPA) axis activity,[42] glucose intolerance,[43] fasting hyper-insulinemia, and hyperglycemia[43] in rat pups. Exposure to cytokines (TNFα, IL-6) is also associated with obesity, alterations in insulin sensitiv-ity,[44,45] hypertension,[45] and dysregulation of the HPA axis.[45]

THE VLBWI

Parallels exist between the epidemiologic observations of Barker et al. and the very low birth weight (VLBW) infant, as up to 40% of preterm infants may be growth restricted at birth,[46] and as many as 100% growth restricted at hospital discharge.[1,47] Even if they were not malnourished *in utero*, most VLBW infants are malnourished after delivery, that is, during the latter part of the second and throughout the whole third trimester.

Parallels also exist with animal data. Global dietary or protein restriction and hormonal intervention are used to study metabolic syndrome in animals. Inadequate intakes are important contributing factors to EUGR in VLBWI. In the study of Embleton et al., the deficit in protein and energy intake accounted for ~50% of vari-ability in EUGR.[2] Body composition data indicate increased/altered adiposity as well as a reduction in lean body mass.[48,49]

Additional risk factors in the VLBWI include:

1. Postnatal administration of steroids; for example, for the treatment of ino-trope-resistant hypotension, prevention/treatment of chronic lung disease, etc.
2. Maternal chorio-amnionitis, a common occurrence with preterm labor, leading to pro-inflammatory cytokine production.
3. Recurrent postnatal stress as occurs with intercurrent illness; for example, sepsis, necrotizing enterocolitis, etc., which increase cortisol secretion and pro-inflammatory cytokine production.

Collectively, these data have been interpreted to indicate that VLBW infants may be at an increased risk of developing insulin resistance and visceral obesity.[50] Mechanistically, increased TNFα and cortisol levels, because of stress/infection, coupled with low protein intakes blunt insulin sensitivity and acutely increase insu-lin levels (Figure 6.4). With recurrent stress and low protein intakes/high-glycemic diet, chronic hyperinsulinemia ensues and there is a down-regulation of β3 visceral adreno-ceptors, reduced visceral lipolysis, and increased visceral mass (Figure 6.4).

Inadequate protein and energy intakes can be directly related to reduced body size and altered body composition. However, whether this is associated with alterations in endocrine, renal, or hepatic function on a temporary or permanent basis is unclear. Further studies are needed to examine these key issues in VLBW infants.

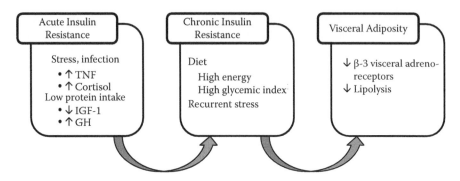

FIGURE 6.4   Schematic representation of the possible progression from acute insulin resistance to chronic insulin resistance, and finally to increased visceral adiposity in the preterm infant precipitated by a combination of stress and nutritional factors.

LONG-TERM METABOLIC EFFECTS OF PREMATURITY AND POSTNATAL GROWTH

In attempting to determine the effects of preterm birth, *in utero* growth restriction (IUGR), EUGR, and subsequent catch-up growth on the risk of the metabolic syndrome, we set ourselves a difficult task. The metabolic syndrome may take many decades to become apparent, and if we wait for such data, our results will no longer be applicable to the then current practice of neonatology. Rather than knowing how to manage our current preterm infants, we will only know how we should have managed preterm infants born, and cared for, several decades earlier. To obtain timely and clinically relevant data, we are forced to use proxy measures of the metabolic syndrome such as body adiposity or biochemical measures of insulin sensitivity, or blood lipids. In order to find any effect that may exist, we need to do the right measurement, at the right time, in the right infants, and carry out the right analysis.

RIGHT MEASUREMENT

Selecting the correct proxy measure is difficult. The total amount of body fat can be analyzed as an absolute number, as a percentage of body mass (e.g., percentage body fat), or normalized to body size (e.g., normalizing to height as in the fat mass index). Describing regionalization of partitioning of fat between different depots is even harder. For example, there are many permutations of body composition that could lead to an increased percentage of body fat being on the trunk, rather than the limbs (i.e., "central" rather than "peripheral"):

1. There may be a general increase in adiposity that is most marked centrally, that is, both the numerator (central fat) and denominator (peripheral fat) are increased, but the ratio remains increased.

2. There may be normal whole body fat mass, but fat is shifted from peripheral to central sites, that is, numerator (central fat) is increased and denominator (peripheral fat) is decreased, leading to an increased ratio.
3. There may be reduced body fat, but the fat is most markedly reduced in peripheral sites, that is, numerator (central fat) is reduced but the denominator (peripheral fat) is reduced more, causing the ratio to be increased.

All three of these examples lead to an increase in central fat as a percentage of total body fat, but the whole body adiposity may be increased, decreased, or normal, the absolute amount of fat in central depots may be increased, decreased, or normal, and the amount of fat in peripheral depots may be increased, decreased, or normal, depending on the individual case. It is unlikely that all such permutations carry the same long-term metabolic risks. The same problem is seen when considering the percentage of fat in subcutaneous tissues, in internal tissues, in the abdomen, etc.

When considering insulin sensitivity, some tests are relatively easy and can be used in large populations (e.g., fasting glucose, fasting insulin, HOMA-IR). Others are more complex and expensive, and so are harder to use in large groups (oral and IV glucose tolerance tests). Finally, tests such as hyperinsulinemic euglycemic clamp are even more difficult and invasive to perform and published data is available only for relatively small samples sizes.

RIGHT TIME

Selecting the correct time is also important. There is evidence from term SGA infants that some proxyl measures (such as body adiposity or insulin sensitivity) may be normal, or indeed more favorable than term SGA infants than term AGA infants, early in life[51] and metabolic derangements only become more apparent with age.[52,53] Results early in life, therefore, may be deceptive. Outcomes at certain time points (e.g., at term corrected age) may be confounded by the rapid changes that occur immediately after delivery in term infants (see later).

RIGHT PATIENT

Many cohorts have been recruited based on their body weight rather than on their gestational age. Although most VLBW (<1.5 kg birth weight) will be preterm, a small number will be term. However, if AGA VLBW are considered, they will all be preterm. If the population selects LBW infants (< 2.5 kg birth weight), the proportion of term infants will be much higher.

Not all preterm infants are likely to be a similar risk. It would be expected that moderately preterm infants would be a less risk (although this is unproven), but cohorts of preterm infants vary in their inclusion criteria, and some will include such infants. This is understandable, as stricter enter criteria and narrower gestational age limits will rapidly reduce the number of potentially eligible infants.

Large, high-quality cohorts are difficult to recruit, require large amounts of work from multiple people, and are extremely expensive. Therefore, the number of such cohorts is very limited. As a result, more than one paper can report related (but distinct) markers of metabolic risk in the same cohort. For example, the excellent Dutch Preterm and Small-for-gestational-age infants (POPS) cohort has been the basis of many of the papers we will review next.[54-62] Although this approach is completely appropriate, and results from one of those papers can support results in another, it should be remembered that the cohorts are either closely related or identical, so the two sets of results are not provide truly *independent* confirmation of each other's results.

RIGHT ANALYSIS

When examining the effects of prematurity, it seems obvious that the comparison group should be term infants. However, up to 50% of preterm infants have IUGR or are diagnosed as SGA. Therefore, should the comparison group be term AGA infants, term SGA infants, or both? Presumably, the most "normal" condition is the term AGA infant (ideally those exclusively fed human milk) but does that result in an impossibly high standard for preterm infants to meet?

Many studies have looked at the effect of postnatal growth on metabolic risk factors. However, it is well known that early catch-up growth is greater in babies who were born SGA. If an analysis examines the effect of the change in weight Z-score between, for example, birth and 3 m corrected age, this is confounded by the effect of birth weight Z-score as infants with lower birth weight Z-scores will have greater catch-up growth early in life. This effect is well known, and most published studies have accounted for it; however, some do not.

Just as the definition of EUGR is open to debate, so is the meaning of catch-up growth or "faster growth." Some studies have discussed "more rapid" and "less rapid" growth in preterm infants in the first two weeks of life. For example, what is the meaning of "greater weight gain" when it refers to a mean population weight gain of 38 g over 2 w (less than 3 g/d or about 2g/kg/d), rather than a mean weight decrease of 122 g over the same period?[63]

COMPONENTS OF THE METABOLIC SYNDROME

The definition of the metabolic syndrome is open to argument,[64-66] and is even more difficult to define in children. This serves to complicate the selection of "right test" in studies of growth and metabolic risk.

However, four components are frequently included in the *clinical* definition of metabolic syndrome:

1. Obesity. This may be defined based on whole body adiposity (typically using the proxy measure of body mass index), or on central adiposity (usually using the proxy measure of waist:hip ratio).
2. Hypertension.
3. Insulin resistance. This is most commonly diagnosed based on fasting blood glucose levels, or on 2-h values from an oral glucose tolerance test.
4. Dyslipidemia. This includes both abnormal cholesterol metabolism and elevated serum triglycerides.

We will now review the evidence linking preterm birth to these outcomes, and any evidence suggesting that the risk of these outcomes in preterm infants can be positively or negatively modified by rates of postnatal growth.

ADIPOSITY

In considering the effects of catch-up growth in preterm infants on later outcomes, such as risk factors for the metabolic syndrome, we need to consider two related questions:

1. What is the effect of preterm birth (and its associated comorbidities) on the outcome?
2. What effect (if any) does catch-up growth (or nutrition or diet) have on the relationship between preterm birth and the outcome?

We can consider these questions using the example of whole body adiposity ("fatness") in preterm infants, and ask the following questions:

1. Are preterm infants fatter or thinner than their term-born peers?
2. Does catch-up growth affect the adiposity of preterm infants?

CONFOUNDING FACTORS

In many studies, body adiposity is presented as percentage body fat (i.e., a percentage of total body mass, or the sum of lean and fat mass). An increase in percentage body fat, therefore, can represent an increase in the amount of fat tissue as a fraction of body mass *or* a decrease in the amount of lean tissue.

Another confounding issue may be the localization of adipose tissue. It is believed that intra-abdominal and specifically intra-hepatic fat may be particular risk factors for development of the metabolic syndrome,[67] MRI,[67,68] and MRS[67] and had led to the identification of the "fat on the inside, thin on the outside" phenotype as a risk factor for metabolic syndrome.

Often this is expressed as a ratio of the intra-abdominal fat to the abdominal subcutaneous fat.[52,67] Once again, an elevated value can represent either an increase in intra-abdominal fat or a decrease in abdominal subcutaneous fat. Whether there two circumstances have the same metabolic effects is unclear.

Both these issues can confound the interpretation of body composition data. In preterm infants, an increased percentage body fat may represent an increase in the amount of adipose tissue or a decrease in the amount of lean tissue. For this reason, the concept of fat mass index (the total body fat mass divided by the height squared) and the fat-free mass index or lean mass index (the total body lean mass divided by the height squared) have gained wider traction.

In addition, a population with reduced adiposity, in whom the reduction in fat is most prominent in subcutaneous tissues, may have the same ratio (%) of intra-abdominal fat to subcutaneous fat as an obese population whose excessive adipose tissue is disproportionately deposited in intra-abdominal sites. Although the two populations have similar percentage of intra-abdominal fat, they differ greatly in total body fat, and in the mass of fat tissue in subcutaneous depots and the amount of fat in intra-abdominal depots. Whether their similar values for percentage of intra-abdominal fat confer the same metabolic risks to the two populations is an open question.

POSTNATAL CHANGES IN ADIPOSITY

In term infants, there is a rapid growth in fat mass in the first few months of life, and the rate of increase in fat exceeds the rate of growth of other tissues.[69–71] As a result, the amount of fat as a percentage of total body weight increases from 11 to 14% at age 2 weeks to approximately 30% at three months of age.[69] The factors leading to this rapid increase are unclear, but presumably could include the changes in nutritional composition (a higher fat-based enteral diet compared to a higher carbohydrate-based transplacental route), a change to episode bolus feeds instead of continuous supply across the placenta leading to periods of fasting, the various neuroendocrine changes associated with birth, and the need to maintain one's own core body temperature *ex utero*. The fetus is known to gain fat rapidly during the third trimester and percentage body fat increases during the later stages of term pregnancy.[72] It is clear, however, is that these early postnatal changes are not simply the continuation of the *in utero* pattern of fat gain—the trajectory of fat accumulation changes dramatically near the time of birth[73] (Figure 6.5).

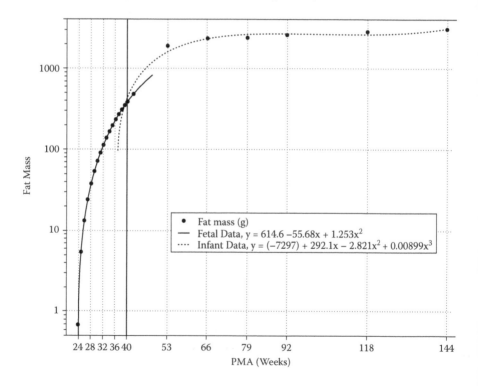

FIGURE 6.5 *In utero* and *ex utero* increases in total body fat in the fetus and term infant. (From Reference 73. With permission.)

Adiposity increases rapidly after birth. Between 1 w and 12 w after birth, males in one study gained 2.6 ± 0.58 kg in weight, of which 47% (1.23 kg ± 0.43) was fat. This resulted in a change in body adiposity from 12.5 ± 4.0% at 1 w to 26.4 ± 5.1% at 12 w.[74] Females in the same study gained 2.3 ± 0.49% (46% was fat), increasing body fat from 13.4 ± 3.7% to 26.3 ± 4.2% between 1 w and 12 w.[74]

EFFECT OF PRETERM BIRTH ON BODY ADIPOSITY

Near Term Corrected Age

Whatever drives the rapid increase in adiposity in term infants also seems to drive a rapid increase in adiposity in preterm infants beginning at birth. By term-corrected age, preterm infants have greater percentage body fat than do term infants.[75,76] This presumably reflects the fact that the preterm infants have had a substantial period of time between their preterm birth and their expected term date to accrete additional fat. Term infants, of the same post-menstrual age, are only a few days old and have not had time to accrete this fat. This would be consistent with data showing that differences in adiposity at term-expected age are greater for infants born more preterm,[75] as they have a long period of postnatal *ex utero* life to accrete fat at the increased *ex utero* rate.

Two things can be drawn from this:

1. Comparison of adiposity at term-corrected age between term and preterm born infants is confounded by the very different length of time spent *ex utero*.
2. This age is probably not helpful in understanding the long-term effects of preterm birth on body fatness.

It is now clear that the higher percentage body fat at term in preterm infants is not just due to increased absolute fat mass; the absolute lean mass is reduced at term in preterm infants compared to term infants and this accentuates the differences in percent body fat.[76] In some studies, there are no differences in fat mass between term and preterm infants, but the relatively lower lean mass in preterm infants leads to a greater calculated fat percentage in preterm infants.[77]

One meta-analysis has shown that both lean mass and fat mass are lower in preterm infants at term-expected age compared to term-born infants.[78] However, the deficit in lean mass (460 g) is much greater than the deficit in fat mass (50 g), leading to a significantly higher percentage fat mass in preterm infants at this age.[78]

Through Infancy and Beyond

The difference seen at term-expected age persists into early infancy. At 1 m corrected age, the percentage body fat of preterm infants remains higher than for term infants, although the relative difference between the groups is much less.[79] By 3 m corrected age, no difference in percent fat is apparent between the term and preterm infants.[79] Another study has demonstrated that the percentage body fat of former preterm infants slowly catches up with their term-born peers through the first year of life,[73] but that preterm infants continue to have lower percentage body fat even at

12 m corrected age.[73] For example, when the whole body adiposity of former preterm infants is assessed at 3 m, 6 m, and 12 m of age, the quartile with the higher weight gain from birth had increased adiposity than the lowest weight gain quartile.[73] However, even the highest weight gain quartile had a lower percentage whole body fat than the reference term infants (Figure 6.6).[73]

These differences persist into school age, when preterm infants have lower BMI, percentage body fat, and lower fat mass index, but normal fat-free mass index.[80] When the partitioning of fat is considered, the largest deficit is in the arms and the legs.[80] There may also be a smaller deficit in truncal fat mass, adjusted for height. The overall result is that former preterm infants have reduced total fat mass, reduced peripheral fat mass (i.e., in the arms), and reduced central fat mass (i.e., in the trunk), but an increased ratio of truncal to limb fat.[80]

At 4.6 y of age, both SGA and AGA preterm infants have body fat levels comparable to term AGA infants.[81] Term SGA infants had higher body adiposity than term AGA, preterm AGA, and preterm SGA infants.[81]

BMI remains lower in preterm infants at 6 to 12 y, compared to term infants.[82] When assessed by DXA, both fat mass and fat-free mass are reduced in preterm infants, but as the reduction in fat mass is disproportionately larger, the overall global percentage fat mass is reduced in preterm infants (20.1 ± 8.3%) compared to term infants (23.3 ± 8.3%, p < 0.005). When the amount of fat-free mass is normalized to height using the fat-free mass index (fat mass/height$^{2.5}$), the two groups are similar (11.4 ± 1.6 vs. 11.6 ± 1.0), but the deficit in fat mass in preterm infants persists (1.56 ± 0.82 vs. 1.81 ± 0.89, p = 0.01).[82]

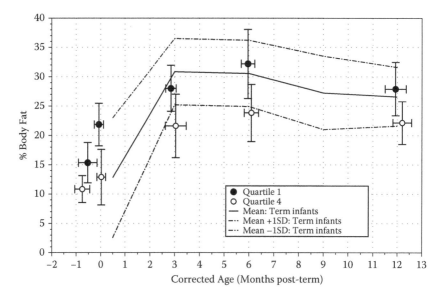

FIGURE 6.6 Whole body adiposity at term, and at 3 m, 6 m, and 12 m corrected age in the fastest and slowest quartile of preterm infants, compared to reference data for term infants. Data for the 1st and 4th growth rate quartiles of preterm infants are shown ±1 SD. (Data is from Reference 73. With permission.)

In Adult Life

There is relatively little data on adiposity in former preterm infants at adult age.

Some studies show no significant differences between preterm and term infants at age 18 to 24 y, either among those with more rapid growth in the first 3 m of life (28.3 ± 9.8% vs. 26.4 ± 9.2%) or those who grew more slowly (21.2 ± 10.4% vs. 19.4 ± 11.6).[83]

In the Dutch POPS cohort, VLBW preterm infants had reduced lean mass and reduced fat mass at age 19 y, than term infants.[84] The differences in lean and fat were similar, however, so that the percentage whole body fat was similar in their term and preterm infants.[84]

Other studies have shown increased percentage fat at 18 to 27 y in former preterm infants by MRI[85] or by DXA at age 18 to 24 y.[86]

Clearly, more follow-up data are needed, especially at older ages. Former preterm infants appear to have lower adiposity than their term peers through the majority of childhood. Limited adult data suggests similar or maybe increased adiposity in early adult life. It should be a matter of some urgency to clarify this issue because if the trend of increasing adipose content in preterm infants relative to term infants continues, it is possible that preterm infants will have substantially increased levels of whole body adiposity later in adult life.

Effect of Growth Rate on the Development of Whole Body Adiposity in the Fetus

The effect of *in utero* growth is best studied for the SGA infant (see Chapter 4).

Some limited *in utero* data suggest that IUGR during fetal life leads to both reduced fetal fat mass and reduced fetal lean mass. A study of 14 IUGR and 14 control fetuses at 30 to 31 w gestation assessed lean and fat masses from ultrasound examination of the fetus.[87] IUGR fetuses had reduced fat mass in the abdomen, subcutaneous tissues, and in the mid-arm, and reduced lean mass in the mid-arm.[87] No differences in fat or lean mass in the fetal arm were seen.[87] A second study assessed fetal lean and fat mass from in utero ultrasound of the fetal thigh.[88] Both lean and fat mass in the mid-thigh were reduced in this study. However, lean mass is disproportionately decreased to calculated percentage fat mass is actually increased.[88]

The adult effects of poor fetal growth based on results of observational cohort studies are contradictory. In the large cohort of infants born during the Dutch Famine, maternal malnutrition during the third trimester led to lower birth weight and a decreased risk of adult obesity, while exposure during the first or second trimester was associated with an increased risk of adult obesity.[89] No such effects on adult obesity were seen in the Leningrad Siege cohort,[89] perhaps because the Dutch Famine cohort had subsequent catch-up growth, while the Leningrad Siege cohort did not.[89]

Both maternal type 1 diabetes and gestational diabetes are associated with increased risk of obesity in offspring in adulthood[89] and it has been estimated that 1 kg increase in birth weight increases adult BMI by 0.5 to 0.7 kg/m^2.[89] Similar effects may be seen without overt disturbances in maternal blood glucose concentration. For example, Sewell et al.[90] compared obese and normal weight mothers, all of whom had normal glucose levels. Maternal overweight tended to increase neonatal birth weight and neonatal fat mass, but had no effect on lean mass. Multivariate analysis is confusing. Among mothers with normal pregravid BMI, maternal weight gain (which was used as a proxy measure of fetal growth) was associated with increased lean mass in infants at birth.[90] In the overweight/obese mothers, maternal weight gain was associated with infant percentage body fat at birth, but not with lean mass.[90]

Fetal growth is strongly associated with percentage body fat at birth, even in a population of predominantly AGA infants.[91] Birth weight (used as a proxy measurement of fetal growth) is significantly positively associated with percentage body fat, and explains 44% of the variability in percentage body fat at birth.[91] Alternatively, prenatal determination of estimated fetal weight or abdominal circumference explains 25% or 30%, respectively, of the variability in percentage body fat at birth.[91]

EFFECT OF GROWTH RATE ON THE DEVELOPMENT OF WHOLE BODY ADIPOSITY IN THE TERM INFANT

The Term SGA Infant

The term SGA infant is reviewed in detail elsewhere. Briefly, adiposity of AGA and SGA infants starts to diverge between 2 and 4 years of age and is related to the amount of catch-up growth[53] and the difference is well established by 6 to 8 years of age.[52,92] Abdominal fat content of AGA and SGA infants also diverges between 2 and 4 years.[53] Percentage body fat in SGA infants is related to the rates of weight gain between 0 and 2 years and between 2 and 4 years.[53] The amount of abdominal fat is related to growth between 0 and 2 years but not growth between 2 and 4 years.[53]

The Term AGA Infant

The effect of birth weight per se on long-term metabolic risk in term AGA infants is unclear.

Higher birth weight may be associated with early increases in fat mass index and BMI at 12 w of age.[93] However, by 11 y birth weight is unrelated to fat mass index, truncal fat, or percentage body fat,[94] although it was positively associated with height in both genders and with fat-free mass index in boys.[94]

Outcomes in Infancy

Childhood weight gain is known to be a heritable characteristic and may be a more important determinant of later metabolic risk than birth weight.[95] Weight gain between birth and 3 m is positively associated with higher fat-mass index and fat-free mass index (lean mass index) at 3 m of age.[93]

Other studies have not identified a significant effect of weight gain, but have identified a significant effect of length gain. In a mixed cohort of AGA and IUGR term infants, more rapid length gain was associated with increased adiposity at 6 w of age.[96] No such effect of weight gain is seen.[96] In this study, the highest body adiposity was seen in the human-milk-fed IUGR infants.[96] As is the case with the preterm infant, it is unknown whether this increased early adiposity is beneficial, detrimental, or of no consequence.

Outcomes in Childhood

In one study, the effect of rapid childhood weight gain (defined as an increase in weight SDS > 0.67 between 0 and 2 y) was associated with an increased BMI and an increased percentage body fat at age 7 y.[97] A similar study on more than 5000 term infants from the Seychelles showed that weight gain during the first year of life was strongly associated with the risk of obesity at 4 to 7 y even when the effect of birth weight was accounted for.[98]

Outcomes in Adult Life

Several studies have looked at the effects of early growth on metabolic risk at 17 to 20 y. In one study,[99] metabolic risk was associated with weight gain during infancy (0 to 6 m) but not during childhood (3 to 6 y).[99] Similar results were seen in a study of 300 African Americans.[83] Approximately 29% of subjects had rapid weight gain between 0 and 4 m (>1 SDS gain in weight), and these infants were at significantly increased risk of obesity at age 20 y.[100] Rapid weight gain between 0 and 4 m increased the odds for adult obesity 5.2-fold, and increased the odds for overweight 6.7-fold.[100]

Kerkhof et al. compared the effects of early weight gain in 162 preterm infants and 217 term infants at age 18 to 24 years old.[83] In term-born infants, rapid weight gain in the first year of life (weight SDS increase >0.67) was associated in increased body fat, truncal fat, increased waist circumference, and decreased insulin sensitivity, but had no effect on blood pressure or serum lipids.[83]

EFFECT OF GROWTH RATE ON THE DEVELOPMENT OF WHOLE BODY ADIPOSITY IN THE PRETERM INFANT

At Term

In preterm infants, whole body adiposity at term-expected age is associated with growth rate, with infants with the most rapid weight gain between birth and term having the highest adiposity,[101] and preterm infants who developed EUGR having lower percentage body fat at term.[102]

These findings are confirmed by MRI data[48] demonstrating that whole body adiposity in preterm infants is significantly related to the rate of *ex utero* weight gain. Although this dataset is a little atypical as it does not identify increased adiposity in preterm infants compared to term infants, rather, in this cohort the percentage total body adiposity was similar in preterm (17.0 ± 4.0%) and term (18.3 ± 2.5%, p = 0.64) infants.[48]

Roggero et al. studied VLBW infants (<1.5 kg at birth) classified based on whether they were below the 10th percentile for weight for age at birth (AGA or SGA) and whether their weight for age Z-score was below or above –2 SD at term-expected age (growth restricted or not growth restricted).[103] Among the AGA infants, those with postnatal growth restriction had lower weight Z-scores at term (by definition) and lower percentage body fat at term. Between term and 3 m corrected age, the growth-restricted AGA infants gained significantly more fat than their non-growth-restricted AGA peers, and had similar adiposity at 3 m corrected age. Between 3 m and 5 m corrected age, the two groups accreted similar amounts of fat and continued to have similar fat percentages at 5 m post-term.[103] At term, the SGA group had similar percentage fat to the growth-restricted AGA infants, and all three groups had similar fat percentages at 3 m and 5 m post-term.[103]

In Infancy and Childhood

As part of the large preterm and SGA infant cohort in Holland, the effects of birth weight Z-score and change in weight Z-score between birth and 3 m corrected age and 3 m and 12 m corrected age were evaluated in 403 preterm infants.[54] Early postnatal growth (birth to 3 m corrected age) was significantly positively associated with both fat mass and fat-free mass; however, the effect of fat mass was larger so that adiposity (either measured as percentage body fat or fat mass index) was greater if growth between birth and 3 m corrected age was greater, even if birth weight Z-score was corrected for.[54] Likewise, even following correction for birth weight Z-score and weight gain between birth and 3 m corrected age, later childhood growth (between 3 m and 12 m corrected age) was significantly associated with fat mass, fat-free mass, percentage body fat, and fat mass index.[54] Waist circumference was independently associated with birth weight Z-score and with weight gain between birth and 3 m, and between 3 m and 12 m corrected age.[54]

We have shown growth rates during the first year of life are associated with adiposity. In a large cohort of preterm infants, the fastest growing quartile of preterm infants had significantly higher whole body adiposity at multiple time points, through to 12 m corrected age[73] (Figure 6.6). What is noteworthy is that the highest growing quartile still has relatively low adiposity compared to term-born peers.[73] Whether one considers these difference in adiposity as "higher adiposity" or "more normal adiposity" in more rapidly growing infants is a matter of perspective.[73]

In one small group of VLBW infants, percentage body fat was significantly positively related to change in weight SD score between birth and 2 w and between birth and 4 w.[104]

Later in Life

In Kerkhof's study (see previously under "Outcomes in Adults, the Term AGA Infant"), more rapid weight gain in preterm infants during the first year of life was associated with increased body fat and increased waist circumference at 18 to 24 y.[83] When the first year was examined in more detail, weight gain between birth and term-expected age and between-term expected age and 3 m corrected age was significantly associated with both percentage body fat and waist circumference at 18 to 24 y.[83]

Similar to the Euser study[54] of 400 infants born before 32 w gestation, follow-up at 19 y demonstrated that weight gain between birth and 3 m corrected age and between 3 m and 12 m corrected age was significantly positively associated with percentage body fat at 19 y (and also BMI, waist circumference, absolute fat mass, and absolute fat mass corrected for height).[54]

FAT PARTITIONING

The literature on fat partitioning in former preterm infants is limited, and the data examining the effect of postnatal growth rates is even more limited.

At Term

Term and preterm born infants were compared at term-corrected age using MRI.[48] The two groups had similar percentage body fat, but the preterm infants had higher subcutaneous and intra-abdominal fat. Weight gain (expressed as change in SD score) was significantly associated with percentage intra-abdominal fat (r = 0.40, p = 0.0014), and with percentage of fat in subcutaneous depots (r = 0.40, p = 0.0012) in the preterm infants. However, these effects were lost on multivariate testing that corrected for birth weight and illness severity (using a proxy measure of the amount of time requiring higher-acuity care).[48] The multivariate analysis showed that the apparent effect of weight gain was probably being driven by illness acuity rather than being a primary effect of growth rate per se. The proxy assessments of illness severity remained the only significant factors explaining the percentage of fat in subcutaneous tissues (p = 0.017) or in intra-abdominal adipose tissue (p = 0.0009), while birth weight, gestational age, and weight gain (p = 0.28 and p = 0.75, respectively) were not significant.[48]

The same group has reported intrahepatocellular lipid using MRI/MRS in 18 preterm infants (gestational age less than 32 w) near the time of their expected date of delivery.[105,106] Comparisons were made to term-born infants and to adult data. The preterm infants had dramatically increased intrahepatocellular lipid (IHCL) than the term-born infants (increased over fivefold; P < 0.003.). There was no significant difference between the term infants and the adults. These findings are striking, but their significance is unclear. Three important factors should be considered:

1. Fat intake was high and the protein intake low in these infants throughout their hospitalization, and IHCL was significantly related to fat intake, especially fat intake in the first week.[105]
2. No data are presented on the relationship, if any, between postnatal growth rates and IHCL.
3. The age of examination (term-corrected age) is a time period that is unrepresentative of the rest of the first year of life and beyond in terms of whole body adiposity (at term-corrected age, preterm have higher percentage fat than their term peers, but lower adiposity for the rest of childhood and on into adulthood).

Finally, the authors found no relationship between postnatal growth and IHCL.[106] Despite these limitations, these provocative data merit further investigation.

In Infancy and Childhood

We have described fat partitioning at term, 3 m, 6 m, and 12 m corrected age based on compartmentalization of DXA (dual X-ray absorptiometry data).[73] Whether central adiposity is expressed as the ratio of the fat mass in the trunk and pelvis divided by that in the arms and legs, or by the ratio of the fat mass in the trunk and pelvis divided by that in the arms, legs, and head, we were unable to identify a relationship between growth rate and central adiposity during the first year of life.[73]

Although preterm infants (both SGA and AGA) had similar adiposity (measured as fat mass index) as term AGA infants at 4.6 y, the distribution of fat mass may be different.[81] In a study comparing SGA and AGA preterm and term infants, the truncal fat mass index differed between the groups with the preterm AGA infants having a higher truncal fat index (3.6, SEM 0.4) than the preterm SGA (2.9 SEM 0.5), term AGA (2.7 SEM 0.1), or term SGA infants (2.4 SEM 0.3).[81] The amount of truncal fat was correlated with weight gain between birth and the time of measurement, but is not clear whether this analysis accounts for the effects of body size at birth (e.g., birth weight Z-score).[81]

Later in Life

Based on DXA data from one study, preterm infants at 18 to 24 y[86] had higher trunk and limb fat mass, although the ratio of the two appears similar between groups. At 18 to 27 y of age, one small MRI/MRS study suggested that internal adipose tissue was significantly increased in males who were preterm compared to males who were born at term, but no such effect was seen in females. Compared to term infants, preterm infants had higher abdominal fat (both subcutaneous and internal), and higher intrahepatocellular (IHCL) and intramyocellular (IMCL) lipid in the tibialis muscle, but there were no differences in non-abdominal fat (either subcutaneous or internal nor in IMCL in the soleus muscle).[85]

EFFECTS OF INTERVENTIONS ON ADIPOSITY IN PRETERM INFANTS

Protein

There is relatively little data on the effect of protein intake on body composition in preterm infants. One randomized controlled study was unable to identify changes in body composition (including percentage body fat) due to three different levels of protein in infants.[107] However, one observational study has demonstrated that higher early protein intakes are associated with higher lean tissue mass, lower fat mass, and lower percentage fat mass.[108]

Follow-on Formulas

Once again, changes in body composition have proven difficult to identify in response to modifications of discharge formulas. Several randomized controlled studies have failed to see any difference in percentage fat mass.[109–112] For example, in one study preterm infants were randomized to receive a preterm formula from discharge to 6 m corrected age, a term formula from discharge to 6 m corrected age, or a preterm formula until their expected date of delivery and then the term formula.[110,113] A non-randomized group of human-milk-fed infants was prospectively followed.[113] Body composition was assessed at discharge, term, and at 3 m, 6 m, and 12 m corrected age.[113] Weight gain through to 12 m corrected age was significantly higher in the preterm formula group (i.e., given preterm formula until 6 m corrected age).[113]

Body composition, assessed by DXA, revealed significantly higher lean tissue mass in the preterm formula group than in the other three groups, and significantly higher fat mass.[113] The result was that percentage fat mass was similar in all four groups.[113] When partitioning of fat mass was examined, central fat mass (trunk, pelvis, or torso) was significantly lower in the crossover group than in the other three groups, and the amount of fat in the legs was significantly higher in the preterm formula group than the other three groups. No between-group differences in the amount of fat on the arms or legs was noted.[113]

In a study of 152 preterm infants, two isocaloric formulas were compared with a non-randomized group of human-milk-fed infants.[114] When the two randomized formula groups were compared, no significant differences in weight, length, or head circumference were noted to 6 m of age,[114] but there the two randomized groups were compared, there were significantly greater gains in lean mass and fat mass in the post-discharge formula (higher energy density and higher protein energy ratio) compared to the term formula group. At 6 m of age, the lean mass index was higher, the fat mass index was lower, and the percentage body fat was lower in the post-discharge formula group compared to the term formula group.[114] A similar study by Roggero confirmed the reduced body fat at 6 m corrected age in AGA preterm infants fed an enriched formula compared to a term formula.[115] No such difference was seen in SGA preterm infants.[115] In a non-randomized cohort study, the use of a protein and DHA enriched formula after hospital discharge in VLBW preterm infants led to a significantly lower percentage body fat at 1 y and 2 y corrected age, and to a significantly lower percentage of body fat deposited on the trunk at the same time points, compared to the regular term formula.[116]

HYPERTENSION

EFFECT OF PRETERM BIRTH

It seems likely that preterm birth is associated with modest elevations in both systolic and diastolic blood pressure (BP) in later life.[57,60,117–119] Although the magnitude of the change is small, it is likely to be significant in population terms. The degree of effect on BP appears to be inversely related to gestational age, with the largest effect seen in the most preterm infants.[117,120] In a recent meta-analysis of 10 trials comparing 1342 preterm and 1738 term infants, preterm birth was associated with an increase in systolic BP of 2.5 mmHg.[120] Among the subset of highest-quality studies, the effect was slightly greater, with a difference of 3.8 mmHg (95% CI 2.6 – 5.0).[120]

The relationship between BP and prematurity can be confounded by the effect of growth restriction. For example, in the EPIcure study of extremely preterm infants (<25 completed weeks gestation), systolic and diastolic BP were both lower in the preterm infants than in their classmates.[121] However, when the small body size of the preterm infants (both weight and BMI) was accounted for, the groups had similar BP.[121]

MODIFYING EFFECT OF POSTNATAL GROWTH

Some studies find no effect of postnatal growth on the risk of hypertension in preterm infants.[83,122] For example, in one small study, preterm infants and term controls were re-evaluated at approximately 24 y of age.[122] As expected, the LBW infants had significantly higher adult BP, and adult BP was inversely correlated with gestational age.[122] Lower birth weight was also inversely correlated with higher adult BP, but by 4 w post-term, no relationship between body size and adult BP was seen, nor was one seen for any 4-w period until 1 y corrected age.[122]

However, several studies find an effect of growth at older ages, but not earlier growth. For example, in a prospective study of over 400 Dutch infants born before 32 w gestation, systolic, mean, and diastolic BP was not affected by birth weight SD score[57] at age 19 y. Nor did change in weight SD score between birth and 3 m, 3 m and 6 m, or 6 m to 12 m have any effect.[57] However, systolic BP was affected by weight gain between 1 and 2 y, 2 and 5 y, 5 and 10 y, and 10 and 19 y, and by height SD score gains between 2 and 5 y, 5 and 10 y, and 10 and 19 y.[57]

In a study by Hack et al., the effect of weight and length at birth, 8 m, and 20 m, and on weight, length, and BMI at 8 y and 20 y was assessed in male and preterm infants.[123] Up to and including 8 m of age, none of the growth measures affected systolic or diastolic BP in either gender. Length at 20 m was positively associated with systolic BP (not diastolic BP) but only in females. In males, weight and BMI SD score at 8 y was associated with diastolic BP, and weight and BMI SD score at 20 y were associated with diastolic and systolic BP. Length was not associated with BP at either age in males. In females, systolic BP was associated with weight and height SD score at 8 y (but not BMI SD score), and with weight SD score (not height or BMI at 20 y).[123]

In a separate cohort of VLBW infants, systolic BP at age 18 to 27 y was 2.4 mmHg higher in preterm infants than in term infants.[124] BP was not related to either weight SD score at birth or at term-expected age.[124] A greater drop in weight SD score between birth and term (i.e., greater EUGR) was associated with an increased systolic and diastolic BP, although this was partly explained by differences in gestational age.[124] Within the VLBW AGA preterm infants, adult BP was unrelated to weight SD score at any time between birth and adulthood.[124]

Finally, in a small group of AGA and SGA preterm infants in young adulthood, the preterm infants in the highest systolic BP quartile had higher height SD scores from 3 m of age to 21 y as well as higher weight SD scores at between 1 y and 21 y, than those in the lowest systolic BP quartile.[59]

INSULIN RESISTANCE

EFFECT OF PRETERM BIRTH

In the last decade, the quality and amount of evidence on the metabolic risk of preterm birth and catch-up growth has increased dramatically. As before, we will examine the evidence for an effect of prematurity first, then the potential modifying role of postnatal growth rate.

Outcomes in Childhood

Several studies have examined the metabolic consequences in childhood of being preterm, either SGA or AGA.

In one study, preterm infants aged approximately 4 y have similar measures of insulin sensitivity and glucose homeostasis (fasting insulin, fasting glucose, and HOMA-IR) to term AGA infants.[81] This was true for both AGA and SGA preterm infants, and metabolic parameters did not differ between the two groups of preterm infants.[81] Term SGA infants at the same age, however, have higher HOMA-IR, glucose, and insulin levels than either term AGA infants or either of the groups of preterm infants.[81]

However, several other studies disagree with this. For example, in two studies carried out at age 4 to 7 y, preterm infants have reduced insulin sensitivity compared to term infants using an intravenous glucose tolerance test[125,126] and reduced acute insulin response.[126]

The effect of SGA status remains controversial, with some studies showing no difference between AGA and SGA preterm infants,[81,126] while others show a disadvantage to SGA status.[127]

Among a population of short SGA, the preterm infants had higher insulin secretion (higher acute insulin release), higher disposal index, but similar insulin sensitivity, fasting glucose, fasting insulin, and HOMA-IR.[128]

Outcomes in Adolescence

Several follow-up studies[17,63,129] have examined the metabolic outcomes of preterm babies at 13 to 16 y of age. The study subjects were initially enrolled in two randomized controlled trials of early diet; one comparing a term infant formula to a preterm formula[130,131] and one comparing unfortified donor human milk to a term formula.[132,133] In both studies, infants were fed their own mother's milk if available. If mother's milk supply was inadequate or absent, the randomized diet was given as a supplement to mother's own milk or as a sole diet. Diets were continued for approximately 1 month. The initial results of the randomized groups were presented for those receiving the formula as a sole diet, for those receiving it as a supplement to mother's milk, and for the two groups combined. Additional analysis was carried out for infants receiving the largest proportion of the study diet.

The developmental results of these studies have been reviewed elsewhere (Chapter 7). In brief, improved developmental outcomes were seen in the groups with the highest growth rates (i.e., higher in the preterm formula than the term formula and higher in the term formula than in donor human milk).

The first of these follow-up studies examined the concentrations of insulin, proinsulin, split 32–33 proinsulin and glucose at 13 to 16 years of age.[17] The most striking results were for the split 32–33 proinsulin. In the two studies separately (preterm formula vs. term formula, and donor human milk vs. term formula), there was a trend for higher split 32–33 proinsulin in the lower nutrient density diet (P = 0.07 for each). When the two trials were combined, the split 32–33 proinsulin concentration was significantly lower in the infants randomized to the lower nutrient density diet.[17] In addition, weight gain between birth and 2 weeks of age was significantly correlated with split 32–33 proinsulin (P = 0.0009) and with serum insulin concentration (P = 0.0001), suggesting a protective effect of lower nutrient intakes during the first 4 w of life in preterm infants, and with poorer weight gain in the first 2 w.[17] When weight gain between birth and 2 w of age was divided into quartiles, there was a significant trend for higher split 32–33 proinsulin levels with higher early weight gain.[17] What is sometimes overlooked is how much weight these infants lost: the lowest quartile lost more than 116 g over 14 d (>8% of birth weight), while the highest quartile gained at least 13 g (1% of birth weight). Furthermore, the cause of the differences in weight is not known. It is possible that the highest weight change quartile had significantly more edema, higher fluid intakes, or reduced urine output, all of which may be markers for severity of illness and have confounded the subsequent data.

Although infrequently discussed, Singhal et al.[17] also followed a comparison group of term infants. When one compares the preterm infants randomized to a higher nutrient diet or a lower nutrient diet to the non-randomized term infants, the preterm infants have serum insulin, proinsulin, and split 32–33 proinsulin more similar to the term infants than to the preterm infants on a lower nutrient diet (Figure 6.7). Although it is possible, it seems implausible that poorer nutrient intake in preterm infants could lead to a more favorable metabolic phenotype than seen in term infants with normal postnatal growth.

Outcomes in Adult Life

In the Dutch POPS study cohort, a variety of measures of insulin sensitivity has been carried out. Results of oral glucose tolerance at 19 y testing demonstrated higher fasting insulin levels, and higher 2-h insulin and glucose levels in preterm infants compared to term infants.[84] When the preterm AGA and SGA infants were considered separately at age 21 y, the preterm AGA infants had similar insulin sensitivity to the term AGA infants.[60] Both AGA groups (preterm and term) had better insulin sensitivity and lower post-prandial insulin than the preterm SGA cohort.[60] Among males, preterm SGA infants had higher post-prandial triglyceride concentrations than the AGA preterm and term infants.[60] These data suggest poorer insulin sensitivity in the preterm SGA compared to control term AGA infants, but normal insulin sensitivity in the preterm AGA infants.[60] More sophisticated testing using a hyperinsulinemic euglycemic clamp in young adults (21 y) produced somewhat different results.[59] Insulin sensitivity was lower in both preterm groups (AGA and SGA) compared to the term infants.[59]

In other studies, several have failed to identify a difference in markers of insulin sensitivity between term and preterm infants.[83,85,134] However, some have identified increased insulin levels or decreased insulin sensitivity in preterm infants at 21 to 23 y,[135] 24 y,[122] or 30 y.[119] One study described similar insulin levels between term and preterm infants but an increased fasting glucose,[122] while another has seen increased insulin concentration and increased fasting glucose once current weight was accounted for.[122]

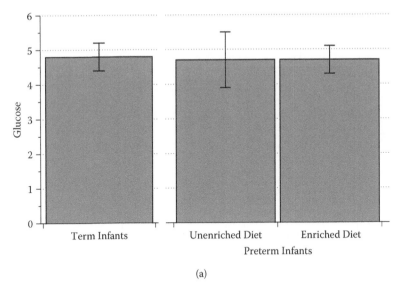

(a)

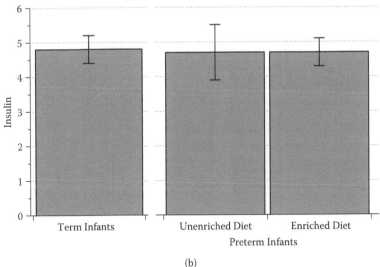

(b)

FIGURE 6.7 Markers of insulin resistance [serum insulin (a), proinsulin (b), split 32–33 proinsulin (c), and glucose (d)] from two combined studies of preterm infants depending on whether they received a lower nutrient diet (donor human milk, or term formula) or a higher nutrient diet (term formula, or a preterm formula), and a non-randomized comparison group of term infants. (Data from Reference 17.)   *(continued)*

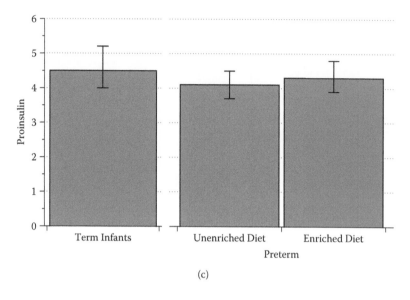

(c)

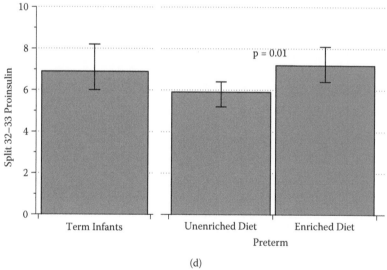

(d)

FIGURE 6.7 (CONTINUED) Markers of insulin resistance [serum insulin (a), proinsulin (b), split 32–33 proinsulin (c), and glucose (d)] from two combined studies of preterm infants depending on whether they received a lower nutrient diet (donor human milk, or term formula) or a higher nutrient diet (term formula, or a preterm formula), and a non-randomized comparison group of term infants. (Data from Reference 17.)

Modifying Effect of Postnatal Growth

The concern that differences in early postnatal growth in the NICU and afterward may predispose to later development of the metabolic syndrome is widespread, and may have changed nutritional practices. Despite this, many reviews find the evidence to be far from complete.[117,136,137]

Outcomes in Childhood

At 4.6 y, insulin sensitivity, measured using the HOMA-IR and insulin AUC correlated with gain in weight Z-score between birth and the expected data of delivery.[81] However, the relationships were lost once the analyses were corrected for birth weight Z-score.[81] In other words, the apparent relationship between early postnatal growth and later insulin sensitivity was due to the fact that *in utero* growth-restricted infants were at highest risk of later impaired insulin sensitivity, and showed catch-up growth between birth and term, and that then there was a direct effect of postnatal growth on insulin sensitivity.[81] Similar results were seen in 60 VLBW at 5.7 y.[127] Although both HOMA-IR and insulin AUC were higher in the infants with most rapid weight gain between birth and term, the effect disappeared once the birth weight Z-score was accounted for.[127] Some associations between markers of insulin sensitivity and instantaneous weight velocities at isolated times after term were seen.[127] The meaning of this is unclear.

Regan et al. showed that more rapid weight gain between term and 12 m was associated with increased risk of insulin resistance at 2 to 6 y, but that growth between birth and term, or after 12 m corrected age was not.[125] However, it is unclear whether these analyses corrected for the effect of birth weight Z-score that was seen in the subjects.[125]

In one large study of 385 preterm infants, the effects of *in utero* and postnatal growth on blood concentrations of split proinsulin and insulin at 9 to 12 y were examined.[138] Growth between 18 m and 9 y had the largest effect on split proinsulin, and growth rate between birth and 18 m had no effect on measures of insulin sensitivity.[138]

The effect of percentile crossing was examined in a mixed cohort of AGA and SGA VLBW infants. Approximately 50% had significant percentile crossing by age 2 y,[139] and this was associated with higher glucose, insulin, and HOMA-IR at follow-up. Weight gain between birth and 12 m (measured as change in Z-score) was significantly associated with BMI Z-score, waist circumference, serum insulin, and HOMA-IR, but not with blood glucose.[139]

Outcomes in Adolescence

As discussed previously, weight gain very early in life (between birth and 2 w of age) was associated with reduced brachial artery flow mediated dilation[63] and higher split 32–33 proinsulin levels in preterm infants.[17]

Outcomes in Early Adult Life

In preterm infants in the POPS cohort, weight Z-score at 3 m and 12 m corrected age has no relationship to C-peptide or HOMA-IR once birth weight was accounted for.[62]

However, higher height Z-score at 1, 2, and 5 y of age, and higher weight Z-score at 2, 5, 10, 19, and 21 y of age *were* associated with reduced insulin sensitivity on hyperinsulinemic euglycemic clamp testing.[59]

Studies have looked for an effect of postnatal growth in other cohorts. Kerkhof measured insulin sensitivity in term and preterm infants at age 21 y.[83] In the term infants, more rapid early growth was associated with reduced insulin sensitivity in adulthood. However, no similar effect could be detected in the preterm infants.[83]

DYSLIPIDEMIA

The literature on adult lipid levels in preterm infants is contradictory. Compared to term infants, many have increased lipoprotein A,[86] increased apoprotein A1,[83,86] decreased apoprotein B,[83] increased LDL,[140] increased[140] or unchanged cholesterol,[119,122,141] unchanged triglycerides,[119,122,134] and unchanged HDL.[122,140]

Data is limited but some evidence suggests that more rapid growth between birth and 3 m is associated with HDL-cholesterol levels, growth between term and 3 m corrected age with total cholesterol and LDL-cholesterol, and between 9 m and 12 m corrected age with total cholesterol and apoprotein B.[83]

The effect birth weight growth between (birth and 3 m corrected age) and later growth have on lipid panels has been examined in preterm infants in the POPS study.[61] As might be expected, current BMI Z-score was associated with total cholesterol, LDL, HDL, HDL/LDL ratio, triglyceride concentration, apoprotein A1, apoprotein B, and the ratio of aporotein A1 to B. However, birth weight Z-score was not associated with any of these parameters.[61] Early weight gain (birth to 3 m) was not associated with any of these lipid measures (cholesterol, HDl, LDL, HDl/LDL, triglycerides, apoprotien B, apoprotein A1, or apoprotein A1/apoprotein B ratio). Later weight gain (3 m to 12 m corrected age) was associated with HDL, but not after correcting for current height.[61]

Former preterm infants may also have reduced arterial dilation compared to term infants[63,142] and increased intimal thickness.[140] Neither early weight gain (birth to 3 m corrected age) or later weight gain (3 m to 12 m corrected age) are associated with carotid intimal thickness.[61]

When serum lipids were examined in follow-up studies of the Lucas cohort, infants on the highest intakes of donor human milk had lower CRP and lower LDL/HDL ratio than those fed formula.[129] This change favors the group with the slower growth rate (donor human milk) rather than that with the higher growth rate (formula).[129] In the other comparison (preterm formula vs. term formula), the same pattern was not seen: the faster-growing preterm formula group tended to have lower LDL/HDL ratios (P = 0.07) and lower ApoB/ApoA1 ratio (P = 0.09) than the slower-growing group.[129] The data was not analyzed by quartile of early weight gain[129] as had been done for other manuscripts by the same authors.[17,63]

SUMMARY OF THE CLINICAL LITERATURE IN PRETERM INFANTS

Whole body adiposity: At term-expected age, whole body adiposity is increased in preterm infants compared to term infants. This is due to deficit in lean mass in preterm infants at this time, rather than to an absolute excess of fat mass. Effects at this age are confounded by the rapid postnatal increase in fat mass that occurs in the weeks immediately after birth, and have yet to occur in the term infant. Throughout infancy and childhood, percentage body fat is lower in preterm infants than in term infants, although more rapid growth preterm infants have adiposity more similar to the term infant. In adolescence, percentage body fat is similar (or perhaps lower) in preterm infants than in term infants. By early adulthood, percentage body fat is similar (or perhaps higher) in preterm infants than in term infants. Where this possible trend of preterm infants approaching (and maybe overtaking) their term counterparts in percentage body fat continues into later adulthood is unknown.

Central adiposity: At term, the proportion of fat mass found centrally is probably normal, although small MRI studies have suggested increased intra-abdominal fat[48] or intrahepatocellular fat.[105,106] This is, however, no evidence that this partitioning is affected by growth rate. The effect of prematurity, and of postnatal growth, on central adiposity is controversial. Once again, small MRI/MRS studies suggest a possible effect of prematurity on intrahepatocellular and intramyocellular adipose, without any effect of *ex utero* growth.

Blood pressure: Systolic BP is increased in preterm infants, and the incidence of hypertension is higher. This effect seems unrelated to growth during the first year of life. However, larger body size or higher growth rates after about 12 to 20 m may be associated with higher BP in preterm infants.

Insulin resistance: Insulin sensitivity is probably reduced in preterm infants during childhood and in to adult life. The effect of postnatal growth remains controversial. However, the POPS study shows that increased body height after 1 y (but not before) and increased body weight after 2 y (but not before) are associated with reduced insulin sensitivity.[59] Those data[59] and those of Fewtrell[138] do not suggest that catch-up growth in the first year of life is likely to have adverse long-term metabolic consequences. There is limited data that reduced nutritional intakes and greater postnatal weight loss in the first 2 w of life may improve markers of cardiovascular morbidity. However, as those same studies showed that reduced nutrient intakes were also associated with poorer neurodevelopment (see Chapter 7), this does not seem to be a prudent approach.

Dyslipidemia: There is some limited evidence that former preterm infants may have an increased risk of dyslipidemia. Early postnatal growth (after 3 m corrected age, or maybe earlier) may worsen the risk of later dyslipidemia, but data is very limited.

CONCLUSION AND IMPLICATIONS

There is evidence that preterm infants may be at increased risk of adverse metabolic outcome later in life. However, the effects of prematurity, low birth weight, early EUGR, and subsequent catch-up growth on metabolic outcomes are extremely difficult to disentangle. The evidence that early postnatal catch-up growth (e.g., within the first year of life) leads to poorer metabolic outcomes is relatively poor, and much weaker than the evidence for beneficial effects of catch-up growth on neurodevelopmental outcomes in the same time period.

REFERENCES

1. Ehrenkranz, R.A., et al., Longitudinal growth of hospitalized very low birth weight infants. *Pediatrics*, 1999. **104**(2 Pt 1): 280–9.
2. Embleton, N.E., N. Pang, and R.J. Cooke, Postnatal malnutrition and growth retardation: an inevitable consequence of current recommendations in preterm infants? *Pediatrics*, 2001. **107**(2): 270–3.
3. Dobbing, J., *Developing Brain and Behaviour,* 1997, San Diego, CA: Academic Press.
4. Ong, K.K., Size at birth, postnatal growth and risk of obesity. *Horm Res*, 2006. **65 Suppl 3**: 65–9.
5. Dulloo, A.G., et al., The thrifty "catch-up fat" phenotype: its impact on insulin sensitivity during growth trajectories to obesity and metabolic syndrome. *Int J Obes* (Lond), 2006. **30 Suppl 4**: S23–35.
6. Dulloo, A.G., et al., Propellers of growth trajectories to obesity and the metabolic syndrome. *Int J Obes* (Lond), 2006. **30 Suppl 4**: S1–3.
7. Dobbing, J., *Early Nutrition and Later Achievement,* 1987, London: Academic Press.
8. Singer, L.T., Methodological considerations in longitudinal studies of infant risk, in *Developing Brain and Behaviour: The Role of Lipids in Infant Formula,* J. Dobbing, Ed., 1997, Academic Press: San Diego. 209–252.
9. Morley, R., et al., Mother's choice to provide breast milk and developmental outcome. *Arch Dis Child*, 1988. **63**(11): 1382–5.
10. Hack, M., et al., Catch-up growth in very-low-birth-weight infants. Clinical correlates. *Am J Dis Child*, 1984. **138**(4): 370–5.
11. Hack, M., et al., The prognostic significance of postnatal growth in very low: birth weight infants. *Am J Obstet Gynecol*, 1982. **143**(6): 693–9.
12. Latal-Hajnal, B., et al., Postnatal growth in VLBW infants: significant association with neurodevelopmental outcome. *J Pediatr*, 2003. **143**(2): 163–70.
13. Dharmaraj, S.T., Postnatal growth retardation, catch-up growth and developmental outcome in preterm infants [Abstract]. *Arch Dis Child*, 2005. **90**: 11A.
14. McCance, R.A. and E.M. Widdowson, The determinants of growth and form. *Proc R Soc Lond B Biol Sci*, 1974. **185**(78): 1–17.
15. Myers, R.E., et al., Fetal growth retardation produced by experimental placental insufficiency in the rhesus monkey. I. Body weight, organ size. *Biol Neonate*, 1971. **18**(5): 379–94.
16. Singhal, A., T.J. Cole, and A. Lucas, Early nutrition in preterm infants and later blood pressure: two cohorts after randomised trials. *Lancet*, 2001. **357**(9254): 413–9.
17. Singhal, A., et al., Low nutrient intake and early growth for later insulin resistance in adolescents born preterm. *Lancet*, 2003. **361**(9363): 1089–97.
18. Barker, D.J., *Fetal and Infant Origins of Adult Disease,* 1992, London: British Medical Journal.
19. Barker, D.J.P., The undernourished baby, in *Babies and Disease in Later Life,* 1994, BMJ Publishing Group: London. 121–139.
20. Bremer, A.A., M. Mietus-Snyder, and R.H. Lustig, Toward a unifying hypothesis of metabolic syndrome. *Pediatrics*, 2012. **129**(3): 557–70.
21. Cornier, M.A., et al., The metabolic syndrome. *Endocr Rev*, 2008. **29**(7): 777–822.
22. Ginsberg, H.N., Insulin resistance and cardiovascular disease. *J Clin Invest*, 2000. **106**(4): 453–8.
23. Kahn, B.B. and J.S. Flier, Obesity and insulin resistance. *J Clin Invest*, 2000. **106**(4): 473–81.
24. Gustafson, B., et al., Inflamed adipose tissue: a culprit underlying the metabolic syndrome and atherosclerosis. *Arterioscler Thromb Vasc Biol*, 2007. **27**(11): 2276–83.

25. Heilbronn, L.K. and L.V. Campbell, Adipose tissue macrophages, low grade inflammation and insulin resistance in human obesity. *Curr Pharm Des*, 2008. **14**(12): 1225–30.
26. Skurk, T., et al., Relationship between adipocyte size and adipokine expression and secretion. *J Clin Endocrinol Metab*, 2007. **92**(3): 1023–33.
27. Boden, G., et al., Mechanisms of fatty acid-induced inhibition of glucose uptake. *J Clin Invest*, 1994. **93**(6): 2438–46.
28. Dresner, A., et al., Effects of free fatty acids on glucose transport and IRS-1-associated phosphatidylinositol 3-kinase activity. *J Clin Invest*, 1999. **103**(2): 253–9.
29. Roden, M., et al., Rapid impairment of skeletal muscle glucose transport/phosphorylation by free fatty acids in humans. *Diabetes*, 1999. **48**(2): 358–64.
30. Ozaki, T., et al., Dietary restriction in pregnant rats causes gender-related hypertension and vascular dysfunction in offspring. *J Physiol*, 2001. **530**(Pt 1): 141–52.
31. Garofano, A., P. Czernichow, and B. Breant, Effect of ageing on beta-cell mass and function in rats malnourished during the perinatal period. *Diabetologia*, 1999. **42**(6): 711–8.
32. Lesage, J., et al., Maternal undernutrition during late gestation induces fetal overexposure to glucocorticoids and intrauterine growth retardation, and disturbs the hypothalamo-pituitary adrenal axis in the newborn rat. *Endocrinology*, 2001. **142**(5): 1692–702.
33. Snoeck, A., et al., Effect of a low protein diet during pregnancy on the fetal rat endocrine pancreas. *Biol Neonate*, 1990. **57**(2): 107–18.
34. Desai, M., et al., Organ-selective growth in the offspring of protein-restricted mothers. *Br J Nutr*, 1996. **76**(4): 591–603.
35. Langley, S.C., R.F. Browne, and A.A. Jackson, Altered glucose tolerance in rats exposed to maternal low protein diets in utero. *Comp Biochem Physiol Physiol*, 1994. **109**(2): 223–9.
36. Gorski, J.N., et al., Postnatal environment overrides genetic and prenatal factors influencing offspring obesity and insulin resistance. *Am J Physiol Regul Integr Comp Physiol*, 2006. **291**(3): R768–78.
37. Thompson, N.M., et al., Prenatal and postnatal pathways to obesity: different underlying mechanisms, different metabolic outcomes. *Endocrinology*, 2007. **148**(5): 2345–54.
38. Unger, R.H., The physiology of cellular liporegulation. *Annu Rev Physiol*, 2003. **65**: 333–47.
39. Abrams, M.E., et al., Hydrops fetalis: a retrospective review of cases reported to a large national database and identification of risk factors associated with death. *Pediatrics*, 2007. **120**(1): 84–9.
40. Benediktsson, R., et al., Glucocorticoid exposure in utero: new model for adult hypertension. *Lancet*, 1993. **341**(8841): 339–41.
41. Lindsay, R.S., et al., Prenatal glucocorticoid exposure leads to offspring hyperglycaemia in the rat: studies with the 11 beta-hydroxysteroid dehydrogenase inhibitor carbenoxolone. *Diabetologia*, 1996. **39**(11): 1299–305.
42. Welberg, L.A., J.R. Seckl, and M.C. Holmes, Inhibition of 11beta-hydroxysteroid dehydrogenase, the foeto-placental barrier to maternal glucocorticoids, permanently programs amygdala GR mRNA expression and anxiety-like behaviour in the offspring. *Eur J Neurosci*, 2000. **12**(3): 1047–54.
43. Nyirenda, M.J., et al., Glucocorticoid exposure in late gestation permanently programs rat hepatic phosphoenolpyruvate carboxykinase and glucocorticoid receptor expression and causes glucose intolerance in adult offspring. *J Clin Invest*, 1998. **101**(10): 2174–81.
44. Dahlgren, J., et al., Prenatal cytokine exposure results in obesity and gender-specific programming. *Am J Physiol Endocrinol Metab*, 2001. **281**(2): E326–34.
45. Samuelsson, A.M., et al., Prenatal exposure to interleukin-6 results in inflammatory neurodegeneration in hippocampus with NMDA/GABA(A) dysregulation and impaired spatial learning. *Am J Physiol Regul Integr Comp Physiol*, 2006. **290**(5): R1345–56.

46. Larsen, T., G. Greisen, and S. Petersen, Prediction of birth weight by ultrasound-estimated fetal weight: a comparison between single and repeated estimates. *Eur J Obstet Gynecol Reprod Biol,* 1995. **60**(1): 37–40.

47. Cooke, R.J., et al., Feeding preterm infants after hospital discharge: growth and development at 18 months of age. *Pediatr Res,* 2001. **49**(5): 719–22.

48. Uthaya, S., et al., Altered adiposity after extremely preterm birth. *Pediatr Res,* 2005. **57**(2): 211–5.

49. Cooke, R.J. and I. Griffin, Altered body composition in preterm infants at hospital discharge. *Acta Paediatr,* 2009. **98**(8): 1269–73.

50. Yeung, M.Y., Postnatal growth, neurodevelopment and altered adiposity after preterm birth: from a clinical nutrition perspective. *Acta Paediatr,* 2006. **95**(8): 909–17.

51. Ibanez, L., et al., Abdominal fat partitioning and high-molecular-weight adiponectin in short children born small for gestational age. *J Clin Endocrinol Metab,* 2009. **94**(3): 1049–52.

52. Ibanez, L., et al., Visceral adiposity without overweight in children born small for gestational age. *J Clin Endocrinol Metab,* 2008. **93**(6): 2079–83.

53. Ibanez, L., et al., Early development of adiposity and insulin resistance after catch-up weight gain in small-for-gestational-age children. *J Clin Endocrinol Metab,* 2006. **91**(6): 2153–8.

54. Euser, A.M., et al., Associations between prenatal and infancy weight gain and BMI, fat mass, and fat distribution in young adulthood: a prospective cohort study in males and females born very preterm. *Am J Clin Nutr,* 2005. **81**(2): 480–7.

55. Finken, M.J., et al., Abdominal fat accumulation in adults born preterm exposed antenatally to maternal glucocorticoid treatment is dependent on glucocorticoid receptor gene variation. *J Clin Endocrinol Metab,* 2011. **96**(10): E1650–5.

56. Finken, M.J., et al., Antenatal glucocorticoid treatment is not associated with long-term metabolic risks in individuals born before 32 weeks of gestation. *Arch Dis Child Fetal Neonatal Ed,* 2008. **93**(6): F442–7.

57. Keijzer-Veen, M.G., et al., Is blood pressure increased 19 years after intrauterine growth restriction and preterm birth? A prospective follow-up study in The Netherlands. *Pediatrics,* 2005. **116**(3): 725–31.

58. Keijzer-Veen, M.G., et al., Microalbuminuria and lower glomerular filtration rate at young adult age in subjects born very premature and after intrauterine growth retardation. *J Am Soc Nephrol,* 2005. **16**(9): 2762–8.

59. Rotteveel, J., et al., Infant and childhood growth patterns, insulin sensitivity, and blood pressure in prematurely born young adults. *Pediatrics,* 2008. **122**(2): 313–21.

60. Rotteveel, J., et al., Abnormal lipid profile and hyperinsulinaemia after a mixed meal: additional cardiovascular risk factors in young adults born preterm. *Diabetologia,* 2008. **51**(7): 1269–75.

61. Finken, M.J., et al., Lipid profile and carotid intima-media thickness in a prospective cohort of very preterm subjects at age 19 years: effects of early growth and current body composition. *Pediatr Res,* 2006. **59**(4 Pt 1): 604–9.

62. Finken, M.J., et al., Preterm birth and later insulin resistance: effects of birth weight and postnatal growth in a population based longitudinal study from birth into adult life. *Diabetologia,* 2006. **49**(3): 478–85.

63. Singhal, A., et al., Is slower early growth beneficial for long-term cardiovascular health? *Circulation,* 2004. **109**(9): 1108–13.

64. Ford, E.S. and C. Li, Defining the metabolic syndrome in children and adolescents: will the real definition please stand up? *Journal of Pediatrics,* 2008. **152**(2): 160–164.

65. Golley, R.K., et al., Comparison of metabolic syndrome prevalence using six different definitions in overweight pre-pubertal children enrolled in a weight management study. *International Journal of Obesity,* 2006. **30**(5): 853–860.

66. O'Sullivan, T.A., et al., Dietary glycaemic carbohydrate in relation to the metabolic syndrome in adolescents: comparison of different metabolic syndrome definitions. *Diabetic Medicine,* 2010. **27**(7): 770–778.
67. Thomas, E.L., et al., The missing risk: MRI and MRS phenotyping of abdominal adiposity and ectopic fat. *Obesity* (Silver Spring), 2012. **20**(1): 76–87.
68. Uthaya, S., J. Bell, and N. Modi, Adipose tissue magnetic resonance imaging in the newborn. *Horm Res,* 2004. **62 Suppl 3**: 143–8.
69. Butte, N.F., et al., Body composition during the first 2 years of life: an updated reference. *Pediatr Res,* 2000. **47**(5): 578–85.
70. Fomon, S.J., et al., Body composition of reference children from birth to age 10 years. *Am J Clin Nutr,* 1982. **35**(5 Suppl): 1169–75.
71. Fomon, S.J. and S.E. Nelson, Body composition of the male and female reference infants. *Annu Rev Nutr,* 2002. **22**: 1–17.
72. Ziegler, E.E., et al., Body composition of the reference fetus. *Growth,* 1976. **40**(4): 329–41.
73. Griffin, I.J. and R.J. Cooke, Development of whole body adiposity in preterm infants. *Early Hum Dev,* 2012. **88 Suppl 1**: S19–24.
74. Eriksson, B., M. Lof, and E. Forsum, Body composition in full-term healthy infants measured with air displacement plethysmography at 1 and 12 weeks of age. *Acta Paediatr,* 2010. **99**(4): 563–8.
75. Gianni, M.L., et al., Adiposity in small for gestational age preterm infants assessed at term equivalent age. *Arch Dis Child Fetal Neonatal Ed,* 2009. **94**(5): F368–72.
76. Ramel, S.E., et al., Body composition changes in preterm infants following hospital discharge: comparison with term infants. *J Pediatr Gastroenterol Nutr,* 2011. **53**(3): 333–8.
77. Simon, L., et al., Effect of sex and gestational age on neonatal body composition. *Br J Nutr,* 2013. **109**(6): 1105–8.
78. Johnson, M.J., et al., Preterm birth and body composition at term equivalent age: a systematic review and meta-analysis. *Pediatrics,* 2012. **130**(3): e640–9.
79. Gianni, M.L., et al., Postnatal catch-up fat after late preterm birth. *Pediatr Res,* 2012. **72**(6): 637–40.
80. Gianni, M.L., et al., Regional fat distribution in children born preterm evaluated at school age. *J Pediatr Gastroenterol Nutr,* 2008. **46**(2): 232–5.
81. Darendeliler, F., et al., Insulin resistance and body composition in preterm born children during prepubertal ages. *Clin Endocrinol* (Oxf), 2008. **68**(5): 773–9.
82. Fewtrell, M.S., et al., Prematurity and reduced body fatness at 8–12 y of age. *Am J Clin Nutr,* 2004. **80**(2): 436–40.
83. Kerkhof, G.F., et al., Health profile of young adults born preterm: negative effects of rapid weight gain in early life. *J Clin Endocrinol Metab,* 2012. **97**(12): 4498–506.
84. Hovi, P., et al., Glucose regulation in young adults with very low birth weight. *N Engl J Med,* 2007. **356**(20): 2053–63.
85. Thomas, E.L., et al., Aberrant adiposity and ectopic lipid deposition characterize the adult phenotype of the preterm infant. *Pediatr Res,* 2011. **70**(5): 507–12.
86. Breukhoven, P.E., et al., Fat mass and lipid profile in young adults born preterm. *J Clin Endocrinol Metab,* 2012. **97**(4): 1294–302.
87. Larciprete, G., et al., Intrauterine growth restriction and fetal body composition. *Ultrasound Obstet Gynecol,* 2005. **26**(3): 258–62.
88. Padoan, A., et al., Differences in fat and lean mass proportions in normal and growth-restricted fetuses. *Am J Obstet Gynecol,* 2004. **191**(4): 1459–64.
89. Wells, J.C., S. Chomtho, and M.S. Fewtrell, Programming of body composition by early growth and nutrition. *Proc Nutr Soc,* 2007. **66**(3): 423–34.
90. Sewell, M.F., et al., Increased neonatal fat mass, not lean body mass, is associated with maternal obesity. *Am J Obstet Gynecol,* 2006. **195**(4): 1100–3.

91. Lee, W., et al., Fetal growth parameters and birth weight: their relationship to neonatal body composition. *Ultrasound Obstet Gynecol,* 2009. **33**(4): 441–6.
92. Ibanez, L., et al., Early development of visceral fat excess after spontaneous catch-up growth in children with low birth weight. *J Clin Endocrinol Metab,* 2008. **93**(3): 925–8.
93. Chomtho, S., et al., Early growth and body composition in infancy. *Adv Exp Med Biol,* 2009. **646**: 165–8.
94. Chomtho, S., et al., Associations between birth weight and later body composition: evidence from the 4-component model. *Am J Clin Nutr,* 2008. **88**(4): 1040–8.
95. Beardsall, K., et al., Heritability of childhood weight gain from birth and risk markers for adult metabolic disease in prepubertal twins. *J Clin Endocrinol Metab,* 2009. **94**(10): 3708–13.
96. Modi, N., et al., Determinants of adiposity during preweaning postnatal growth in appropriately grown and growth-restricted term infants. *Pediatr Res,* 2006. **60**(3): 345–8.
97. Karaolis-Danckert, N., et al., Rapid growth among term children whose birth weight was appropriate for gestational age has a longer lasting effect on body fat percentage than on body mass index. *Am J Clin Nutr,* 2006. **84**(6): 1449–55.
98. Stettler, N., et al., Prevalence and risk factors for overweight and obesity in children from Seychelles, a country in rapid transition: the importance of early growth. *Int J Obes Relat Metab Disord,* 2002. **26**(2): 214–9.
99. Ekelund, U., et al., Association of weight gain in infancy and early childhood with metabolic risk in young adults. *J Clin Endocrinol Metab,* 2007. **92**(1): 98–103.
100. Stettler, N., et al., Rapid weight gain during infancy and obesity in young adulthood in a cohort of African Americans. *Am J Clin Nutr,* 2003. **77**(6): 1374–8.
101. Roggero, P., et al., Is term newborn body composition being achieved postnatally in preterm infants? *Early Hum Dev,* 2009. **85**(6): 349–52.
102. Gianni, M.L., et al., Body composition in newborn infants: 5-year experience in an Italian neonatal intensive care unit. *Early Hum Dev,* 2012. **88 Suppl 1**: S13–7.
103. Roggero, P., et al., Rapid recovery of fat mass in small for gestational age preterm infants after term. *PLoS One,* 2011. **6**(1): e14489.
104. Hernandez, M.I., et al., Leptin and IGF-I/II during the first weeks of life determine body composition at 2 years in infants born with very low birth weight. *J Pediatr Endocrinol Metab,* 2012. **25**(9–10): 951–5.
105. Vasu, V., et al., Early nutritional determinants of intrahepatocellular lipid deposition in preterm infants at term age. *Int J Obes* (Lond), 2013.
106. Thomas, E.L., et al., Neonatal intrahepatocellular lipid. *Arch Dis Child Fetal Neonatal Ed,* 2008. **93**(5): F382–3.
107. Embleton, N.D. and R.J. Cooke, Protein requirements in preterm infants: effect of different levels of protein intake on growth and body composition. *Pediatr Res,* 2005. **58**(5): 855–60.
108. Roggero, P., et al., Influence of protein and energy intakes on body composition of formula-fed preterm infants after term. *J Pediatr Gastroenterol Nutr,* 2008. **47**(3): 375–8.
109. Wauben, I.P., et al., Growth and body composition of preterm infants: influence of nutrient fortification of mother's milk in hospital and breastfeeding post-hospital discharge. *Acta Paediatr,* 1998. **87**(7): 780–5.
110. Cooke, R.J., et al., Body composition of preterm infants during infancy. *Arch Dis Child Fetal Neonatal Ed,* 1999. **80**(3): F188–91.
111. De Curtis, M., C. Pieltain, and J. Rigo, Body composition in preterm infants fed standard term or enriched formula after hospital discharge. *Eur J Nutr,* 2002. **41**(4): 177–82.
112. Aimone, A., et al., Growth and body composition of human milk-fed premature infants provided with extra energy and nutrients early after hospital discharge: 1-year follow-up. *J Pediatr Gastroenterol Nutr,* 2009. **49**(4): 456–66.

113. Cooke, R.J., I.J. Griffin, and K. McCormick, Adiposity is not altered in preterm infants fed with a nutrient-enriched formula after hospital discharge. *Pediatr Res,* 2010. **67**(6): 660–4.

114. Amesz, E.M., et al., Optimal growth and lower fat mass in preterm infants fed a protein-enriched postdischarge formula. *J Pediatr Gastroenterol Nutr,* 2010. **50**(2): 200–7.

115. Roggero, P., et al., Growth and fat-free mass gain in preterm infants after discharge: a randomized controlled trial. *Pediatrics,* 2012. **130**(5): e1215–21.

116. Pittaluga, E., et al., Benefits of supplemented preterm formulas on insulin sensitivity and body composition after discharge from the neonatal intensive care unit. *J Pediatr,* 2011. **159**(6): 926–32 e2.

117. Lapillonne, A. and I.J. Griffin, Feeding preterm infants now for later metabolic and cardiovascular outcomes. *J Pediatr,* 2013. **162**: S7–16.

118. Kistner, A., et al., Increased systolic daily ambulatory blood pressure in adult women born preterm. *Pediatr Nephrol,* 2005. **20**(2): 232–3.

119. Dalziel, S.R., et al., Cardiovascular risk factors at age 30 following pre-term birth. *Int J Epidemiol,* 2007. **36**(4): 907–15.

120. de Jong, F., et al., Systematic review and meta-analysis of preterm birth and later systolic blood pressure. *Hypertension,* 2012. **59**(2): 226–34.

121. Bracewell, M.A., et al., The EPICure study: growth and blood pressure at 6 years of age following extremely preterm birth. *Arch Dis Child Fetal Neonatal Ed,* 2008. **93**(2): F108–14.

122. Irving, R.J., et al., Adult cardiovascular risk factors in premature babies. *Lancet,* 2000. **355**(9221): 2135–6.

123. Hack, M., et al., Blood pressure among very low birth weight (<1.5 kg) young adults. *Pediatr Res,* 2005. **58**(4): 677–84.

124. Hovi, P., et al., Ambulatory blood pressure in young adults with very low birth weight. *J Pediatr,* 2010. **156**(1): 54–59 e1.

125. Regan, F.M., et al., The impact of early nutrition in premature infants on later childhood insulin sensitivity and growth. *Pediatrics,* 2006. **118**(5): 1943–9.

126. Hofman, P.L., et al., Premature birth and later insulin resistance. *N Engl J Med,* 2004. **351**(21): 2179–86.

127. Bazaes, R.A., et al., Determinants of insulin sensitivity and secretion in very-low-birth-weight children. *J Clin Endocrinol Metab,* 2004. **89**(3): 1267–72.

128. Willemsen, R.H., et al., Independent effects of prematurity on metabolic and cardiovascular risk factors in short small-for-gestational-age children. *J Clin Endocrinol Metab,* 2008. **93**(2): 452–8.

129. Singhal, A., et al., Breastmilk feeding and lipoprotein profile in adolescents born preterm: follow-up of a prospective randomised study. *Lancet,* 2004. **363**(9421): 1571–8.

130. Lucas, A., et al., Early diet in preterm babies and developmental status at 18 months. *Lancet,* 1990. **335**(8704): 1477–81.

131. Lucas, A., et al., Randomized trial of nutrient-enriched formula versus standard formula for postdischarge preterm infants. *Pediatrics,* 2001. **108**(3): 703–11.

132. Lucas, A., et al., Early diet in preterm babies and developmental status in infancy. *Arch Dis Child,* 1989. **64**(11): 1570–8.

133. Lucas, A., et al., Multicentre trial on feeding low birthweight infants: effects of diet on early growth. *Arch Dis Child,* 1984. **59**(8): 722–30.

134. Kistner, A., et al., IGFBP-1 levels in adult women born small for gestational age suggest insulin resistance in spite of normal BMI. *J Intern Med,* 2004. **255**(1): 82–8.

135. Rotteveel, J., M.M. van Weissenbruch, and H.A. Delemarre-Van de Waal, Decreased insulin sensitivity in small for gestational age males treated with GH and preterm untreated males: a study in young adults. *Eur J Endocrinol,* 2008. **158**(6): 899–904.

136. Greer, F.R., Post-discharge nutrition: what does the evidence support? *Semin Perinatol,* 2007. **31**(2): 89–95.

137. Thureen, P.J., The neonatologist's dilemma: catch-up growth or beneficial undernutrition in very low birth weight infants-what are optimal growth rates? *J Pediatr Gastroenterol Nutr,* 2007. **45 Suppl 3**: S152–4.

138. Fewtrell, M.S., et al., Effects of size at birth, gestational age and early growth in preterm infants on glucose and insulin concentrations at 9–12 years. *Diabetologia,* 2000. **43**(6): 714–7.

139. Bo, S., et al., Insulin resistance in pre-school very-low-birth weight pre-term children. *Diabetes Metab,* 2006. **32**(2): 151–8.

140. Lazdam, M., et al., Elevated blood pressure in offspring born premature to hypertensive pregnancy: is endothelial dysfunction the underlying vascular mechanism? *Hypertension,* 2010. **56**(1): 159–65.

141. Mortaz, M., et al., Cholesterol metabolism in 8 to 12-year-old children born preterm or at term. *Acta Paediatr,* 2003. **92**(5): 525–30.

142. Evensen, K.A., et al., Effects of preterm birth and fetal growth retardation on cardiovascular risk factors in young adulthood. *Early Hum Dev,* 2009. **85**(4): 239–45.

7 Postnatal Growth in Preterm Infants
Neurodevelopmental Effects

Ian J. Griffin and Jennifer Scoble

ABBREVIATIONS

AGA: Appropriate for gestational age
BPD: Bronchopulmonary dysplasia
CP: Cerebral palsy
ELBW: Extremely low birth weight (<1 kg at birth)
IVH: Intraventricular hemorrhage
LBW: Low birth weight
MDI: Mental development index
NEC: Necrotizing enterocolitis
PDI: Psychomotor development index
PVL: Periventricular leukomalacia
ROP: Retinopathy of prematurity
SGA: Small for gestational age
VLBW: Very low birth weight (<1.5 kg at birth)

INTRODUCTION

Preterm birth disrupts the supply of nutrients to the developing fetus and significantly impacts the orderly process of fetal growth. The peak period of head growth occurs in the fetus at approximately 20 weeks gestation (Figure 7.1),[1] and this peak is considerably earlier than the peak rate of weight or length gain.[2] Growth in weight of the human brain is largely complete by 2 years of age, and growth in brain cell number is mostly complete by 1 to 2 years.[3] Any adverse physiological conditions during this critical time could affect brain growth and development. As growth is most rapid during the third trimester, disruptions during this period may have the most significant impact on brain formation.

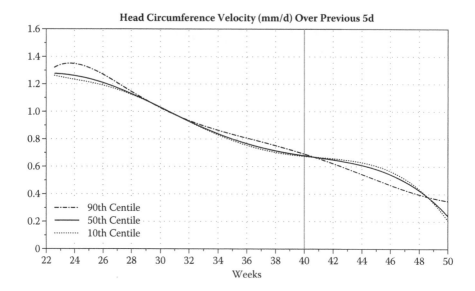

FIGURE 7.1 Head circumference velocity over the preceding 5 days calculated from fits of the Fenton growth data (see Chapter 11). Velocities are for hypothetical subjects growing along the 10th, 50th, and 90th percentiles, and are expressed as mm/d.

DEVELOPMENT OF PRETERM INFANTS

RISK FACTORS FOR ADVERSE DEVELOPMENT

Neurodevelopmental impairment is common in extremely preterm infants, and is a major concern to both caregivers and to parents. Prematurity is the major risk factor for cerebral palsy (CP) and for neurodevelopmental impairment, but other risk factors include male sex, severe intraventricular hemorrhage (IVH, Grade III or IV), periventricular leukomalacia (PVL), chronic lung disease, necrotizing enterocolitis (NEC), retinopathy of prematurity (ROP), postnatal steroid use, and lower maternal education levels.[4–8] Antenatal steroids reduced the risk of adverse outcome.[5]

For example, Mikkola et al.[5] assessed neurodevelopmental outcomes in extremely low birth weight (ELBW, birth weight < 1 kg) Finnish infants, at age 5 years and found that severe IVH, ROP requiring treatment, and lack of antenatal steroids were risk factors for major disability (which included blindness, deafness, CP, or convulsions). Chronic lung disease, perforated NEC, lack of antenatal steroids, and hospital of birth were associated with cognitive impairment at age 5 years, as was decreasing gestational age.[5] These data are not unique. In Swedish infants aged 24 to 28 weeks gestation, male gender, higher stages of ROP, BPD, and maternal socio-economic status have been associated with death or moderate to severe neurodevelopmental disability.[9]

TEMPORAL TRENDS IN NEURODEVELOPMENTAL OUTCOME

Fanaroff et al.[10] evaluated 18,153 very low birth weight (VLBW, birth weight <1500 g) infants from the NICHD network from three time intervals, one from 1990 to 1991 (immediate post-surfactant era), another from 1995 to 1996 (reflecting antenatal steroid use), and a third from 1997 to 2002. Mortality declined from 20% in the first cohort to 16% in the second, and then to 15% in the third. However, there was no significant decrease in morbidities associated with neurodevelopmental impairment such as severe IVH, BPD, or NEC. In fact, these complications increased from the first to the second cohort (likely due to an increase in survival of the smallest infants), and then remained relatively stable from the second to the third cohort.[10] However, despite many of the risk factors of neurodevelopmental impairment remaining common, there is evidence of improving neurodevelopmental outcomes in preterm infants. Moore et al. compared neurodevelopmental outcomes of infants born in England at 22 to 25 weeks gestation in 1995 to those born in 2006. Survival improved from 39% to 52% between the two time periods. However, survival without disability also increased significantly, from 23% to 34%. Improved intact survival (survival without major impairment) was most apparent among the 24- and 25-week gestational infants.[11] Similarly, a cohort of preterm infants in Sweden (24 to 27 weeks gestation) born between 2000 and 2008, demonstrated decreasing mortality from 44% in 2000–2002, to 32% in 2003–2005, and to 28% in 2006–2008. Survival without moderate to severe disability also improved from 27% in the first cohort, to 36% in the second, and to 39% in the third.[9]

It is intriguing to see that neurodevelopmental outcome may be improving without an improvement in the co-morbidities (such as BPD and NEC) associated with adverse developmental outcome. One possible explanation for this is suggested by Enhrenkranz.[12] He demonstrated that ELBW infants who were more critically sick were at increased risk of subsequently developing CP, or having an MDI score < 70 or a PDI score < 70.[12] More critically sick infants also had lower intakes of energy and protein during days 1 to 7, 8 to 14, and 15 to 21.[12] However, in a complex multivariate analysis he was able to show that the adverse effect of critical illness on neurodevelopment was in part due to decreased energy intake in the first week of life.[12] Therefore, improved nutrition may reduce the effects of co-morbidities, such as NEC and BPD, on long-term developmental outcomes.

GROWTH AS A RISK FACTOR FOR LATER NEURODEVELOPMENT

It is almost self-evident that brain size would have some relationship to brain function. It is not surprising, therefore, that an abnormally small head circumference would be a risk factor for impaired neurodevelopment.[13] In one series, microcephaly (i.e., an occipitofrontal head circumference more than 2 standard deviations below the mean) was seen in 15% of patients referred to a child development center.[13] Although the majority of microcephalic children have normal development, they are much more likely than normocephalic children to have moderate mental retardation (10.3% vs. 3.3%, p < 0.001) or severe mental retardation (11.0% vs. 2.0%, p < 0.01).[13]

However, it is not just *in utero* head growth that is important; *ex utero* growth is also critical. Among very low birth weight infants (BW < 1500 g) the presence of microcephaly at birth is associated with poor neurodevelopmental outcomes.[14] Subsequent poor postnatal head circumference growth is also associated with lower Bayley MDI scores at 6 months of age than seen in infants with greater postnatal head growth, both in the infants born microcephalic (63 ± 14 vs. 85 ± 16, p < 0.01) *and* in the normocephalic infants (79 ± 16 vs. 100 ± 15, p < 0.01).[14]

The timing of *ex utero* changes in growth is also important. Hack et al. followed a cohort of very low birth weight infants over many years, and they were classified as being microcephalic (head circumference more than 2 SD below the mean-for-age) at birth, 8 months, and 20 months of age.[15–17] Sixty-six infants had normal head circumferences at birth, but subsequently fell below 2 SD. The 37 infants whose head circumferences caught-up by 8 months had significantly better developmental scores at 20 months than those who did not catch up (neonatal onset, Figure 7.2). Similarly, of the 68 infants with small head circumferences at birth, catch-up in head circumference by 8 months tended to be associated with better developmental scores (prenatal onset, Figure 7.2). Finally, 43 infants with previously normal head circumferences developed microcephaly after the neonatal period. Those in whom this occurred before 8 months scored more poorly on developmental scores at 20 months than those who developed microcephaly after 8 months (post-neonatal onset,

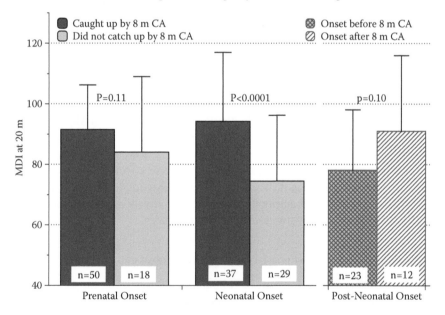

FIGURE 7.2   Left Panel: Developmental scores at 20 months for VLBW infants with prenatal or neonatal onset of microcephaly, and by whether they did (black bars) or did not (grey bars) catch up to a normal head circumference by 8 months. Data are summarized from Table 4 in Reference 16. Right Panel: Developmental scores at 20 months for VLBW infants with post-neonatal onset of microcephaly, depending on whether this occurred before or after 8 months of age. Data are summarized from Table 4 in Reference 16.

Figure 7.2). Irrespective of the time of onset, therefore, restoration of normal head circumference size by 8 months (or maintenance of normal head circumference until 8 months) was associated with better developmental outcome.[16]

GROWTH AND LATTER NEURODEVELOPMENT—THE PRESENT LITERATURE

There is a large amount of literature on the effect of early growth or body size on later neurodevelopment, both in preterm [6–8, 14–16, 18–35] and term infants.[22, 36–50] As would be expected, these studies differ in the specific assessments of growth they consider (weight, length, head circumference, etc.), the study population considered (ELBW, VLBW, preterm, etc.), the proportion of SGA (small-for-gestational-age) infants enrolled, the ages at which growth and development are assessed, and the specific developmental assessments carried out.

Perhaps the major distinction between studies is whether they assess the effects of body size or the effects of growth. Body size is a single measurement carried out at a specified time point, and is the integrated result of all of the growth that has occurred up to that time point. Subjects tend to track along percentile lines, such that subjects who are larger at earlier time points are usually also larger at later time points. Simple assessments of body size, therefore, cannot allow the identification of "critical periods" where early differences in growth may have long-lasting effects on neurodevelopment.

Growth (or growth rate, growth velocity), in contrast, is a dynamic measurement made between two time points. Nutritional interventions or other events may lead to changes in growth velocity that are restricted to specific time intervals. An obvious example is the case of preterm birth itself, where early postnatal growth is poor, but subsequent growth is often increased (if catch-up growth occurs) or normal (if catch-up growth does not occur). Studies that consider growth velocity are most useful for identifying "critical periods" when changes in growth are most related to subsequent development. Body size can be expressed in many ways, for example, as continuous data (e.g., weight in grams or length as a Z-score for age), as binomial categories (e.g., microcephaly or normocephaly, or weight above or below the 10th percentile for age), or as nominal data (e.g., in quartiles of body weight). Similarly, growth rate can be expressed in a multitude of ways, for example, weight growth could be expressed as a change in grams between two time periods, in terms of g/d or g/kg/d, as a change in weight-for-age Z-score, or as quartiles of weight gain. Despite all of these differences in study design and data analysis, a number of very clear patterns emerge from the published literature. We will now review that literature.

GROWTH AND NEURODEVELOPMENT IN PRETERM INFANTS

IN-HOSPITAL GROWTH

The best-known recent study on the effect of growth on long-term outcome is the data of Ehrenkranz et al.[21] Data for 495 very low birth weight (BW < 1500 g) infants from the NICHD network born between 1994 and 1995 were examined.[21] Growth velocity was calculated from the time birth weight was regained to the time of discharge (or

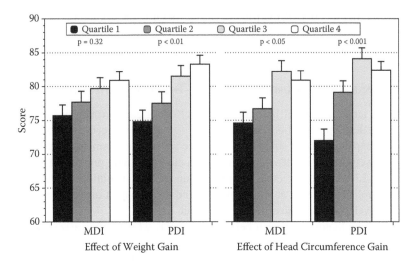

FIGURE 7.3 Bayley MDI and PDI scores by quartiles of weight (left panel) and head circumference (right panel) growth for preterm infants during their initial hospitalization. (From the data of Ehrenkranz et al.[21])

transfer to another institution, or reaching a weight of 2 kg, or age 120 days, whichever came first) and infants were divided into quartiles based on their rates of growth. The weight velocity of the slowest growing quartile was 12.0 g/kg/d (SD 2.1), length velocity was 0.82 cm/wk (SD 0.3) and head circumference velocity was 0.77 cm/wk (SD 0.2). The fastest growing quartile gained weight 75% faster (21.2 g/kg/d [SD 2.0]) and gained length and head circumference approximately 35% faster (1.11 cm/wk [SD 0.2] and 1.07 cm/wk, respectively). Development was assessed at 18 to 22 months using the Bayley scales of infant development.[21] The more rapidly growing quartile of weight gain was associated with a significantly increased PDI score at 18 to 22 months, but there was no effect on MDI scores (Figure 7.3, left panel). If head circumference growth was considered, the effect was more marked and both PDI and MDI scores were significantly associated with more rapid growth (Figure 7.3, right panel). More rapid weight gain was associated with a reduced risk of cerebral palsy (p < 0.01), a reduced risk of an MDI score less than 70 (p < 0.01), and a reduced risk of a PDI score less than 70 (p < 0.001). These associations were more significant for head circumference growth, with more rapid growth being associated with a reduced risk of all three adverse outcomes (p < 0.001 for each comparison).

Neubauer reported a geographically based cohort study in 135 ELBW infants from Hanover.[6] Major neurodevelopmental impairment at school-age was associated with higher grades of intraventricular hemorrhage, PVL, male gender, bronchopulmonary dysplasia, necrotizing enterocolitis, the presence of a patent ductus arteriosus, prolonged mechanical ventilation, prolonged parenteral nutrition, and with lower in-hospital growth in weight and head circumference. By stepwise logistic regression, only three factors were independently associated with adverse school-age outcome:[6]

1. The need for prolonged (>14 days) mechanical ventilation
2. The need for prolonged (>41 days) parenteral nutrition
3. Growth in head circumference between birth and discharge of less than 6 mm/wk

Infants with slower growth in head circumference had almost four times higher odds of abnormal school-age outcome. Normal school-age outcomes were seen in 61% of infants who received parenteral nutrition for less than 28 days, but in only 22% of those that required parenteral nutrition for more than 42 days or more.[6]

In a second German cohort, this time from Ulm, the effect of in-hospital growth on outcomes at 5 years was examined in 219 VLBW infants (birth weight less than 1500 g). Slower growth, either of weight or head circumference (expressed as a change in weight-for-age Z-score between birth and discharge), was significantly associated with an increased risk for a mildly or severely abnormal neurological examination at 5.4 years of age.[7] Other significant risk factors were the presence of higher grades of intraventricular hemorrhage or periventricular leukomalacia, higher grades of retinopathy of prematurity, and maternal education.[7]

LONGER-TERM GROWTH

If in-hospital growth has longer-term neurological associations, what about the effects of body size or growth after hospital discharge?

Body Size after Hospital Discharge

In the Ulm cohort,[7] the effects of growth between discharge and follow-up at 5.4 years (expressed as a change in weight or head circumference Z-score for age between discharge from the NICU and follow-up), and of birth size (expressed as weight or head circumference Z-score at birth) on neurodevelopmental outcomes were also examined.[7] Neither lower birth weight nor a smaller head circumference at birth was a risk factor for having an abnormal neurological examination at a 5-year follow-up or for abnormal mobility at follow-up. However, poor weight growth between birth and discharge was a risk factor for an abnormal neurological examination, and poor head circumference gain during the same period was a risk factor for both an abnormal neurological examination or for abnormal mobility at follow-up.[7] For other outcome measures, both prenatal and postnatal growth had effects. Scores on a mental processing composite were associated with size at birth, when expressed as body weight (p = 0.005) and less so when expressed as head circumference at birth (p = 0.06). Mental processing composite was also affected by weight gain between birth and discharge, but not between discharge and follow-up, and by head circumference gain between discharge and follow-up, but not between birth and discharge.[7]

The effect of body size at different ages is summarized in Table 7.1 (for cohorts containing both SGA and AGA preterm infants), Table 7.2 (for cohorts of only AGA preterm infants), and Table 7.3 (for cohorts containing only SGA preterm infants). There is general agreement among the studies that body size at birth is not related to later neurodevelopment in preterm infants. For example, among the 14 comparisons between birth weight and later neurodevelopment (Tables 7.1, 7.2, and 7.3) from eight

TABLE 7.1

Effect of Body Size on Neurodevelopmental Outcome from Studies Examining Mixed Cohorts of SGA and AGA Preterm Infants

Author	Year	n =	Criteria	% SGA	Birth	Disc	8 m	12 m	24 m	8 y	Assessment
							Weight				
Wocadio	1994	266	GA <30 w	38				Y			1 y, NDI
Franz	2009	219	ELBW	12	n						5.4 y, Abnormal neurological examination
Franz	2009	219	ELBW	12	Y						5.4 y, Mental processing
Franz	2009	219	ELBW	12	n						5.4 y, Abnormal mobility
Kan	2008	179	GA <28 w	2	n	n			n	n	8 y, WISC-III IQ
Kan	2008	179	GA <28 w	2	Y	n			Y	n	8 y, Wide Range Achievement Test (Reading)
Kan	2008	179	GA <28 w	2	n	n			Y	n	8 y, Wide Range Achievement Test (Spelling)
Kan	2008	179	GA <28 w	2	n	n			n	n	8 y, Wide Range Achievement Test (Arithmetic)
Kan	2008	179	GA <28 w	2	n	Y			n	n	8 y, Movement ABC
Kon	2010	38	VLBW	53		Y					1.5 y, PDI
Kon	2010	38	VLBW	53		n					1.5 y, MDI
							Height/Length				
No studies identified											
							Head Circumference				
Kuban	2009	958	GA <28 w	?	n				Y		2 y, MDI
Kuban	2009	958	GA <28 w	?	n				Y		2 y, PDI
Kuban	2009	958	GA <28 w	?	n				Y		2 y, CP

(continued)

TABLE 7.1 (CONTINUED)

Effect of Body Size on Neurodevelopmental Outcome from Studies Examining Mixed Cohorts of SGA and AGA Preterm Infants

Author	Year	n =	Criteria	% SGA	Birth	Disc	8 m	12 m	24 m	8 y	Assessment
† Hack	1989	481	VLBW	21		n	Y				1.7 y, MDI
† Hack	1989	481	VLBW	21		n	Y				1.7 y, NDI
Franz	2009	219	ELBW	12	n						5.4 y, Abnormal neurological examination
Franz	2009	219	ELBW	12	n						5.4 y, Abnormal mobility
Franz	2009	219	ELBW	12	n						5.4 y, Mental processing
Kan	2008	179	GA <28 w	2	n				Y	Y	8 y, WISC–III IQ
Kan	2008	179	GA <28 w	2	n				Y	Y	8 y, Wide Range Achievement Test (Reading)
Kan	2008	179	GA <28 w	2	n				Y	Y	8 y, Wide Range Achievement Test (Spelling)
Kan	2008	179	GA <28 w	2	n				n	n	8 y, Wide Range Achievement Test (Arithmetic)
Kan	2008	179	GA <28 w	2	n				Y	Y	8 y, Movement ABC
Kitchen	1992	162	VLBW	?						Y	8 y, IQ

Note: GA = Gestational age

ELBW = Extremely low birthweight (BW < 1 kg)

VLBW = Very low birthweight (BW < 1.5 kg)

† AGA and SGA cohorts also shown separately.

Note: The effect of *body size* on neurodevelopment in mixed cohorts of AGA and SGA preterm infants. If body size (weight, length, or head circumference) is significantly associated with neurodevelopment, it is noted as "Y"; if not, as "n." Also shown are the proportion of SGA infants in the cohort, the sample size, the neurodevelopmental assessment used, and the age at which neurodevelopmental testing was carried out. Cohorts also shown in Table 7.2 and 7.3 are marked †. Data are given in decreasing order of sample size and are from References 7, 16, 23, 25, 26, 34.

TABLE 7.2

Effect of Body Size on Developmental Outcome from Studies Examining Cohorts of AGA Preterm Infants

Author	Year	n =	Criteria	Birth	Disc	1 m	3 m	4 m	6 m	8 m	9 m	12 m	24 m	36 m	8 y	Assessment
Weight																
Latal-Hajnal	2003	125	VLBW	n									n			2 y, MDI
Latal-Hajnal	2003	125	VLBW	n									Y			2 y, PDI
Latal-Hajnal	2003	125	VLBW	n									Y			2 y, CP
Ross	1983	86	VLBW			n	Y		Y		Y	Y				1 y, NDI
Ross	1985	86	VLBW											n		3 y, Stanford-Binet IQ
Ross	1985	86	VLBW											n		3 y, NDI
Height/Length																
Latal-Hajnal	2003	125	VLBW	n									n			2 y, MDI
Latal-Hajnal	2003	125	VLBW	n									Y			2 y, PDI
Latal-Hajnal	2003	125	VLBW	n									Y			2 y, CP
Ross	1983	86	VLBW			n	Y		Y		Y	Y				1 y, NDI
Ross	1985	86	VLBW											n		3 y, Stanford-Binet IQ
Ross	1985	86	VLBW											Y		3 y, NDI
Ramel	2012	62	VLBW	n	n			Y				Y	n			2 y, BSID-III Cognitive scale
Ramel	2012	62	VLBW	n	n			n				n	n			2 y, BSID-III Motor scale
Ramel	2012	62	VLBW	Y	Y			n				n	n			2 y, BSID-III Speech scale
Head Circumference																
† Hack	1989	379	VLBW		n					Y						1.7 y, MDI
† Hack	1989	379	VLBW		n					Y						1.7 y, NDI
Latal-Hajnal	2003	125	VLBW	n									n			2 y, MDI

(continued)

TABLE 7.2 (CONTINUED)

Effect of Body Size on Developmental Outcome from Studies Examining Cohorts of AGA Preterm Infants

Author	Year	n =	Criteria	Birth	Disc	1 m	3 m	4 m	6 m	8 m	9 m	12 m	24 m	36 m	8 y	Assessment
Latal-Hajnal	2003	125	VLBW	n									Y			2 y, PDI
Latal-Hajnal	2003	125	VLBW	n									n			2 y, CP
Ross	1983	86	VLBW			Y	Y		Y		Y	Y				1 y, NDI
Ross	1985	86	VLBW											Y		3 y, Stanford-Binet IQ
Ross	1985	86	VLBW											Y		3 y, NDI
						Composite Diagnosis of "Failure to Thrive"										
Casey	2006	544	VLBW											Y		8 y, WISC Total
Casey	2006	544	VLBW											Y		8 y, WISC Performance
Casey	2006	544	VLBW											Y		8 y, WISC Verbal
Casey	2006	544	VLBW											n		8 y, Peabody Picture test
Casey	2006	544	VLBW											n		8 y, VMI
Casey	2006	544	VLBW											n		8 y, Woodcock-Johnson Broad Math
Casey	2006	544	VLBW											n		8 y, Woodcock-Johnson Broad Reading

Note: VLBW = Very low birth weight (BW < 1.5 kg).

† Also shown as combined AGA and SGA cohorts.

Note: The effect on *body size* on neurodevelopment in cohorts of AGA preterm infants. If body size (weight, length, head circumference, or a diagnosis of failure to thrive) is significantly associated with neurodevelopment, it is noted as "**Y**"; if not, as "**n**". Also shown are the sample size, the neurodevelopmental assessment used, and the age at which neurodevelopmental testing was carried out. Cohorts also shown in Tables 7.1 and 7.3 are marked †. Data are given in decreasing order of sample size and are taken from References 16, 20, 27, 30–32.

TABLE 7.3

Effect of Body Size on Developmental Outcome from Studies Examining Cohorts of SGA Preterm Infants

Author	Year	n =	Criteria	Birth	Disc	8 m	12 m	24 m	36 m	Assessment
						Weight				
Latal-Hajnal	2003	94	VLBW	n				n		2 y, MDI
Latal-Hajnal	2003	94	VLBW	n				Y		2 y, PDI
Latal-Hajnal	2003	94	VLBW	n				Y		2 y, CP
						Height/Length				
Latal-Hajnal	2003	94	VLBW	n				n		2 y, MDI
Latal-Hajnal	2003	94	VLBW	n				Y		2 y, PDI
Latal-Hajnal	2003	94	VLBW	n				Y		2 y, CP
						Head Circumference				
† Hack	1989	102	VLBW		n	Y				1.7 y, MDI
† Hack	1989	102	VLBW		n	Y				1.7 y, NDI
Latal-Hajnal	2003	94	VLBW	n				n		2 y, MDI
Latal-Hajnal	2003	94	VLBW	n				n		2 y, PDI
Latal-Hajnal	2003	94	VLBW	n				n		2 y, CP
Ochiai	2008	56	SGA *				n			3 y, Verbal IQ
Ochiai	2008	56	SGA *				n			3 y, Performance IQ
Ochiai	2008	56	SGA *				Y			3 y, Total IQ
Ochiai	2008	56	SGA *				Y			6 y, Verbal IQ
Ochiai	2008	56	SGA *				Y			6 y, Performance IQ
Ochiai	2008	56	SGA *				Y			6 y, Total IQ
Brandt	2003	46	VLBW				Y			0.5 y, Griffiths DQ
Brandt	2003	46	VLBW				Y			0.75 y, Griffiths DQ

(continued)

TABLE 7.3 (CONTINUED)
Effect of Body Size on Developmental Outcome from Studies Examining Cohorts of SGA Preterm Infants

Author	Year	n =	Criteria	Birth	Disc	8 m	12 m	24 m	36 m	Assessment
Brandt	2003	46	VLBW				Y			1 y, Griffiths DQ
Brandt	2003	46	VLBW				Y			1.25 y, Griffiths DQ
Brandt	2003	46	VLBW				Y			1.5 y, Griffiths DQ
Brandt	2003	46	VLBW				Y			2 y, Cattrell DQ
Brandt	2003	46	VLBW				Y			3 y, Cattrell DQ
Brandt	2003	46	VLBW				Y			4 y, Stanford-Binet IQ
Brandt	2003	46	VLBW				Y			5 y, Stanford-Binet IQ
Brandt	2003	46	VLBW				Y			6 y, Stanford-Binet IQ
Brandt	2003	46	VLBW				Y			"Adult," Manneheimer IQ
					Composite Diagnosis of "Failure to Thrive"					
Casey	2006	109	VLBW						Y	8 y, WISC Total
Casey	2006	109	VLBW						Y	8 y, WISC Performance
Casey	2006	109	VLBW						n	8 y, WISC Verbal
Casey	2006	109	VLBW						Y	8 y, Peabody Picture test
Casey	2006	109	VLBW						n	8 y, VMI
Casey	2006	109	VLBW						Y	8 y, Woodcock-Johnson Broad Math
Casey	2006	109	VLBW						n	8 y, Woodcock-Johnson Broad Reading

Note: VLBW = Very low birth weight (BW < 1.5 kg); SGA = Small for gestational age

† Also shown as combined AGA and SGA cohorts.

Note: The effect of *body size* on neurodevelopment in cohorts of AGA and SGA preterm infants. If *body size* (weight, length, head circumference, or a diagnosis of failure to thrive) is significantly associated with neurodevelopment, it is noted as "Y"; if not, as "n." Also shown are the sample size, the neurodevelopmental assessment used, and the age at which neurodevelopmental testing was carried out. Cohorts also shown in Tables 7.1 and 7.2 are marked †. Data are given in decreasing order of sample size and are taken from References 16, 19, 20, 27, 29.

different studies,[7, 23, 25, 27, 31, 32, 34] only two show significant associations. One of these is from Franz et al.[7] where one of three neurodevelopmental assessments at 5.4 years was correlated with birth weight, and the other from Kan et al. where one out of five neurodevelopmental assessments at 8 years was related to birth weight.[23] Data for other measures of body size at birth are no more compelling, with none of 18 measures of neurodevelopment being associated with head circumference at birth, and only one of nine comparisons between birth length and later neurodevelopment being significant (Tables 7.1, 7.2, and 7.3).

Most studies that have compared the effects of body size at birth (a proxy for *in utero* growth) and of postnatal growth have shown postnatal growth to be a more important determinant of neurodevelopmental outcome. In a matched-cohort study[34] comparing preterm infants (less than 30 weeks gestation) born SGA or AGA, neurodevelopmental impairment occurred at the same rate in the two cohorts (22% vs. 22%, p > 0.99). However, infants who were small at the time of assessment at age 1 year had a much higher rate of adverse neurological outcome than those who were larger at age 1 year (27% vs. 9%, p < 0.0001). In a similar study by Latal-Hajnal, 219 VLBW infants were categorized as being SGA or AGA at birth (weight < or ≥ 10th percentile for age) or small or not at 2 years of age (weight < or ≥ 10th percentile for age).[27] Being SGA at birth had no effect on PDI or MDI scores at 2 years or on the risk of cerebral palsy. However, larger body size (either as body weight or as body length) at 2 years was associated with a reduced risk of cerebral palsy and higher PDI scores at 2 years. This effect was seen in infants born SGA and in those born AGA.[27] Head circumference at 2 years was less associated with outcomes than weight or length. Head circumference was not associated with the rate of cerebral palsy in either SGA or AGA infants, and was only associated with PDI score in AGA infants but not in SGA infants.[27]

Effects of Postnatal Growth

Latal-Hajnal also assessed the effect of growth between birth and 2 years on neurodevelopmental outcomes. PDI score at 2 years was significantly associated with weight gain between birth and 2 years in SGA and AGA infants, as was length gain between birth and 2 years in SGA and AGA infants, and head circumference gain between birth and 2 years in AGA, but not SGA, infants. Higher rates of weight gain between birth and 2 years were associated with lower rates of cerebral palsy in AGA and SGA infants. Greater rates of length gain, or head circumference gain, between birth and 2 years were associated with reduced risk of cerebral palsy in AGA infants, but not SGA infants.[27] None of the measures of body size, or of growth rate, were associated with MDI at 2 years.[27]

Figures 7.4, 7.5, and 7.6 summarize the current literature on the effect of growth and later development for cohorts comprising both AGA and SGA infants (Figure 7.4), or cohorts of only AGA infants (Figure 7.5) or only SGA infants (Figure 7.6). Periods where the effect of growth velocity, or growth rate, or change in body size were assessed between two identified times are shown as horizontal bars that span that time interval. Bars that are shaded (grey) represent time intervals where growth rates were significantly related to subsequent neurodevelopment in that cohort; time intervals where no significant effect was seen are shown as open (white) bars.

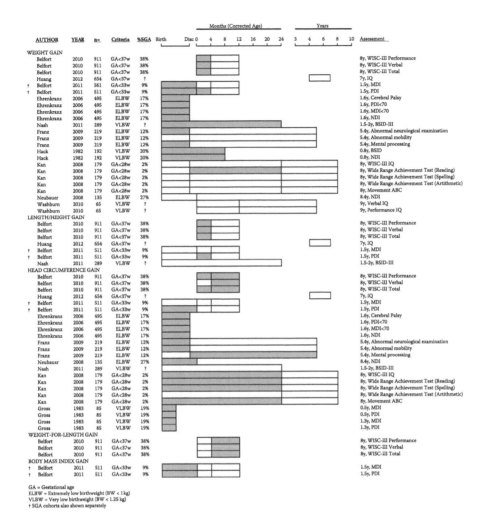

FIGURE 7.4 The effect of *growth* on neurodevelopment in mixed cohorts of AGA and SGA preterm infants. If growth (gain in weight, length, head circumference, body mass index, or weight-for-length between two time points) is significantly associated with neurodevelopment, it is shown as a shaded horizontal bar between those two time points. If growth between two time points was found not to be associated with neurodevelopment, it is shown as an open horizontal bar. Also shown are the proportion of SGA infants in the cohort, the sample size, the neurodevelopmental assessment used, and the age at which neurodevelopmental testing was carried out. Cohorts also shown as separate AGA or SGA cohorts as well are marked †. Data are given in decreasing order of sample size and are from References 6–8, 14, 15, 18, 21–23, 28.

Many of the studies in Figures 7.4, 7.5, and 7.6 examine multiple time periods. For example, the Franz dataset,[7] discussed previously, shows that an abnormal neurological examination at 5.4 years was associated with poorer weight gain between discharge and term (so that bar is shaded grey under "Weight gain" in Figure 7.4) but not with growth between discharge and 5 years (so that bar in Figure 7.4 is not shaded).

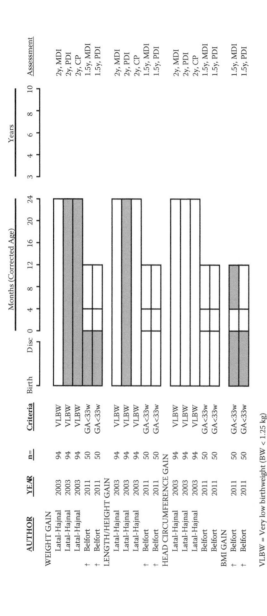

FIGURE 7.5   The effect of *growth* on neurodevelopment in AGA preterm infants. If growth (gain in weight, length, head circumference, body mass index, or weight-for-length between two time points) is significantly associated with neurodevelopment, it is shown as a shaded horizontal bar between those two time points. If growth between two time points was found not to be associated with neurodevelopment, it is shown as an open horizontal bar. Also shown are the sample size, the neurodevelopmental assessment used, and the age at which neurodevelopmental testing was carried out. Cohorts also shown as combined AGA and SGA cohorts are marked †. Data are given in decreasing order of sample size and are from References 8 and 27.

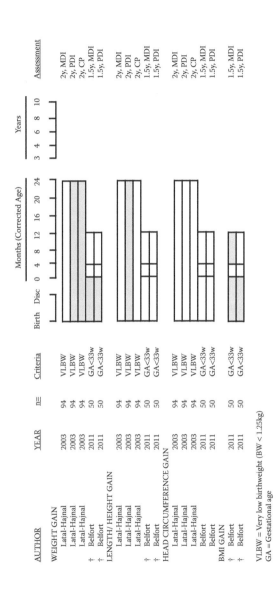

FIGURE 7.6 The effect of *growth* on neurodevelopment in SGA preterm infants. If growth (gain in weight, length, head circumference, body mass index, or weight-for-length between two time points) is significantly associated with neurodevelopment, it is shown as a shaded horizontal bar between those two time points. If growth between two time points was found not to be associated with neurodevelopment, it is shown as an open horizontal bar. Also shown are the sample size, the neurodevelopmental assessment used, and the age at which neurodevelopmental testing was carried out. Cohorts also shown as combined AGA and SGA cohorts are marked †. Data are given in decreasing order of sample size and are from References 8 and 27.

Looking at the studies *in toto*, the highest density of data is for the period beginning at birth, continuing until hospital discharge or to near term-corrected age. The majority of studies (6/8) examining weight gain during this period find a significant association with at least one measure of later neurodevelopment[7, 8, 15, 21, 28, 35] and only two studies fail to identify an effect during this period.[6, 23] Likewise, five of the seven studies examining head circumference gain over this period show a significant effect on growth,[6–8, 14, 21] and two do not.[23, 28] The data on length gain restricted to this period are more limited, and neither of the two published studies finds an association with neurodevelopment.[8, 28]

After discharge, growth continues to be associated with neurodevelopment. Some studies showing an effect of growth cover a relatively long period from discharge, for example, the paper of Franz,[7] which measures growth from discharge to 5.4 years or that of Latal-Hajnal,[27] which assesses it between term and 2 years. Such wide age ranges make it difficult to focus on a small "critical window," although they do support the importance of later growth on neurodevelopment.

In other studies, growth in weight,[8, 18] length,[8, 18] and head circumference[18] between discharge and 4 months corrected age is associated with neurodevelopment. These studies also examine the period between 4 and 12 months post-term as well. During the later time period, weight gain and length gain are not associated with neurodevelopment,[8,18] but gains in head circumference and in body mass index are.[8,18] Some studies find significant associations with growth between birth and 2 years of age,[27, 28] or discharge and 2 years of age,[23] and neurodevelopment. However, none of the studies we have identified (Figures 7.4 to 7.6) identify a time period beginning *after* 12 months post-term that is associated with later neurodevelopment in preterm infants.

Although the data is heterogeneous, we believe that there are some broad conclusions that can be drawn:

1. Relative body size at birth has little effect on long-term neurodevelopment (especially once corrected for gestational age), but an association is very likely for body size later in the first 12 to 24 months of life.
2. More rapid growth between birth and discharge (i.e., in-hospital growth) is associated with improved neurodevelopmental outcome. This effect is seen most strongly for weight gain and head circumference gain.
3. Growth rate after hospital discharge is also associated with improved neurodevelopmental outcome. This is most clearly seen for the period extending to 4 months post-term, but is also seen until 12 months post-term. Again, this is true for weight growth and head circumference growth.
4. There is little evidence that growth rate after 12 months post-term has any significant long-term neurodevelopmental associations in preterm infants, although few studies have examined this time period.

The SGA Preterm Infant

SGA status is often considered to be a risk factor for poor neurodevelopmental outcome, especially in term infants,[51, 52] and SGA infants are over-represented in the preterm population.[53]

In our analysis, body weight at birth has little apparent effect on later neuro-development. This would imply that SGA status *itself* has a limited effect as well. Whether this is correct depends on to which group SGA preterm infants are com-pared: either to infants of similar birth weight (who will be more premature) or to infants of a similar gestational age (who will be heavier).

Several studies have compared preterm SGA infants to *birth weight*-matched pre-term infants, and found no significant difference in neurodevelopmental outcome between the groups[54–56] and one study even showed a lower risk of an abnormal neurological outcome in the SGA infants,[54] presumably as they were of higher ges-tational age than the weight-matched comparison group.[54] Casey,[20] for example, compared 434 preterm LBW infants who were AGA and 68 similar SGA infants; none had postnatal failure to thrive. SGA status did not affect a range of measures of neurodevelopmental outcome at age 8 years, even though the SGA group had significantly lower birth weights than the AGA infants.[20] This is consistent with our analysis earlier that birth weight has no significant impact on later neurodevelopment even in cohorts containing both AGA and SGA infants (Table 7.1).

When SGA infants are compared to preterm infants of the same gestation age, the literature is less clear. Some studies see no differences in outcome,[34,55,57] while oth-ers see worse developmental outcome in SGA infants,[54,56] although sometimes only in the most severely affected and in females.[58]

Other points to come from these studies are that the body size of SGA infants does not catch up with that of their AGA peers, at least not during the preschool years.[54,57] Furthermore, even though SGA status at birth is not a risk factor for neurodevelopmental impairment, small size later in life is, whether this is being "short" (lower length/height)[59] or microcephalic (lower head circumference).[55]

Finally, whatever the effects of SGA status per se on neurodevelopment, SGA infants seem to show a similar effect of later body size (Table 7.4) and early growth velocity (Figure 7.6) on subsequent neurodevelopment as other preterm infants.

LIMITATIONS OF THE CURRENT LITERATURE

The data we have at present is, of course, imperfect. The major weakness is that it is largely the result of observational cohort studies. As such, they can only demon-strate an association between growth and body size, and later development; they cannot demonstrate a causal relationship. The relationship between growth and later outcome may be mediated by other factors. For example, sicker preterm infants may grow more poorly, and may have poor neurodevelopment because of their greater illness burden. One NICHD cohort study seems to demonstrate just that: less sick preterm infants had greater nutritional intakes during the first three weeks of life, better short-term outcomes (improved growth, and lower rates of bronchopulmonary dysplasia, late-onset sepsis, or death), and better neurodevelopmental outcome at 18 to 22 m.[12] The effect of severity of illness on these outcomes appeared to be medi-ated, in part, by energy intake during the first week of life.[12] In another study, energy intake between postnatal day 2 and 10 has been shown to be significantly associated with developmental outcome.[19]

Data from animal models[60] or from intervention studies in humans would support a causal link between growth (or body size) and neurodevelopment. Alternatively, the demonstration of a similar relationship between growth (or body size) and neurodevelopment in a less sick group of infants, for example, healthy term infants, would suggest that the effects on growth (or body size) and neurodevelopment are not explained by the effects of illness severity.

GROWTH AND NEURODEVELOPMENT IN TERM AGA INFANTS

The effect of body size[36, 38, 41, 42, 45–50] or of growth rate[22, 37, 39, 41, 42, 45, 46, 48, 50] on neurodevelopment in healthy term infants has been examined in a large number of studies.

For example, Silva et al. studied a cohort of 11,244 British children, and carried out five different developmental assessments at 10 years of age.[49] Developmental scores were lower in the VLBW infants and in the low birth weight infants (LBW, birth weight < 2.5 kg).[49] However, developmental scores continued to increase as a function of birth weight even in those infants weighing more than 2.5 kg at birth (Figure 7.7).[49] Even in AGA infants, a higher birth weight was associated with better developmental outcome.[49]

Another study of 3483 infants born in the 1950s and 1960s showed that IQ at 7 years increased as a linear function of birth weight and that this was seen in both males and in females.[47] Compared with infants born weighing between 3.0 and 3.499 kg, a birth weight of 3.5 to 3.999 kg was associated with a significantly higher IQ (mean difference 2.2 for males, 1.5 for females), while a birth weight of 2.5 to 2.999 kg was associated with a significantly lower IQ (mean difference –2.2 for males, –2.1 for females).[47] In a cohort of 2913 infants born in Singapore, an additional 1-kg birth weight led to an additional 2.2 IQ points at 7 to 9 years, an additional 1-cm birth length led to a gain of 0.5 IQ points, and an additional 1 cm in head circumference at birth resulted in a gain of 0.6 IQ points.[38]

Table 7.4 summarizes the effect of body size at birth on later development.[36, 38, 41, 42, 45–50] Most of the larger studies show a significant relationship between birth weight,[36, 38, 42, 47–50] length,[38, 42, 48, 50] or head circumference[38, 41, 42, 48, 49] at birth and later development. Only two studies failed to see a difference and they were much smaller in size, studying only 108[45] or 83[46] subjects. This suggests that these negative findings may be the result of inadequate statistical power.

The literature for term infants is different from that for preterm infants, where body size at birth does not appear to have a significant effect on neurodevelopment. However, body size at (or near) the preterm infants *expected* term date does show a positive relationship with neurodevelopment.

Growth failure after birth is also clearly important. For example, term infants diagnosed with failure to thrive have reduced long-term development.[61] However, the effect of later body size is questionable. Few studies (Table 7.4) have addressed this issue and there is little convincing data. It should also be noted that Silva found subjects with higher weights at 10 years to have *lower* neurodevelopment, although greater height was associated with better development.[49]

Even in the absence of failure to thrive, postnatal growth rates are associated with developmental outcome in term infants (Figure 7.8). Emond studied a cohort of 5771 infants from the Avon Longitudinal Study of Parents and Children.[39] IQ at age 8

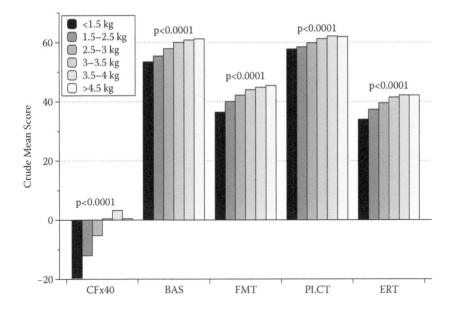

FIGURE 7.7 The effect of birth weight strata on developmental scores at age 10 years in 11,244 British children. Results of all developmental scores increase with increasing birth weight, even once birth weight is > 2.5 kg. CF = cognitive function, BAS = British Ability Scale, FMT = Friendly Maths Test, PLCT = Pictorial Language Comprehension Test, ERT = Shortened Edinburgh Reading Test. The scores for cognitive functioning are multiplied by 40 in order for them to be plotted on the same axis as the other tests.

years was significantly associated with birth weight, but also with conditional weight gain between birth and 9 months of age.[39] When this interval was examined in more detail, weight gain between birth and 8 weeks was significantly associated with IQ (p = 0.002), with higher IQ scores seen in those infants with the most rapid growth. No such effect was seen between 8 weeks and 9 months of age.[39] In a Finnish cohort, rates of weight, body mass index, and head circumference gain between birth and 5 months were important for long-term development, as were head circumference gains between 5 and 26 months, and length gains between 5 to 26 months and 26 to 50 months.[42]

The largest such cohort to date studied almost 12,000 children, all of whom were term (≥ 37 weeks gestation) and weighed > 2.5 kg at birth.[50] Gains in weight during the first 5 years of life were significantly associated with IQ at 6.5 years of age. The largest effect was seen between birth and 3 months (where a 1 standard deviation difference led to a difference of 0.77 IQ points), with smaller effects seen for growth between 3 and 12 months and between 1 and 5 years (where 1 standard deviation in weight gain was associated with a 0.29 and 0.40 improvement in IQ, respectively).[50]

GROWTH AND NEURODEVELOPMENT IN TERM SGA INFANTS

Finally, we will consider the SGA term infant. Relatively little data is available compared to that for the AGA term infant, either relating to the effect of body size (Table 7.5, References 40, 43, 44, 46) or growth rate (Figure 7.8, References 37 and 46).

TABLE 7.4
Effect of Body Size on Developmental Outcome from Studies Examining Cohorts of AGA Term Infants

Author	Year	n =	Birth	4 m	6 m	2 y	5 y	10 y	Developmental Assessment
					Weight				
Yang	2011	11,899	Y						6.5 y, Full-scale IQ
Yang	2011	11,899	Y						6.5 y, Verbal IQ
Yang	2011	11,899	Y						6.5 y, Performance IQ
Silva	2006	11,244	Y					Y	10 y, British Ability Scale
Silva	2006	11,244	Y						10 y, Cognitive Functioning
Silva	2006	11,244	Y						10 y, Friendly Maths Test
Silva	2006	11,244	Y						10 y, Pictorial Language Comprehension
Silva	2006	11,244	Y						10 y, Shortened Edinburgh Reading Test
Broekman	2009	2913	Y						7–9 y, IQ
Matte	2001	1670	Y						7 y, IQ
Heinonen	2008	1056	Y						4.7 y, General reasoning
Heinonen	2008	1056	Y						4.7 y, Visual motor functioning
Heinonen	2008	1056	n						4.7 y Verbal functioning
Heinonen	2008	1056	n						4.7 y, Language functioning
Belfort	2008	872	Y		n				3 y, PPVT-III
Belfort	2008	872	n		n				3 y, WRAVMA
Pongchareon	2012	560	n						9 y, Full-scale IQ
Pongchareon	2012	560	n						9 y, Verbal IQ
Pongchareon	2012	560	Y						9 y, Performance IQ
Li	2004	108	n			n			Adult educational achievement

(continued)

TABLE 7.4 (CONTINUED)

Effect of Body Size on Developmental Outcome from Studies Examining Cohorts of AGA Term Infants

Author	Year	n =	Birth	4 m	6 m	2 y	5 y	10 y	Developmental Assessment
					Height/Length				
Yang	2011	11,899	Y						6.5 y, Full-scale IQ
Yang	2011	11,899	Y						6.5 y, Verbal IQ
Yang	2011	11,899	Y						6.5 y, Performance IQ
Silva	2006	11,244					n	Y	10 y, British Ability Scale
Broekman	2009	2913	Y						7–9 y, IQ
Heinonen	2008	1056	Y						4.7 y, General reasoning
Heinonen	2008	1056	Y						4.7 y, Visual motor functioning
Heinonen	2008	1056	Y						4.7 y Verbal functioning
Heinonen	2008	1056	Y						4.7 y, Language functioning
Pongchareon	2012	560	Y						9 y, Full-scale IQ
Pongchareon	2012	560	n						9 y, Verbal IQ
Pongchareon	2012	560	Y						9 y, Performance IQ
Li	2004	108	n			Y			Adult educational achievement
					Head Circumference				
Silva	2006	11,244					Y	Y	10 y, British Ability Scale
Broekman	2009	2913	Y						7–9 y , IQ
Heinonen	2008	1056	Y						4.7 y, General reasoning
Heinonen	2008	1056	Y						4.7 y, Visual motor functioning
Heinonen	2008	1056	Y						4.7 y, Verbal functioning
Heinonen	2008	1056	n						4.7 y, Language functioning

(continued)

TABLE 7.4 (CONTINUED)

Effect of Body Size on Developmental Outcome from Studies Examining Cohorts of AGA Term Infants

Author	Year	n =	Birth	4 m	6 m	2 y	5 y	10 y	Developmental Assessment
Gale	2006	633	Y						4 y, Full-scale IQ
Gale	2006	633	Y						4 y, Verbal IQ
Gale	2006	633	Y						4 y, Performance IQ
Gale	2006	633	n						8 y, Full-scale IQ
Gale	2006	633	n						8 y, Verbal IQ
Gale	2006	633	n						8 y, Performance IQ
Pongchareon	2012	560		Y					9 y, Full-scale IQ
Pongchareon	2012	560		Y					9 y, Verbal IQ
Pongchareon	2012	560		Y					9 y, Performance IQ
Li	2004	108	n			Y			Adult educational achievement
Lira	2010	81	n						8 y, Full-scale IQ
Lira	2010	81	n						8 y, Verbal IQ
Lira	2010	81	n						8 y, Performance IQ
					Body Mass Index				
Heinonen	2008	1056	n						4.7 y, General reasoning
Heinonen	2008	1056	Y						4.7 y, Visual motor functioning
Heinonen	2008	1056	n						4.7 y, Verbal functioning
Heinonen	2008	1056	n						4.7 y, Language functioning

Note: The effect of *body size* on neurodevelopment in cohorts of AGA term infants: If body size (weight, length, head circumference, or body mass index) is significantly associated with neurodevelopment, it is noted as "**Y**"; if not, as "**n**." Also shown are the sample size and the neurodevelopmental assessment used, and the age at which neurodevelopmental testing was carried out. Data are given in decreasing order of sample size and are taken from References 36, 38, 41, 42, 45–50.

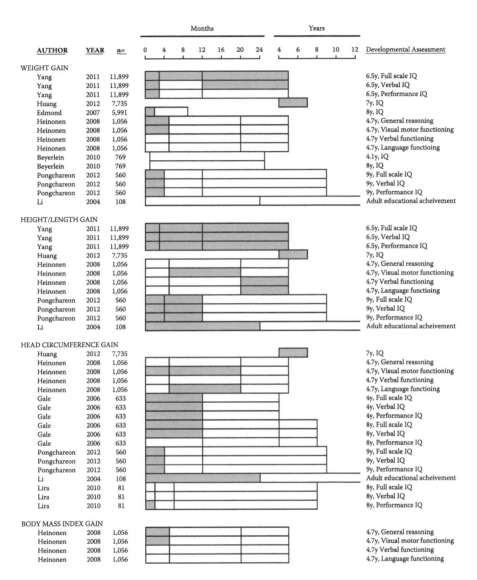

FIGURE 7.8 The effect of *growth* on neurodevelopment in AGA term infants. If growth (gain in weight, length, head circumference, or body mass index between two time points) is significantly associated with neurodevelopment, it is shown as a shaded horizontal bar between those two time points. If growth between two time points was found not to be associated with neurodevelopment, it is shown as an open horizontal bar. Also shown are the sample size, the neurodevelopmental assessment used, and the age at which neurodevelopmental testing was carried out. Data are given in decreasing order of sample size and are from References 22, 37, 39, 41, 42, 45, 46, 48, 50.

TABLE 7.5

Effect of Body Size on Developmental Outcome from Studies Examining Cohorts of SGA Term Infants

Author	Year	n =	Birth	6 m	1 y	2 y	3 y	6 y	10 y	Developmental Assessment
Weight										
Fattal-Valevski	2009	136			Y	Y		Y	Y	9–10 y, NDI
Fattal-Valevski	2009	136			n	Y		Y	Y	9–10 y, IQ
Leitner	2007	123	Y							9–10 y, WISC-III IQ
Leitner	2007	123	Y						Y	9–10 y, NDI
Fattal-Valevski	1999	85	Y							3 y, NDI
Leitner	2000	81						Y		6 y, NDI
Leitner	2000	81						n		6 y, IQ
Length/Height										
Fattal-Valevski	2009	136			Y	Y		n	n	9–10 y, NDI
Fattal-Valevski	2009	136			Y	n		n	n	9–10 y, IQ
Fattal-Valevski	1999	85					Y			3 y, NDI
Leitner	2000	81						Y		6 y, NDI
Leitner	2000	81						n		6 y, IQ

(continued)

TABLE 7.5 (CONTINUED)
Effect of Body Size on Developmental Outcome from Studies Examining Cohorts of SGA Term Infants

Author	Year	n =	Birth	6 m	1 y	2 y	3 y	6 y	10 y	Developmental Assessment
					Head Circumference					
Fattal-Valevski	2009	136			Y	n		Y	Y	9–10 y, NDI
Fattal-Valevski	2009	136			Y	Y		Y	Y	9–10 y, IQ
Leitner	2007	123	Y			Y		Y	Y	9–10 y, WISC-III IQ
Leitner	2007	123	Y						Y	9–10 y, NDI
Fattal-Valevski	1999	85	Y							3 y, NDI
Lira	2010	83	n							8 y, Full-scale IQ
Lira	2010	83	n							8 y, Verbal IQ
Lira	2010	83	n							8 y, Performance IQ
Leitner	2000	81						n		6 y, NDI
Leitner	2000	81						Y		6 y, IQ
				Other Measures (Catch-up in Wt, L, and HC)						
Leitner	2007	123				Y			Y	9–10 y, WISC-III IQ
Leitner	2007	123				Y			Y	9–10 y, NDI

Note: The effect of *body size* on neurodevelopment in cohorts of SGA term infants: If body size (weight, length, head circumference, or body mass index) is significantly associated with neurodevelopment, it is noted as "**Y**"; if not, as "**n**." Also shown are the sample size and the neurodevelopmental assessment used, and the age at which neurodevelopmental testing was carried out. Data are given in decreasing order of sample size and are taken from References 40, 43, 44, 46.

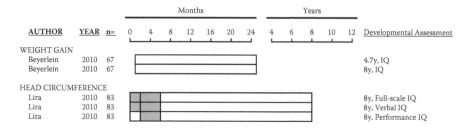

FIGURE 7.9 The effect on growth on neurodevelopment in SGA term infants: If growth (gain in weight, or head circumference between two time-points) is significantly associated with neurodevelopment it is shown as a shaded horizontal bar between those two time points. If growth between two time points was found not to be associated with neurodevelopment it is shown as an open horizontal bar. Also shown are the sample size, and the neurodevelopmental assessment used, and the age at which neurodevelopmental testing was carried out. Data are given in decreasing order of sample size and is from References 37,46.

Most studies suggest that both birth weight and later measures of body size are positively associated with neurodevelopment (Table 7.5 and Figure 7.9). Those studies that identify an effect of body size after birth usually identify it by age 1 to 2 years.

The data on growth is poorer, with only two small studies published. One examines the effect of weight gain, and finds no effect.[37] The other examines the effect of head circumference gain and found a positive association on neurodevelopment between gains in head circumference in early life (birth to 2 months, and 2 months to 6 months).[46]

Specific Intervention, Growth, and Neurodevelopment

Several different interventions have been studied aiming to improve the growth of preterm infants. We will now consider a selection of them, and examine whether they lead to improved neurodevelopment.

"Aggressive" Nutrition

"Aggressive" nutrition involves a range of interventions, including higher amino acid, lipid, and energy intakes, the earlier start of enteral feeds and their more rapid advancement, and the use of insulin to maintain targeted glucose infusion rates.[62] As its goals are to ensure an infant receives an adequate nutritional intake in as timely a manner as possible, it should perhaps be considered "appropriate" nutrition rather than "aggressive" nutrition.[63]

Several observational cohort studies have suggested that individual components of "aggressive" nutrition may be associated with improved neurodevelopment. Prolonged periods of low energy intake are associated with poorer development at age 1 year.[64] Higher energy intakes between day 2 and day 10[19] or during the first week of life[65] have been associated with improved development between 12 and 18 months of age. The poorer developmental outcome of infants on mechanical ventilation more than 14 days appears to be partly explained by lower energy intakes in the first week of life.[12] Early administration of lipids may also have developmental benefits. In one cohort study, cumulative intake of lipids during the first 14 days of life was positively associated with developmental quotient at 1 year of age.[35] No such relationship with development was seen for the cumulative energy or protein intake in the first 14 d.[35]

Studies of appropriate nutrition (compared to less appropriate nutrition) show improved nutrient intakes[66–70] and better growth parameters.[66–70] However, these studies either have not assessed long-term neurodevelopment[66–68, 70] or have failed to find a relationship with the provision of "aggressive" nutrition.[71]

IN-HOSPITAL DIET

Mother's Own Milk

It is difficult to assess the effect of mother's own milk on neurodevelopment in preterm infants, as the population is largely self-selected. It has been known since the 1980s that mothers who decide to give their low birth weight infants their own milk, and are successful in doing so, are significantly older, better educated, and more likely to be primiparous.[72] Given the optimum "best case" combination of circumstances, a mother is almost 1000-times more likely to provide her own milk than under the "worst case" scenario.[72] This has changed little over the following 30 years, with breastfeeding mothers of preterm infants being significantly older, better educated, better insured, having higher incomes, lower parity, and being more likely to be Caucasian.[73]

Preterm infants whose mother are successfully able to provide them mother's own milk have improved development at 18 months[73,74] and at 30 months[75] of age. In one study, an 8-point advantage in IQ was seen, although this fell to 4.3 points once known confounding variables were accounted for. The remaining difference, may be due to a variety of factors. To quote one of the original authors:

> It is possible that our failure to "adjust out" the advantage seen in babies whose mothers chose to provide breast milk was due to some extent to our failure to identify all relevant demographic factors...Alternatively we have considered the possibility that fresh maternal milk might contain a factor or factors, hitherto unrecognised, which promote brain growth or maturation in the period of rapid growth preterm....Finally, it is possible that the advantage is related to the mother's decision to provide milk, rather than to the consumption of breast milk itself.[74]

RANDOMIZED TRIALS USING HUMAN MILK

In order to overcome the confounding effect of self-selection, randomized controlled trials must be carried out. However, it is not possible to randomize children to receive their own mother's milk or not, if such milk is available. However, randomized controlled trials using donor human milk are possible. Alan Lucas's group has carried out two studies that have been very influential in the debate about optimum growth rates in preterm infants. We will review those studies, concentrating on the intriguing *development* results they present.

Both studies had similar designs. Preterm infants during their initial hospitalization were randomized to one of two feeding types. In one case, banked donor milk was compared to a preterm formula, in the other a term formula was compared to a preterm formula. If mothers did not provide breast milk, the randomized diet was given as a sole diet ("Trial A"), if they did provide breast milk, the randomized diet was given as a supplement if breast milk supply was inadequate (Trial B). Data were analyzed for Trials A and B separately, for both combined, and for a select group of infants who had the highest intake of the randomized diets.

DONOR HUMAN MILK VS. PRETERM FORMULA

In the first multicenter study, preterm infants weighing less than 1850 g birth weight were recruited between 1982 and 1984, and randomized to diets of either unfortified donor human milk or a preterm formula either as a sole diet (Trial A) or as a supplement to mother's own milk should supply be inadequate (Trial B). The study intervention lasted a median of 30 days. Interim analysis of in-hospital growth data (n = 194) showed significantly better weight and length gain in the preterm formula group (in both Trial A and in Trial B), and significantly greater head circumference gain (in Trial A only).[76] If the associations between growth and development described previously were valid, development would be expected to have been better in the preterm formula group. The expected difference in developmental quotient was indeed seen at 9 months (n = 400).[77] Developmental quotient was three points higher in infants receiving preterm formula (p < 0.025) than in infants receiving donor human milk (Trials A and B combined).[77] In the subgroup of infants who received >50% of their enteral intake from the randomized diet, there was a 3.6-point advantage for preterm formula (p < 0.01).[77] The difference was larger in infants born growth retarded (5.3 points) and larger in males (3.3 points) compared to female (1.7 points).[77] By 18 months of age, no differences in developmental outcome were seen.[78]

TERM FORMULA VS. PRETERM FORMULA

In the second study, preterm infants weighing less than 1850 g at birth were randomized to a term formula or a preterm formula either as a supplement to mothers own milk (Trial B) or as a sole diet (Trial A).[79] Diets were given for a median of approximately 4 weeks[79] and 344 infants had follow-up at 18 months. Weight gain was significantly greater in infants receiving the preterm formula (in both Trial A and in Trial B, and in the two trials combined) at 18 months. Head circumference growth was better in the infants receiving preterm formula, but only in those in Trial A.[79] Bayley PDI scores at 18 months of age were significantly higher in infants receiving the preterm formula than the term formula (difference 6.2 points, in Trials A and B combined). This was even more marked in Trial A where the formulas were given as the sole enteral diet (difference 14.5 points).[79] In infants on the highest intakes of the randomized diet, both PDI and MDI were increased in those receiving preterm formula.[79] There were significant increases in the odds ratio of a PDI < 86 in infants receiving the term formula, both in the whole cohort (OR 1.8) as well as in selected infants on the highest intakes of the randomized diets (OR 3.4). Similarly, odds ratios for an MDI < 86 in infants receiving the term formula were 1.4 for the whole cohort and 1.9 in selected infants on the highest intakes of the randomized diets, although these did not reach statistical significance.[79] Once again, the randomized group with the highest in-hospital growth rates had the higher developmental scores.

Subjects were re-evaluated at 7 to 8 years of age (n = 360).[80] The rate of cerebral palsy was significantly lower in infants receiving the preterm formula (1.5% vs. 12%, p = 0.03).[80] There were no significant differences in IQ when the genders were analyzed together, even in those on the highest intakes of the randomized diet. However, infants fed the preterm formula were significantly less likely to have a verbal IQ <85 compared to those fed term formula (14% vs. 31%, p = 0.022). Verbal IQ and overall IQ were higher in boys receiving the preterm formula than boys receiving the term formula. The combined outcome of cerebral palsy or a verbal IQ less than 70 was significantly less common in those receiving the preterm formula (15%) than in those receiving the term formula (38%, p = 0.003).[80]

SUMMARY OF LUCAS STUDIES

The two Lucas studies demonstrate that nutritional intervention that affects in-hospital growth also significantly affects developmental outcome, even though the interventions only lasted a median of 4 weeks.

In both studies, the intervention group with the more rapid in-hospital weight gain also had improved developmental outcome. In the comparison of donor human milk and preterm formula, the developmental advantages of the more rapidly growing group (preterm formula) were clearly seen at 9 months,[77] but not at 18 months.[78] In the comparison of term and preterm formulas, the developmental advantages of the more rapidly growing group (preterm formula) were clearly seen at 18 months.[80] Benefits persisted to 7 to 8 years of age, where they were seen in both genders, but they were most clear in males.[80]

Perhaps the last word on these studies should go to the investigators, "our previous observation that improved nutrition in this same period may have beneficial effects on long-term development remains an important incentive to pay close attention to nutrition in hospitalized preterm infants."[81]

POST-DISCHARGE FORMULAS

In contrast to the case of in hospital interventions, the literature assessing the developmental sequelae of post-discharge nutritional interventions, either post-discharge "follow on" formulas or low birth weight formulas, is limited. Although several studies have suggested growth advantages to these interventions,[82–87] none of the studies that have assessed longer-term development have identified advantages to the enriched formula.[85–87]

SUMMARY AND CONCLUSIONS

Larger physical size and more rapid body growth in term and preterm infants is associated with improved neurodevelopmental outcomes.

In term infants, physical size at birth is clearly associated with better neurodevelopment. This appears to be true at older ages as well in SGA term infants, although the evidence for AGA term infants at older ages is less clear.

In preterm infants, size at birth has little effect on later neurodevelopment. However, closer to term-corrected age (or the time of hospital discharge) a clear association between later neurodevelopment and body size is demonstrated. This relationship appears to persist for 1 to 3 years, perhaps longer.

The beneficial association of larger body size in term and preterm infants is seen across the entire range of body sizes, and well into the "normal" range, and they are observed for differences in body weight and in body length, not just for head circumference.

Growth rate (or velocities) in early life is also associated with improved neurodevelopment. In term AGA, the benefits are seen most for higher growth rates in the first year of life, but the same benefit may be present for higher growth rates much later in life as well. In preterm infants, the benefit is most clear between birth and 4 months corrected age. However, it is also seen for growth rates through to 1 year post-term, maybe to 2 years post-term. There is little evidence for associations between growth rate and neurodevelopment beyond that period in preterm infants.

These associations are supported both by limited animal studies[60] and by data relating higher nutritional intakes in early life and later neurodevelopment.

Finally, the large cohort study of Lucas from the 1980s shows that preterm infants randomized to nutritional regimens that improved early growth showed improved neurodevelopmental outcome in later life. In one of the two studies, benefits remained until 7 to 8 years of age.

We conclude the following: The evidence demonstrating that more *rapid* growth is associated with improved neurodevelopment in preterm infants is far more compelling, both in quantity and in quality, than the data suggesting later metabolic advantages to *slower* early growth. Although the data are imperfect and incomplete, a simple risk–benefit calculation would suggest that more rapid early growth is to be much preferred compared to slower growth.

REFERENCES

1. Milani S, Bossi A, Bertino E, et al. Differences in size at birth are determined by differences in growth velocity during early prenatal life. *Pediatr Res* 2005;57:205–10.
2. Fok TF, Hon KL, So HK, et al. Fetal growth velocities in Hong Kong Chinese infants. *Biol Neonate* 2005;87:262–8.
3. Dobbing J, Sands J. Quantitative growth and development of human brain. *Arch Dis Child* 1973;48:757–67.
4. Vohr BR, Wright LL, Dusick AM, et al. Neurodevelopmental and functional outcomes of extremely low birth weight infants in the National Institute of Child Health and Human Development Neonatal Research Network, 1993–1994. *Pediatrics* 2000;105:1216–26.
5. Mikkola K, Ritari N, Tommiska V, et al. Neurodevelopmental outcome at 5 years of age of a national cohort of extremely low birth weight infants who were born in 1996–1997. *Pediatrics* 2005;116:1391–400.

6. Neubauer AP, Voss W, Kattner E. Outcome of extremely low birth weight survivors at school age: the influence of perinatal parameters on neurodevelopment. *Eur J Pediatr* 2008;167:87–95.

7. Franz AR, Pohlandt F, Bode H, et al. Intrauterine, early neonatal, and postdischarge growth and neurodevelopmental outcome at 5.4 years in extremely preterm infants after intensive neonatal nutritional support. *Pediatrics* 2009;123:e101–9.

8. Belfort MB, Rifas-Shiman SL, Sullivan T, et al. Infant growth before and after term: effects on neurodevelopment in preterm infants. *Pediatrics* 2011;128:e899–906.

9. Schlapbach LJ, Adams M, Proietti E, et al. Outcome at two years of age in a Swiss national cohort of extremely preterm infants born between 2000 and 2008. *BMC Pediatr* 2012;12:198.

10. Fanaroff AA, Stoll BJ, Wright LL, et al. Trends in neonatal morbidity and mortality for very low birthweight infants. *Am J Obstet Gynecol* 2007;196:147 e1–8.

11. Moore T, Hennessy EM, Myles J, et al. Neurological and developmental outcome in extremely preterm children born in England in 1995 and 2006: the EPICure studies. *BMJ* 2012;345:e7961.

12. Ehrenkranz RA, Das A, Wrage LA, et al. Early nutrition mediates the influence of severity of illness on extremely low birth weight infants. *Pediatr Res* 2011;69:522–9.

13. Watemberg N, Silver S, Harel S, Lerman-Sagie T. Significance of microcephaly among children with developmental disabilities. *J Child Neurol* 2002;17:117–22.

14. Gross SJ, Oehler JM, Eckerman CO. Head growth and developmental outcome in very low-birth-weight infants. *Pediatrics* 1983;71:70–5.

15. Hack M, Merkatz IR, Gordon D, Jones PK, Fanaroff AA. The prognostic significance of postnatal growth in very low birth weight infants. *Am J Obstet Gynecol* 1982;143:693–9.

16. Hack M, Breslau N, Fanaroff AA. Differential effects of intrauterine and postnatal brain growth failure in infants of very low birth weight. *Am J Dis Child* 1989;143:63–8.

17. Hack M, Breslau N, Weissman B, Aram D, Klein N, Borawski E. Effect of very low birth weight and subnormal head size on cognitive abilities at school age. *N Engl J Med* 1991;325:231–7.

18. Belfort MB, Martin CR, Smith VC, Gillman MW, McCormick MC. Infant weight gain and school-age blood pressure and cognition in former preterm infants. *Pediatrics* 2010;125:e1419–26.

19. Brandt I, Sticker EJ, Lentze MJ. Catch-up growth of head circumference of very low birth weight, small for gestational age preterm infants and mental development to adulthood. *J Pediatr* 2003;142:463–8.

20. Casey PH, Whiteside-Mansell L, Barrett K, Bradley RH, Gargus R. Impact of prenatal and/or postnatal growth problems in low birth weight preterm infants on school-age outcomes: an 8-year longitudinal evaluation. *Pediatrics* 2006;118:1078–86.

21. Ehrenkranz RA, Dusick AM, Vohr BR, Wright LL, Wrage LA, Poole WK. Growth in the neonatal intensive care unit influences neurodevelopmental and growth outcomes of extremely low birth weight infants. *Pediatrics* 2006;117:1253–61.

22. Huang C, Martorell R, Ren A, Li Z. Cognition and behavioural development in early childhood: the role of birth weight and postnatal growth. *Int J Epidemiol* 2012.

23. Kan E, Roberts G, Anderson PJ, Doyle LW. The association of growth impairment with neurodevelopmental outcome at eight years of age in very preterm children. *Early Hum Dev* 2008;84:409–16.

24. Kitchen WH, Doyle LW, Ford GW, Callanan C, Rickards AL, Kelly E. Very low birth weight and growth to age 8 years. II: Head dimensions and intelligence. *Am J Dis Child* 1992;146:46–50.

25. Kon N, Tanaka K, Sekigawa M, et al. Association between iron status and neurodevelopmental outcomes among VLBW infants. *Brain Develop* 2010;32:849–54.

26. Kuban KC, Allred EN, O'Shea TM, et al. Developmental correlates of head circumference at birth and two years in a cohort of extremely low gestational age newborns. *J Pediatr* 2009;155:344–9 e1–3.

27. Latal-Hajnal B, von Siebenthal K, Kovari H, Bucher HU, Largo RH. Postnatal growth in VLBW infants: significant association with neurodevelopmental outcome. *J Pediatr* 2003;143:163–70.

28. Nash A, Dunn M, Asztalos E, Corey M, Mulvihill-Jory B, O'Connor DL. Pattern of growth of very low birth weight preterm infants, assessed using the WHO Growth Standards, is associated with neurodevelopment. Applied physiology, nutrition, and metabolism = *Physiologie appliquee, nutrition et metabolisme* 2011;36:562–9.

29. Ochiai M, Nakayama H, Sato K, et al. Head circumference and long-term outcome in small-for-gestational age infants. *J Perinat Med* 2008;36:341–7.

30. Ramel SE, Demerath EW, Gray HL, Younge N, Boys C, Georgieff MK. The relationship of poor linear growth velocity with neonatal illness and two-year neurodevelopment in preterm infants. *Neonatology* 2012;102:19–24.

31. Ross G, Krauss AN, Auld PA. Growth achievement in low-birth-weight premature infants: relationship to neurobehavioral outcome at one year. *J Pediatr* 1983;103:105–8.

32. Ross G, Lipper EG, Auld PA. Physical growth and developmental outcome in very low birth weight premature infants at 3 years of age. *J Pediatr* 1985;107:284–6.

33. Washburn L, Nixon P, Snively B, Tennyson A, O'Shea TM. Weight gain in infancy and early childhood is associated with school age body mass index but not intelligence and blood pressure in very low birth weight children. *Journal of Developmental Origins of Health and Disease* 2010;1:338–46.

34. Wocadlo C, Rieger I. Developmental outcome at 12 months corrected age for infants born less than 30 weeks gestation: influence of reduced intrauterine and postnatal growth. *Early Hum Dev* 1994;39:127–37.

35. dit Trolli SE, Kermorvant-Duchemin E, Huon C, Bremond-Gignac D, Lapillonne A. Early lipid supply and neurological development at one year in very low birth weight (VLBW) preterm infants. *Early Hum Dev* 2012;88 Suppl 1:S25–9.

36. Belfort MB, Rifas-Shiman SL, Rich-Edwards JW, Kleinman KP, Oken E, Gillman MW. Infant growth and child cognition at 3 years of age. *Pediatrics* 2008;122:e689–95.

37. Beyerlein A, Ness AR, Streuling I, Hadders-Algra M, von Kries R. Early rapid growth: no association with later cognitive functions in children born not small for gestational age. *Am J Clin Nutr* 2010;92:585–93.

38. Broekman BF, Chan YH, Chong YS, et al. The influence of birth size on intelligence in healthy children. *Pediatrics* 2009;123:e1011–6.

39. Emond AM, Blair PS, Emmett PM, Drewett RF. Weight faltering in infancy and IQ levels at 8 years in the Avon Longitudinal Study of Parents and Children. *Pediatrics* 2007;120:e1051–8.

40. Fattal-Valevski A, Toledano-Alhadef H, Leitner Y, Geva R, Eshel R, Harel S. Growth patterns in children with intrauterine growth retardation and their correlation to neuro-cognitive development. *J Child Neurol* 2009;24:846–51.

41. Gale CR, O'Callaghan FJ, Bredow M, Martyn CN. The influence of head growth in fetal life, infancy, and childhood on intelligence at the ages of 4 and 8 years. *Pediatrics* 2006;118:1486–92.

42. Heinonen K, Raikkonen K, Pesonen AK, et al. Prenatal and postnatal growth and cognitive abilities at 56 months of age: a longitudinal study of infants born at term. *Pediatrics* 2008;121:e1325–33.

43. Leitner Y, Fattal-Valevski A, Geva R, et al. Six-year follow-up of children with intrauterine growth retardation: long-term, prospective study. *J Child Neurol* 2000;15:781–6.

44. Leitner Y, Fattal-Valevski A, Geva R, et al. Neurodevelopmental outcome of children with intrauterine growth retardation: a longitudinal, 10-year prospective study. *J Child Neurol* 2007;22:580–7.
45. Li H, DiGirolamo AM, Barnhart HX, Stein AD, Martorell R. Relative importance of birth size and postnatal growth for women's educational achievement. *Early Hum Dev* 2004;76:1–16.
46. Lira PI, Eickmann SH, Lima MC, Amorim RJ, Emond AM, Ashworth A. Early head growth: relation with IQ at 8 years and determinants in term infants of low and appropriate birthweight. *Dev Med Child Neurol* 2010;52:40–6.
47. Matte TD, Bresnahan M, Begg MD, Susser E. Influence of variation in birth weight within normal range and within sibships on IQ at age 7 years: cohort study. *BMJ* 2001;323:310–4.
48. Pongcharoen T, Ramakrishnan U, DiGirolamo AM, et al. Influence of prenatal and postnatal growth on intellectual functioning in school-aged children. *Arch Pediatr Adolesc Med* 2012;166:411–6.
49. Silva A, Metha Z, O'Callaghan F J. The relative effect of size at birth, postnatal growth and social factors on cognitive function in late childhood. *Annals of Epidemiology* 2006;16:469–76.
50. Yang S, Tilling K, Martin R, Davies N, Ben-Shlomo Y, Kramer MS. Pre-natal and post-natal growth trajectories and childhood cognitive ability and mental health. *Int J Epidemiol* 2011;40:1215–26.
51. Bos AF, Einspieler C, Prechtl HFR. Intrauterine growth retardation, general movements, and neurodevelopmental outcome: a review. *Developmental Medicine & Child Neurology* 2001;43:61–8.
52. de Bie HM, Oostrom KJ, Delemarre-van de Waal HA. Brain development, intelligence and cognitive outcome in children born small for gestational age. *Horm Res Paediatr* 2010;73:6–14.
53. Groom KM, Poppe KK, North RA, McCowan LM. Small-for-gestational-age infants classified by customized or population birthweight centiles: impact of gestational age at delivery. *Am J Obstet Gynecol* 2007;197:239 e1–5.
54. Sung IK, Vohr B, Oh W. Growth and neurodevelopmental outcome of very low birth weight infants with intrauterine growth retardation: comparison with control subjects matched by birth weight and gestational age. *J Pediatr* 1993;123:618–24.
55. Amin H, Singhal N, Sauve RS. Impact of intrauterine growth restriction on neurodevelopmental and growth outcomes in very low birthweight infants. *Acta Paediatr* 1997;86:306–14.
56. McCarton CM, Wallace IF, Divon M, Vaughan HG, Jr. Cognitive and neurologic development of the premature, small for gestational age infant through age 6: comparison by birth weight and gestational age. *Pediatrics* 1996;98:1167–78.
57. Gortner L, van Husen M, Thyen U, Gembruch U, Friedrich HJ, Landmann E. Outcome in preterm small for gestational age infants compared to appropriate for gestational age preterms at the age of 2 years: a prospective study. *Eur J Obstet Gynecol Reprod Biol* 2003;110 Suppl 1:S93–7.
58. Streimish IG, Ehrenkranz RA, Allred EN, et al. Birth weight- and fetal weight-growth restriction: impact on neurodevelopment. *Early Hum Dev* 2012;88:765–71.
59. Ranke MB, Vollmer B, Traunecker R, et al. Growth and development are similar in VLBW children born appropriate and small for gestational age: an interim report on 97 preschool children. *J Pediatr Endocrinol Metab* 2007;20:1017–26.
60. Jou M-Y, Lonnerdall BL, Griffin IJ. Effects on early postnatal growth restriction and subsequent catch-up growth on body composition, insulin sensitivity and behavior in neonatal rats. *Pediatr Res* 2013; In Press.

61. Rudolf MC, Logan S. What is the long term outcome for children who fail to thrive? A systematic review. *Arch Dis Child* 2005;90:925–31.

62. Ehrenkranz RA. Early, aggressive nutritional management for very low birth weight infants: what is the evidence? *Semin Perinatol* 2007;31:48–55.

63. Lapillonne A, Griffin IJ. Feeding preterm infants today for later metabolic and cardiovascular outcomes. *J Pediatr* 2013;162:S7–16.

64. Georgieff MK, Hoffman JS, Pereira GR, Bernbaum J, Hoffman-Williamson M. Effect of neonatal caloric deprivation on head growth and 1-year developmental status in preterm infants. *J Pediatr* 1985;107:581–7.

65. Stephens BE, Walden RV, Gargus RA, et al. First-week protein and energy intakes are associated with 18-month developmental outcomes in extremely low birth weight infants. *Pediatrics* 2009;123:1337–43.

66. Wilson DC, Cairns P, Halliday HL, Reid M, McClure G, Dodge JA. Randomised controlled trial of an aggressive nutritional regimen in sick very low birthweight infants. *Arch Dis Child Fetal Neonatal Ed* 1997;77:F4–11.

67. Dinerstein A, Nieto RM, Solana CL, Perez GP, Otheguy LE, Larguia AM. Early and aggressive nutritional strategy (parenteral and enteral) decreases postnatal growth failure in very low birth weight infants. *Journal of Perinatology* 2006;26:436–42.

68. Maggio L, Cota F, Gallini F, Lauriola V, Zecca C, Romagnoli C. Effects of high versus standard early protein intake on growth of extremely low birth weight infants. *J Pediatr Gastroenterol Nutr* 2007;44:124–9.

69. Tan MJ, Cooke RW. Improving head growth in very preterm infants–a randomised controlled trial I: neonatal outcomes. *Arch Dis Child* 2008;93:F337–F41.

70. Can E, Bulbul A, Uslu S, Comert S, Bolat F, Nuhoglu A. Effects of aggressive parenteral nutrition on growth and clinical outcome in preterm infants. *Pediatrics International: Official Journal of the Japan Pediatric Society* 2012;54:869–74.

71. Tan M, Abernethy L, Cooke R. Improving head growth in preterm infants: a randomised controlled trial II: MRI and developmental outcomes in the first year. *Arch Dis Child* 2008;93:F342–F6.

72. Lucas A, Cole TJ, Morley R, et al. Factors associated with maternal choice to provide breast milk for low birthweight infants. *Arch Dis Child* 1988;63:48–52.

73. Vohr BR, Poindexter BB, Dusick AM, McKinley LT, Wright LL, Langer JC. Beneficial effects of breast milk in the neonatal intensive care unit on the developmental outcome of extremely low birth weight infants at 18 months of age. *Pediatrics* 2006;118:e115–23.

74. Morley R, Cole T, Powell R, Lucas A. Mother's choice to provide breast milk and developmental outcome. *Arch Dis Child* 1988;63:1382–5.

75. Vohr BR, Poindexter BB, Dusick AM, et al. Persistent beneficial effects of breast milk ingested in the neonatal intensive care unit on outcomes of extremely low birth weight infants at 30 months of age. *Pediatrics* 2007;120:e953–9.

76. Lucas A, Gore SM, Cole TJ, et al. Multicentre trial on feeding low birthweight infants: effects of diet on early growth. *Arch Dis Child* 1984;59:722–30.

77. Lucas A, Morley R, Cole TJ, et al. Early diet in preterm babies and developmental status in infancy. *Arch Dis Child* 1989;64:1570–8.

78. Lucas A, Morley R, Cole T, Gore S. A randomised multicentre study of human milk versus formula and later development in preterm infants. *Arch Dis Child* 1994;70:F141–F6.

79. Lucas A, Morley R, Cole TJ, et al. Early diet in preterm babies and developmental status at 18 months. *Lancet* 1990;335:1477–81.

80. Lucas A, Morley R, Cole TJ. Randomised trial of early diet in preterm babies and later intelligence quotient. *BMJ* 1998;317:1481–7.

81. Morley R, Lucas A. Randomized diet in the neonatal period and growth performance until 7.5-8 y of age in preterm children. *Am J Clin Nutr* 2000;71:822–8.

82. Lucas A, Bishop NJ, King FJ, Cole TJ. Randomised trial of nutrition for preterm infants after discharge. *Arch Dis Child* 1992;67:324–7.
83. Cooke RJ, Griffin IJ, McCormick K, et al. Feeding preterm infants after hospital discharge: effect of dietary manipulation on nutrient intake and growth. *Pediatr Res* 1998;43:355–60.
84. Carver JD, Wu PY, Hall RT, et al. Growth of preterm infants fed nutrient-enriched or term formula after hospital discharge. *Pediatrics* 2001;107:683–9.
85. Lucas A, Fewtrell MS, Morley R, et al. Randomized trial of nutrient-enriched formula versus standard formula for postdischarge preterm infants. *Pediatrics* 2001;108:703–11.
86. Cooke RJ, Embleton ND, Griffin IJ, Wells JC, McCormick KP. Feeding preterm infants after hospital discharge: growth and development at 18 months of age. *Pediatr Res* 2001;49:719–22.
87. Young L, Morgan J, McCormick FM, McGuire W. Nutrient enriched formula versus standard term formula for preterm infants following hospital discharge. *Cochrane Database Syst Rev* 2012;14:CD004696.

Section II Conclusions

The risks of obesity and metabolic disorders (e.g., insulin resistance or hypertension) are associated both with body size at birth and with whether the infant was at either extreme of the normal range; either small for gestational age (SGA) or large for gestational age (LGA).

In term infants, larger birth weight is associated with an increased risk of obesity in later life. However, SGA term infants are also at increased risk of obesity. Conversely, smaller birth size is generally a risk factor for hypertension and insulin resistance, but SGA and LGA infants are at increased risk as well. Simplistically, the risks of obesity might be considered to have a J-shaped relation to birth size, and the risk of hypertension and insulin resistance have a reversed-J shape (Figure II.1). The data for preterm infants is less clear (Table II.1).

Larger size at birth is associated with improved long-term neurodevelopment in appropriate for gestational age (AGA) and SGA term infants, and larger size by term-expected age is associated with improved neurodevelopment in preterm infants (Table II.1). Poor weight gain in the hospital may therefore worsen developmental outcome, although the benefits in terms of a reduced risk of metabolic syndrome are unclear.

In term AGA infants, more rapid growth in the first 1 to 3 years after birth is associated with an increased risk of obesity, hypertension, and insulin resistance (although there are differences between retrospective and prospective studies). During the same time period, catch-up growth in term SGA infants, or the absence of catch-down growth in term LGA infants, is associated with an increased risk of obesity, hypertension, or insulin resistance. Conversely, more rapid growth in the first 1 to 2 years after birth is associated with improved neurodevelopment in term infants (Table II.2). In preterm infants, there is little evidence that catch-up growth in the first year post-term has any metabolic consequences, but slower growth during this period does appear to worsen neurodevelopmental outcome (Table II.2).

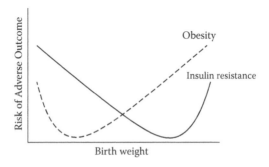

FIGURE II.1 J-shaped relationship between obesity and birth weight, and reversed-J shaped relationship between insulin resistance and birth weight.

TABLE II.1

Effects of Size at Birth (or at term-expected age) for Term AGA, SGA, and LGA Infants, and for Preterm Infants

Group	Long-Term Benefits of Smaller Birth Size	Long-Term Benefits of Larger Birth Size
Term AGA	Dec risk of obesity	Dec risk of insulin resistance
		Dec risk of hypertension
		Dec risk of mortality
		Improved developmental outcome
Term SGA[a]	—	Improved developmental outcome[a]
Term LGA[b]	[b]	—
Preterm[c]	Larger size near term-expected date = Unclear[d]	Larger size near term-expected date = Improved developmental outcome[e]

[a] Being born SGA associated with increased risk of obesity, insulin resistance, and hypertension.

[b] Being born LGA associated with increased risk of obesity, insulin resistance, and hypertension.

[c] Preterm birth associated with increased risk of hypertension, possibly insulin resistance, and obesity unclear.

[d] Limited data that very slow growth for the first few weeks may improve metabolic outcomes.

[e] Based on body size at time of discharge, or at term-corrected age.

TABLE II.2

Effects of Infantile Growth (from birth to age 2 to 3 years) for Term AGA, SGA, and LGA infants, and for Preterm Infants

Group	Long-Term Benefits of Faster Infantile Growth	Long-Term Benefits of Slower Infantile Growth
Term AGA	Improved development[a]	Dec obesity
		Dec insulin resistance
		Dec hypertension
Term SGA	Improved development[a]	Dec obesity
		Dec insulin resistance
		Dec hypertension
Term LGA	–	Dec obesity
		Dec insulin resistance
		Dec hypertension
Preterm	Improved development[b]	Dec insulin resistance[c]
		Dec hypertension[c]

[a] Until 12 months or 24 months of age.

[b] Until 4 months or 6 months of age.

[c] Only for catch-up occurring after ≈ 12 months of age.

Childhood growth (beginning 2 to 3 years after birth) is also positively associated with the risk of obesity, hypertension, or insulin resistance, just as infantile growth (between birth and 2 to 3 years of age, Table II.1) is. This appears to be true for both term and preterm infants. There is limited evidence of any beneficial effects of more rapid growth on neurodevelopmental outcomes during this period.

So what does this information mean in practice for preterm infants? First, it seems clear that *ex utero* growth restriction in preterm infants should be avoided if possible

It is associated with significant reductions in long-term cognitive outcomes and with an increased risk of neurodevelopmental impairments such as cerebral palsy. It this goal could be achieved, we would probably not have to worry about the benefits and risks of catch-up growth in infancy or childhood. However, at present we must balance the benefits of any on-going catch-up growth on neurodevelopment against the risk of catch-up growth. Early catch-up (within the first 12 months after term-expected age) does not seem to be associated with adverse metabolic outcomes in preterm infants, and so should be actively encouraged. After 2 to 3 years of age, the benefits of ongoing catch-up growth are more difficult to identify, and the metabolic risks are clearer. Therefore, it seems prudent to avoid significant upward percentile crossing after 2 to 3 years of age in preterm babies, *just as it is in term-born infants.* The correct balance during the intervening period, between approximately 1 year post-term and approximately 3 years post-term, is harder to determine, although it is the editor's opinion that the benefits of catch-up growth in that period probably continue to outweigh the risks.

Section III

Can We Be Better? Reducing Ex Utero Growth Restriction in Preterm Infants

INTRODUCTION

Ex utero growth restriction (EUGR) is clearly associated with poorer long-term development and one of our goals as neonatologists should be to prevent it. A major modifiable cause of EUGR is inadequate nutrient intakes (Chapter 3), and improving nutrient intake should be a focus.

In this section, we will review how the current recommended intakes for preterm infants are derived, and the uncertainty surrounding them (Chapter 8); how we can optimize nutrient intakes for preterm infants (Chapters 9, 10, and 11), including new methods to customize the fortification of human milk (Chapter 11); and finally, as our ultimate goal is to approximate *in utero* growth rates, we will see how the newest generation of neonatal growth references allows better monitoring of growth using Z-scores statistical trend analysis (Chapter 12).

8 Assessing Nutritional Requirements for Preterm Infants

Frank R. Greer

INTRODUCTION

It should come as no surprise to the reader that the information base with which to support the methods of determining the dietary requirements of preterm infants is limited. This nonhomogeneous population includes the late preterm infant (34 to 37 weeks gestation, birth weight usually >2000 g), the low birth weight infant (birth weight <2000 g), the very low birth weight infant (birth weight <1500 g), and the extremely low birth weight infant (birth weight <1000 g). In addition to the broad range of postconceptional age (23 to 37 weeks) and birth weight, preterm infants have genetic and epigenetic differences, varying rates of growth and energy metabolism, alternative methods of nutrient delivery (parenteral vs. enteral) and variable absorption rates of key nutrients. Any of these could affect the typically rapid growth trajectories of a preterm infant. There are also significant differences in degrees of illness and associated co-morbidities, which have a large impact on nutritional requirements and nutrient utilization. Thus, assessing the dietary requirements of this diverse population of preterm infants is not an easy task, and it is clear that "one size" cannot possibly fit all.

DETERMINING DIETARY REQUIREMENTS FOR PRETERM INFANTS

A dietary requirement is defined as the intake level that will meet specified criteria of nutritional adequacy, while preventing risk of both deficit and excess. The Dietary Reference Intakes (DRIs) are reference values that are generally used for a healthy population and healthy individuals. Utilizing the DRIs for the heterogeneous population of preterm infants with varying degrees of illness to determine the appropriate nutrient intakes is problematic. The DRIs include the Estimated Average Requirement (EAR), the Recommended Dietary Allowance (RDA), the Adequate Intake (AI), and the Tolerable Upper Intake Level (UL) of a given nutrient.[1]

The EAR is the nutrient intake value that is estimated to meet the requirement of 50% of the individuals in a life stage and gender group as predefined by a specified indicator of adequacy such as a biomarker. The EAR is then used to establish the

RDA, which does not apply to a population but to individuals. The RDA is the average dietary intake level that is sufficient to meet the nutrient requirements of 97 to 98% of individuals in a population and it is set at 2 SD above the EAR of a population.

For the premature infant population, it is not possible to calculate the EAR or the RDA for any nutrient. Using an RDA would clearly lead to an excess of nutrients for some preterm infants who are already at risk for the metabolic syndrome. The alternative AI is based on observed or experimentally determined estimates of average nutrient intake of a group of healthy people. For the healthy term infant for whom human milk is the sole source of food, the AI is based on the estimated daily mean nutrient intake supplied by human milk. But again, preterm infants are not a healthy population and human milk alone will not meet their nutrient needs, and cannot be utilized to determine the AI. Nor can the needs of "sick" preterm infants be extrapolated from "healthy" term or preterm infants, as the scientific basis for which to adjust nutrient intakes based on the effects of disease and co-morbidities is not available.

Thus, for describing the dietary requirements for the preterm infant, we often utilize what some have called the "RRI"—the Recommended Range of Intake for a given nutrient.[2] The RRI by definition is the range of average daily intakes derived from observational or randomized trials that appear to sustain adequate nutrition (growth), based on the absence of abnormal clinical signs, symptoms, or biochemical measurements. The RRI would ideally lie in-between the lower limit associated with deficiency and the upper limit associated with toxicity for a given nutrient, and the range would be wide enough to take into account the likelihood that there are significant differences for individual preterm infants within the range of intakes, even for infants of the same weight or postconceptional age. It has also been suggested that the lower limit of the RRI, in theory, should not be less than the EAR and not exceed the UL when and if these values become available for a given nutrient.

These concepts can be visualized in the proposed model in Figure 8.1. As nutritional intake increases, the risk of deficiency (on the left) decreases, but with further increasing intake the risk of excess intake and toxicity begins to increase. Somewhere in the mid-range is the RRI.

One can speculate that for the smallest and most preterm infants, the RRI would be narrower than for the older, less preterm infants given that the most preterm infants have the highest needs per unit of body weight and are more susceptible to deficits as well as excesses of any given nutrient. Thus, the so-called therapeutic window of many nutrients would be narrower for the ELBW infant compared to the late preterm infant. In an ideal world, the RRI would also be defined by the intakes that prevent subclinical adverse effects whether from a deficit or excess of a given nutrient. Additionally, the RRI may be narrower for the initial parenteral feeding goals, which then gradually increase during the transition from parenteral to full enteral feedings, in order to meet the needs for optimal growth and development. Thus, for the individual preterm infant, the RRI for a given nutrient is a moving (or sliding) target, which makes it difficult to decide which infant needs more or less of a given nutrient (Figure 8.1). It would be ideal if there were appropriate biomarkers to use in setting the RRI, such as BUN for protein or alkaline phosphatase for calcium, but these proposed biomarkers lack specificity.

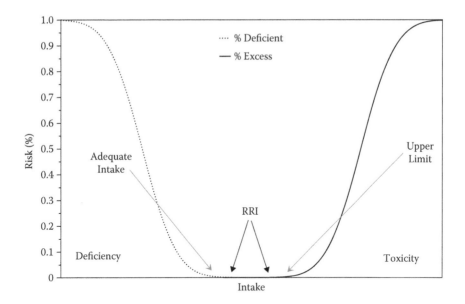

FIGURE 8.1 The cumulative risks of inadequate nutrient intake (deficiency, broken line) and excessive nutrient intake (toxicity, solid line) as nutritional intake changes. Approximate position for the adequate intake and upper limit and for the RRI are shown.

It has been generally agreed upon that the ideal growth rate for the preterm infant should match the *in utero* growth curve for the fetus of the same postconceptional age. Ideally, this would also include body composition when practical measures of assessment become available and the goals for the ideal body composition have been determined for a preterm infant after birth.[3,4] For the healthy preterm infant, growth rate can be determined from the percentile of the birth weight. To achieve this growth rate after birth, two approaches have been used to estimate the intakes for individual nutrients for preterm infants. One approach involves setting a goal for the ideal intake of a given nutrient based on the fetal content of the nutrient at the same gestational age, the so-called factorial approach. The second approach, the empirical approach, is to set a goal to achieve an outcome, such as the amount of protein that optimizes growth rate or the amount of calcium that optimizes bone mineral content.

FACTORIAL APPROACH

As nutrient accretion by the fetus accounts for a large proportion of nutrient intake, the factorial approach is useful for the preterm infant where the underlying principle is that the body composition of the infant should resemble that of the fetus at the same postconceptional age.

The body composition of more than 169 human fetuses has been chemically described in the literature.[5] However, there are many concerns regarding the quality of the reports, as described by Sparks[5] and Ziegler.[6] These include:

1. The fetal gestational age reported was not accurately known.
2. The fetuses came to autopsy for reasons that may have altered growth or nutrient accretion (major congenital anomalies, infants of diabetic or malnourished mothers).
3. The analyzed fetuses may not conform to norms for growth of fetuses in the general population (were still born or expired more than 48 hours priory delivery, were SGA, etc.).
4. The fetuses analyzed were not selected randomly from the general population.
5. The fetuses were not analyzed soon after death, using accurate, precise, and modern methods.

In fact, in constructing "the reference fetus" Ziegler eliminated all but 22 of the fetuses analyzed in the literature as being unsatisfactory.[6] Despite this, there were additional limitations in that the reported data was not always sex specific and the 22 fetuses were skewed toward the more growth retarded, and all but 2 were less than the 50th percentile for weight. Although none were less than the 5th percentile, 7 were less than the 10th percentile for weight. Gestational age ranged from 24 to 40 weeks and birth weights ranged from 690 to 3450 g.[6]

Thus, the factorial approach is subject to major limitations for preterm infants and does not take into account individual variations in nutrient requirements. These are dependent on variations in absorption rate, in nutrient intake, and sources of nutrients including parenteral nutrition. Enteral feedings range from human milk to special formulas for low birth weight infants. The intakes determined by the factorial method should take into account the concept of nutrient retention, including the inevitable losses (dermal, urinary, intestinal), and the need for growth and tissue stores of nutrients. Table 8.1 is an estimate for major mineral and electrolyte intakes needed to achieve fetal weight gain using the factorial approach.[4,7] However, in the preterm infant there remains some uncertainty about the urinary and intestinal losses of these minerals that may be influenced by many factors.[7] Of note, no range

---

TABLE 8.1

Requirements for Major Minerals and Electrolytes Determined by the Factorial Method (per kg/day)

	Body Weight					
	500–1000 g		1000–1500 g		1500–2000 g	
	Accretion	Required Intake	Accretion	Required Intake	Accretion	Required Intake
Ca, mg	102	184	99	178	96	173
P, mg	66	126	65	124	63	120
Mg, mg	2.8	6.9	2.7	6.7	2.5	6.4
Na, mEq	1.54	3.3	1.37	3.0	1.06	2.6
K, mEq	0.78	2.4	0.72	2.3	0.63	2.2
Cl, mEq	2.26	2.8	0.99	2.7	0.74	2.5

of intakes is given in Table 8.1 that could be used to determine an RRI using the factorial approach.

A potential problem with the factorial approach is that although it provides an estimate for any nutrient for which the content of the fetus is known, it does not take into consideration the requirements for catch-up growth. This requires additional information about the degree and speed of catch-up growth desired. Thus, for a fetus born at 24 weeks, who for various reasons does not regain birth weight before 27 weeks, a higher nutrient requirement would be needed than that based on a gestational age of 24 weeks if the fetal rate of growth was to be achieved. Thus, using the factorial approach, "one size" does not really fit all.

EMPIRICAL APPROACH

The empirical approach, sometimes referred to as the functional approach, has largely been used in preterm infants to determine protein and energy requirements. This approach utilizes feedings of varying energy and protein content to maximize nitrogen balance and growth outcomes taking into account nutrient retention and losses (dermal, urinary, and intestinal). Nutrient requirements using this approach are largely dependent on body size rather than gestational age, and biomarkers would be important. Thus, in a feeding study by Kashyap et al., gains in weight and length of preterm infants were greater when protein intake from an infant formula was 3.8 g/kg/d compared to an intake of 2.8 g/kg/d.[9] Similarly, in a feeding study by Polberger et al., infants fed human milk fortified with human milk protein providing 3.6 g/kg/d of protein showed marked increased gains in weight and length compared to infants fed unfortified human milk with a protein intake of 2.1 g/kg/d.[10] Table 8.2 depicts the requirements for protein intake based on the empirical approach.

TABLE 8.2
Protein Intakes Needed To Achieve Fetal Weight Gain Using the Empirical Approach[9, 10]

	Body Weight					
	500–700 g	700–900 g	900–1000 g	1200–1500 g	1500–1800 g	1800–2000 g
Fetal Weight Gain						
g/d	13	16	20	24	29	29
g/kg/d	21	20	19	18	16	14
Protein Balance						
Losses (g/kg/d)	1.0	1.0	1.0	1.0	1.0	1.0
Growth (g/kg/d)	2.5	2.5	2.5	2.4	2.2	2.0
Requirement						
Parenteral (g/kg/d)	3.5	3.5	3.5	3.4	3.2	3.0
Enteral (g/kg/d)	4.0	4.0	4.0	3.9	3.6	3.4

The empirical approach lends itself to determining the needs for catch-up growth, as protein intake by this method may exceed that determined by the factorial approach and the resultant increased rate of growth can be construed as catch-up growth.[7] However, again, this approach does not adequately define a range of protein intakes that would meet the needs of the majority of the population of preterm infants. As infants grow and advance in postconceptional age, the amount of protein intake needed changes, and again one size does not fit all.

Other nutrient requirements may also be determined by the empirical approach. Thus, calcium and vitamin D intakes can be related to maximizing bone health using various medical imaging techniques and biochemical measures of collagen synthesis and bone turnover.

New measures of body composition by medical imaging techniques or air-displacement plethysmography can allow for measures of lean body mass and fat mass and their response to varying dietary intakes of energy, fat, or protein as well. In the future, it can even be anticipated that measures of gene expression as a biomarker may be utilized to determine the amount of a specific nutrient required to trigger a specific mRNA response in a given tissue

DETERMINING A RECOMMENDED RANGE OF INTAKES FOR THE PRETERM INFANT

It should be noted that neither the factorial approach nor the empirical approach allows one to determine a recommended *range* of intakes for the preterm infant, given the degree of individual variation within this mixed population of subjects. As noted, this population has a high prevalence of adverse events and co-morbidities, an expected rapid rate of growth, as well as very limited stores. The limited stores make absorption and retention of nutrients very important. All of these factors make it difficult to establish a recommended range of intakes in the preterm infant, particularly for the micronutrients.

RELATIONSHIP BETWEEN INTAKE, ABSORPTION, AND RETENTION

In a population of healthy, non-growing adults, the relationships between intake, absorption, and retention are relatively simple, assuming a normal distribution within a population. At suboptimal intakes of a given nutrient, requirements exceed the amount absorbed from the diet and the deficit must be made up from stores, or deficiency occurs assuming the absorption rate remains constant. On the other hand, if net absorption exceeds needs, a positive balance results with the excess sequestered into storage pools. If storage mechanisms are exceeded, toxicity may result. However, homeostatic mechanisms allow for a broader intake range over which adequate balance is maintained, minimizing the risks of deficiency or excess. Thus, in times of a deficient intake, up-regulation of absorption may occur, and in times of excess intake, down-regulation of absorption may occur.

For any individual within a population, as nutrient intake rises the risk of deficiency falls. At higher intakes the risk of nutrient excess or toxicity rises. The position of individuals on the intake-balance curve will be different, again assuming a normal distribution (Figure 8.2) For example, individuals with "poor absorption"

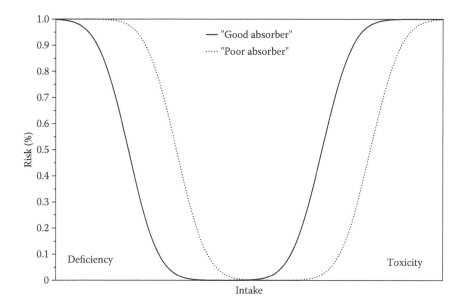

FIGURE 8.2 Different positions on the intake-risk (deficiency/excess) curve between a "good absorber" and a "poor absorber."

(broken line in Figure 8.2) or "good absorption" (solid line in Figure 8.2) will occupy different points on the intake balance curve with different ranges of reasonable intakes. At low intakes, the "good absorbers" are lower risk of nutrient deficiency, but at higher intakes, they are at increased risk of nutrient excess. Thus, the ideal intake-balance curve will be shifted to the left for the "good absorbers" and to the right for "poor absorbers." (Figure 8.2) On the other hand, the reasonable range of intake on the intake-balance continuum would be expected to be larger for any individual within it, than for the entire population (Figure 8.3).

VARIATIONS IN INTAKE, ABSORPTION, AND RETENTION IN THE PREMATURE INFANT

Applying the recommended range of intake concept to the intake-balance continuum to the premature infant within a broad range of weights, gestational ages, and co-morbidities is problematic. The precision with which absorption can be measured and nutrient requirements estimated is less than ideal. To demonstrate the difficulty in establishing a reasonable range of intakes for the preterm infant, the published measurements of zinc intake and zinc retention will be reviewed, acknowledging the fact there is no reliable biomarker for zinc deficiency in individuals.[12]

In a recent review article, published measurements of zinc intake and zinc retention were reviewed for 22 groups of formula-fed infants (n = 342).[13] There was a good correlation between zinc intake and zinc retention (r = 0.56, r^2 = 0.31, p = 0.0043). This correlation increased when a single outlier from these studies was eliminated (r = .64, r^2 = 0.41, p = 0.001, Figure 8.4). The requirement for retained zinc in preterm

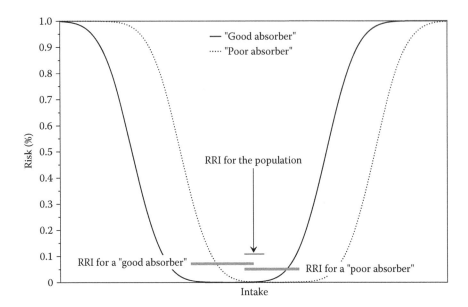

FIGURE 8.3 Approximate RRI for the "good absorber" and "poor absorber" and for the entire population.

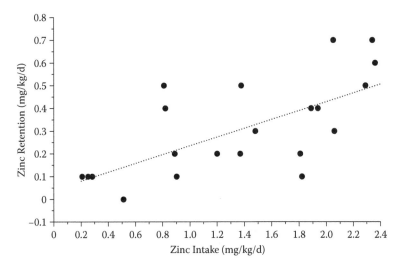

FIGURE 8.4 Relationship between zinc intake and zinc retention in published studies in formula fed intakes (see Reference 13).

infants with a birth weight from 1500 to 2000 g (30 to 32 weeks postconceptional age) has been estimated to be approximately 400 mcg/kg/d.[14] From Figure 8.4, the zinc intake required to achieve this retention can be estimated from the regression line to be 1.85 mg/kg/d. However, the 95% confidence interval around this point estimate of zinc intake would be 1.47 – 2.63 mg/kg/day, or 79 to 142% of the point estimate.

TABLE 8.3
Dietary Zinc Requirements

Weight (kg)	Gestational Age (weeks)	Zinc Requirement for Retention (mcg/kd/d)	Required Zinc Intake from Formula (mcg) (95% CI)
< 1.0	< 28	500	2273 (1379–6465)
1.0–2.0	28–34	400	1818 (1103–5172
2.0–3.5	35-40	300	1364 (828–3879)

Table 8.3 gives the estimated requirements for absorbed zinc by birth weight and gestational age from Figure 8.4. The last column gives the 95% confidence interval for range of zinc intake for each confidence interval. In each case, the confidence interval is between 60 and 280% of the single best estimate. It is also of note that both the estimate of zinc retention and the required zinc intake from infant formula decreases with increasing birth weight, again making it difficult to estimate a reasonable range of intakes for the preterm infant.[14] Note that the zinc data for the preterm infant does not include data on enough infants to estimate values for a birth weight below 750 g (Table 8.3)

For a given individual preterm infant, it is obvious that both the requirement for zinc retention as well as the range of intake required to achieve this retention has a tremendous variation (Table 8.3), but both decrease with increasing weight and increasing postconceptional age. This can be shown for many micronutrients including protein.

SUMMARY

This chapter began with a discussion of the DRIs and how the present determination of these is very difficult for the preterm infant at this time. There was considerable discussion regarding the "RRI," yet the subsequent discussion of the factorial and empirical determinations generally resulted in a single nutrient value, not a recommended range of intakes. The paucity of fetuses used to determine the body composition of the reference fetus (n = 22) hardly lends itself to the discussion of a recommended range of intakes using this method. The empirical method has largely been limited to the determination of the requirement for protein intake. As discussed, many factors affect the determination of the required nutrient intake regardless of whether the factorial or empirical method is used. This includes the variable requirement for growth, absorption, metabolism, and transport of nutrients, as well as nutrient losses (dermal, urinary, and intestinal), deposition, and interaction with other nutrients (e.g., zinc and iron). Published consensus statements generally include a range of intakes as determined by a panel of experts using the observational and limited randomized studies published in the literature.[8] These contain a range of intakes as shown in Table 8.4.

Perhaps one could consider an "individualized" empirical approach to assess adequate nutrient intake in the NICU. That is, assuming a preterm infant is appropriately

TABLE 8.4

Recommended Dietary Intakes (Enteral) for Growing Preterm Infants in Stable Clinical Condition Recommended by Expert Panel

	Consensus Recommendations <1000g	Consensus Recommendations 1000–1500g
Energy, kcal/kg/d	130–150	110–130
Protein, g/kg/d	3.8–4.4	3.4–4.2
Calcium mg/kg/d	100–220	100–220
Phosphorus, mg/kg/d	60–140	60–140
Magnesium, mg/kg/d	7.9–15	7.9–15
Sodium, mg/kg/d	69–115	69–115
Potassium, mg/kg/d	78–117	78–117
Chloride, mg/kg/d	107–249	107–249

** See reference 8

grown at birth and a birth percentile has been established and the goal is to maintain the infant on this percentile while in the NICU, monitoring daily weight and weekly assessments of length and occipitofrontal circumference (OFC) could determine what the protein intake should be. Unfortunately, there are no readily available practical measures of body composition that would be needed in the ideal situation, but it is possible that the BMI curve could be used as a proxy for body composition. These curves are presently being developed for the NICU.[11] Traditionally, NICUs have not measured growth in length as an assessment of growth and this needs to changed especially if weight relative to length is to be accurately determined. Use of electronic medical records easily tracks measures of growth against intakes of various nutrients including protein and energy. Intakes can be varied relatively easily with parenteral nutrition (less so with infant formula) without increasing or decreasing total energy, as the needs for other nutrients change. Human milk can now be analyzed and the protein and caloric content can be adjusted with fortifiers (see Chapter 11). However, there are no vitamin solutions that can be varied in TPN to satisfactorily meet the needs of all preterm infants.

CONCLUSIONS

In conclusion, although most current dietary intake recommendations for preterm infants utilize mostly a range of intakes determined by a panel of experts, they are best guesses.[3,8] More research and clinical studies are needed, including the development of appropriate biomarkers, to assess the nutrient requirements of preterm infants.

REFERENCES

1. Dietary Reference Intakes. In: *Dietary Reference Intakes for Calcium, Phosphorus, Magnesium, Vitamin D and Fluoride.* Institute of Medicine, National Academy Press, Washington, DC; 1997: 21–37

2. Uauy R, Tsang R, Koletzko B, Zlotkin SH. Concepts, definition and approaches to define nutritional needs of LBW infants. In: Tsang RC, Uauy R, Koletzko B, Zlotkin SH, Eds. *Nutrition of the Preterm Infant.* Digital Educational Publishing, Inc, Cincinnati, Ohio; 2005: 1–21

3. Kleinman RE, Greer FR, Eds. Nutritional needs of the preterm infant. In: *Pediatrics Nutrition,* 7th ed., American Academy of Pediatrics, Elk Grove Village, IL; 2013. pp 83–121.

4. Ziegler EE. Meeting the nutritional needs of the low-birth-weight infant. *Ann Nutr Metab.* 2011;58(suppl 1):8–18.

5. Sparks JW. Human intrauterine growth and nutrient accretion. *Seminars in Perinatology.* 1984;9(2):74–93

6. Ziegler EE, O'Donnel AM, Nelson SE, Fomon SJ. Body composition of the reference fetus. *Growth.* 1976;40:329–341.

7. Ziegler EE. Nutrient requirements of premature infants. In: Cooke RJ, Vandenplas Y, Wahn U, Eds. Nutrition support for infants and children at risk. *Nestle Nutr Workshop Ser Pediatr Program.* 2007;59:161–176.

8. Tsang RC, Uauy R, Koletzko B, Zlotkin SH. *Nutrition of the Preterm Infant.* Appendix #3 Summary of reasonable nutrient intakes for preterm infants. Digital Educational Publishing, Inc, Cincinnati, Ohio; 2005:415-416.

9. Kashyap S, Schulze KF, Forsyth M, Zucker C, Dell RB, Ramakrishnan R, Heird WC. Growth, nutrient retention, and metabolic response in low birth weight infants fed varying intakes of protein and energy. *J Pediatr* 1988;113:713–721.

10. Polberger SKT, Axelson IA, Raiha NCE. Growth of very low birth weight infants on varying amounts of human milk protein. *Pediatr Res* 1989;25:414–419.

11. Olsen I, Clark R et al. Pediatrix database personal communication.

12. Kleinman RE, Greer FR, Eds. Trace elements. In: *Pediatric Nutrition*, 7th ed., American Academy of Pediatrics, Elk Grove Village, IL, 2013. pp 463–484.

13. Bhatia J, Griffin I, Anderson D, Kler N, Domellof M. Selected macro/micronutrient needs for the routine preterm infant. *J Pediatr* 2013:161:S48–55.

14. Klein CL, Ed. Nutrient requirements for preterm infant formulas. *J Nutr* 2002;132:1478S–1482S.

9 Meeting Nutritional Goals
Computer-Aided Prescribing of Enteral and Parenteral Nutrition

Magnus Domellöf and Dirk Wackernagel

INTRODUCTION

Many patients in neonatal intensive care units (NICUs) are at high risk of malnutrition and poor growth. The majority of patients at risk of malnutrition are preterm infants, but other groups are also at risk including patients with cardiac failure, severe gastrointestinal disease, hepatic disorders, and those who have undergone abdominal surgery.

Recommendations for enteral and parenteral nutrient intakes of preterm and term infants are available[1,2] and the reason for malnutrition of NICU patients is often non-compliance with these guidelines.[3] Since calculation of enteral and parenteral nutrient intakes is complicated and time-consuming in the clinical setting, there is a need for improved tools to aid neonatologists in prescribing enteral and parenteral nutrition and to reduce errors in order to optimize growth, development, and later health of NICU patients.

NUTRITION AND GROWTH OF SMALL, PRETERM INFANTS

A number of studies from different countries during the last decade have shown that nutrition and growth of very low birth weight (VLBW) infants is suboptimal. A population-based study has been performed of all extremely preterm infants (<27 weeks) born between 2004 and 2007 in Sweden (the EXPRESS-study) showing a high 1-year survival rate: 70% of liveborns.[4] We have assessed nutrient intakes and growth in the same cohort, including all 531 infants alive at 24 hours after birth.[5] Mean gestational age of these infants was 25.3 weeks (SD 1.1) and mean birth weight was 765 g (SD 170).

The clinical routine at Swedish hospitals during this time period was to initiate parenteral nutrition and minimal enteral feeds on the first day of life and then increase enteral feeds as tolerated. The average proportion of enteral intake in relation to total fluid intake increased from 28% during the first week to 69% on Days 8 to 28 and to

94% on Days 29 to 70 of life, implicating that most of these infants received a combination of enteral and parenteral nutrition during the first 28 days of life.

The mean energy intake of these infants was 66 kcal/kg/d during the first week of life, 114 kcal/kg/d at Days 8 to 28 and 132 kcal/kg/d at Days 29 to 70 of life. Mean protein intake during the first week of life was 2.1 g/kg/d and 3.3 g/kg/d at Days 8 to 28 and 29 to 70 of life. These intakes were considerably below recommended intakes, which are 130 to 150 kcal/kg/day and 3.8 to 4.4 g/kg/d, respectively, for growing, enterally fed preterms with birth weights below 1000 g.[1]

During the first 4 weeks of life, mean standard deviation scores (Z-scores) for weight, length, and head circumference (HC) decreased by 2.1, 2.6, and 1.4, respectively, as assessed using a Swedish growth reference.[6]

Taking gestational age, baseline anthropometrics, CRIB score, duration of mechanical ventilation, and postnatal steroid and antibiotic treatments into account, lower energy intake correlated with less gain in weight (r = +0.315, p < 0.001), length (r = +0.215, p < 0.001), and HC (r = +0.218, p < 0.001). In addition, lower protein intake also predicted poor growth in all anthropometric measures, and low fat intake was associated with slower HC growth.

In conclusion, extremely preterm infants born from 2004 to 2007 in Sweden received lower energy and protein intakes than recommended and showed suboptimal postnatal growth. Nutrient intakes were independent predictors of growth even when considering disease-related factors such as mechanical ventilation and postnatal corticosteroid therapy. This implies that optimized nutrition may improve growth and possibly also development and later health of extremely preterm infants.

AVAILABLE COMPUTERIZED SUPPORT
FOR NICU NUTRITION PRESCRIPTIONS

It has been estimated that 750,000 neonatal parentenal nutrition (PN) orders are prescribed each year in the United States.[7] Calculations of TPN composition are time consuming and fraught with the possibility of error.

One approach to simplifying the ordering of parenteral nutrition is to use a small number of stock solutions, rather than developing an individualized solution for each infant. However, individualizing parenteral nutrition composition in order to meet standard goals for nutrient intake may lead to higher amino acid intakes and higher micromineral intakes than standardized use of stock PN solutions.[8] For example, mean daily protein intakes increased from 1.36 g/kg/d to 1.94 g/kg/d.[8] Although both intakes are disappointing, protein intakes (as well as calcium and phosphate intakes) were higher with individualized PN compositions.[8] Another option is to use standard solutions in a flexible way, allowing for daily individualization, which has been shown to result in adequate nutrition and growth.[9] However, this also requires daily calculations of nutrient intakes.

So, how are we to safely achieve customization of PN in a busy NICU when time is limited? Computers have been used to assist in this process for over 30 years,[10, 11] dating back to the era of programmable calculators[12] and the BASIC programming language.[13] A number of older systems for parenteral nutrition have been described, beginning at the dawn of the home computer revolution.[10, 11, 13–15] Reported benefits of computer-supported prescribing of PN include reduced time required,[11] improved metabolic control,[14] and improved growth measures such as reduced early weight loss[14] and higher weight gain.[16]

In recent years, systems that are more sophisticated have been described, all concentrating on the prescription of PN, and many focused on the NICU population. Homegrown calculation spreadsheets are widely used for prescription of total parenteral nutrition in NICUs.[7] Simple, free, web-based calculators are also available. Results of these newer tools are encouraging.

Although some computer-supported systems shift some of the time burden of PN ordering from the physician to the pharmacist,[17] the total time spent on preparation of the PN order is significantly reduced by computer-supported systems,[18] maybe by as much as two-thirds.[17]

Such systems also led to reduced errors,[7, 19,22] as well as to better intakes of protein,[18–20] energy,[18–20] calcium[18,19,22] and phosphate,[18, 19] and more rapid achievement of protein and energy intake goals.[18] In one study, a computer-supported system improved protein intakes during the first week of life, and lipid, glucose, and energy intakes of the first two weeks of life. Over the entire 4-week study period, parenteral energy intakes were higher (118 ± 6 kcal/kg/d vs. 106 ± 12) but parenteral protein intakes were similar (3.7 ± 0.3 vs. 3.5 ± 0.3).[20]

Computer-supported systems also led to improved biochemistry (e.g., a lower alkaline phosphatase concentration)[18] and reduced the risk of osteopenia.[22]

They have also led to improved weight gain,[19, 20] and perhaps to earlier hospital discharge.[19] In one example, preterm infants receiving PN using a computer-supported system *gained* weight on PN (+44 g SD 114), while those in whom PN was prescribed by physicians without computer support lost 53 g (SD 156) while on PN.[19]

As PN ordering requires more mathematical calculations, it is unsurprising that computer-supported systems have first addressed the prescribing of parenteral nutrition. However, preterm infants receive enteral nutrition for much longer than they receive parenteral nutrition, and in-hospital growth continues to falter at a time when most preterm infants would be expected to be receiving all, or almost all, of their nutrient intake enterally.[21]

Only a few of these calculators have included enteral nutrition[20] and these have not considered different sources of breast milk (own mother's or donor milk), breast milk fortifiers, and enteral supplements. A disadvantage with most computer-supported nutrition systems is therefore that they fail to correctly account for enteral intakes, as they do not consider enteral nutrition at all. This is a potentially critical limitation, especially as it is increasingly recommended that enteral nutrition be initiated on the first day of life. Furthermore, the risk period for malnutrition in extremely preterm infants extends throughout the entire hospitalization, not just the period of parenteral nutrition administration. For example, the NICHD dataset of Ehrenkranz[21] shows that preterm infants continue to diverge from the intrauterine growth curves even at 36 weeks post-menstrual age, an age by which most infants would be entirely on enteral nutrition (see also Figure 12.11, Chapter 12). Any system that does not include enteral nutrition will overlook a large time period in which infants receive the majority of their nutrition via the enteral route, and remain at high risk of *ex utero* growth restriction (EUGR).

This is the first study we are aware of that describes the effects of a computer-supported nutritional ordering system that was specifically designed to include all aspects of both parenteral and enteral nutrition.

DEVELOPMENT OF A NEW SYSTEM FOR COMPUTER-AIDED NICU NUTRITION (NUTRIUM™)

Prompted by the poor nutritional situation among Swedish VLBW infants, the practical difficulties in performing individual, daily, manual nutrition calculations, and the absence of a freely or commercially available system that would consider both enteral and parenteral nutrition, we developed a new system for computer-aided NICU nutritional prescribing.

The system was developed in 2005–2007 using Java Web Start (Oracle Corporation, Redwood City, California). Since 2007, the system (called Nutrium) has been commercially available and is currently being used in routine care at 12 Swedish NICUs. The functionality has been continuously improved. Up to now, more than 60,000 nutrition calculations have been performed using the system. Very few of these have been calculations of total parenteral nutrition alone; many have been a combination of enteral and parenteral nutrition and many have also concerned only enteral nutrition.

The home screen of the Nutrium system is a patient list including all current patients at the local neonatal unit. All data pertaining to previously discharged patients is also available and can easily be exported in spreadsheet format for quality control or research purposes.

The system contains extensive data on more than 30 nutrients, more than 200 nutritional products (Table 9.1) and their nutrient contents, several alternative nutrient references, and several alternative growth references. The system allows mixes of products including individual PN prescriptions as well as standard PN mixes. The system also supports breast milk macronutrient analyses, which are routinely used in Sweden. Furthermore, Nutrium saves data on growth and nutrition for each patient and presents growth charts, nutrition charts for individual patients, and statistics for groups of patients for quality improvement and research purposes.

THE NUTRIUM GRAPHICAL USER INTERFACE

In addition to the advanced calculation algorithms and the extensive built-in databases, an appreciated feature of the Nutrium system is the modern graphical user interface. To perform a prescription, the user enters the planned intakes of enteral and parenteral nutrition products and other fluids, chosen from menus or based on the intakes of the previous day. The system has a graphical interface that gives the user an immediate, visual feedback on how the current prescription conforms to recommended intakes for 31 nutrients (Figure 9.1). A traffic light system of colors is used, so a red bar to the left means "much lower than the recommended intake," a yellow bar to the left means "slightly below the recommended intake," and a green

TABLE 9.1

Categories of Nutritional Products Included in the Nutrium™ Database

Type of Product	Number
Enteral products	
Breast milk categories	7
Infant formulas	4
Preterm formulas	7
Special formulas	14
Other enteral food products	2
Breast milk fortifiers	13
Vitamin supplements	19
Mineral supplements	20
Other enteral supplements	4
Total	90
Parenteral products	
Commercial PN products	28
Local PN products	64
Salt/colloid/flush solutions	10
Parenteral additives	16
Blood products	5
Drug infusions	5
Total	128

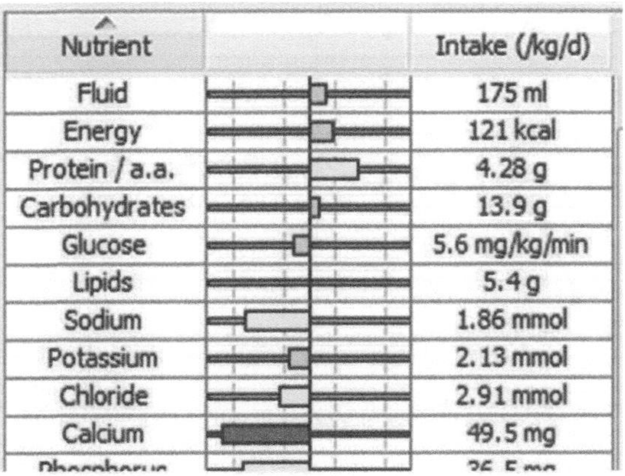

Nutrient		Intake (/kg/d)
Fluid		175 ml
Energy		121 kcal
Protein / a.a.		4.28 g
Carbohydrates		13.9 g
Glucose		5.6 mg/kg/min
Lipids		5.4 g
Sodium		1.86 mmol
Potassium		2.13 mmol
Chloride		2.91 mmol
Calcium		49.5 mg
Phosphorus		26.5 mg

FIGURE 9.1 Detail from the prescription screen in Nutrium, showing the nutrient intakes resulting from the current prescription and indicating how this compares to recommended intakes. As the prescribed intake deviates further from the recommended intake, the slider bar changes color from green, to yellow, to red. The example is from a combined enteral and parenteral nutrition prescription. (Nutrium and all screen images associated with it are copyright of the authors, all rights reserved. Screen image is copyright of the authors, and is used with permission.)

bar signifies that the intake is within the recommended range. Similarly, bars to the right signify intakes above the recommended intake. The ranges are calculated individually, based on the infant's gestational age at birth, postnatal age, current weight, and the proportion of enteral to parenteral intake for each nutrient. Based on the visual feedback, the user can change the prescription and this will have an immediate effect on the colored bars. The user can also invoke a decision support function in which the system gives suggestions of how to optimize the current nutrition in order to better conform to recommended intakes. There are also safety limits of composition of parenteral solutions to prevent precipitation and limits on enteral fortifiers and supplements to prevent intestinal complications.

In addition to regular growth charts and Z-score growth charts, the system also presents "nutrition charts" showing intakes of different nutrients over time, compared to recommended intakes (Figure 9.2). These charts have proved to be very informative and make it possible to identify infants who may be developing accumulated nutrient deficiencies due to suboptimal intakes for an extended period.

EVALUATION OF THE NUTRIUM SYSTEM

In 2009, we conducted a study to evaluate the effect of computer-aided prescription of enteral and parenteral nutrition on the growth of preterm infants, using the Nutrium system on a daily basis. Our aim was to achieve the nutrition recommendations issued by the ESPGHAN[2] and Tsang.[1] We intended to test the hypotheses that the computer-aided prescription would lead to increased nutrient intakes and improved postnatal growth in preterm infants. The study was performed at a Swedish level II NICU (Eskilstuna Hospital) in the Södermanland province of Sweden. The inclusion criteria was infants born before the gestational age of 32 weeks. The study

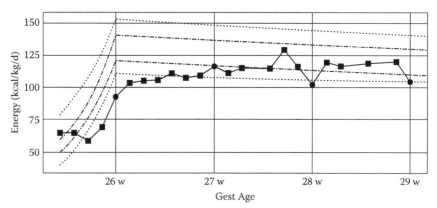

FIGURE 9.2 Nutrition chart from Nutrium, in this case showing energy intake over time in an infant born at a gestation age of 25 weeks + 3 days. Dotted lines show recommended energy intake (corresponding to the color zones of the prescription screen). In this case, the infant received less than recommended energy intakes during the first 1 to 2 weeks of life. (Nutrium and all screen images associated with it are copyright of the authors, all rights reserved. Screen image is copyright of the authors, and is used with permission.)

was designed as a comparison of nutrition and growth before and after the start of using the computer-aided prescription system for all enteral and parenteral nutrition. Retrospectively, we evaluated all infants born < 32 gestational weeks treated at the Eskilstuna NICU from January 2008 to December 2010, divided in two groups: The control group ("control"), born before June 2009, and the intervention group ("Nutrium"), born after June 2009 when the Nutrium system was introduced. Included in the study were 78 infants: 35 infants in the control group and 43 infants in the Nutrium group.

Mean (±SD) birth weight in the Nutrium and control groups were 1413.8 (±431.5) g and 1281.4 (±419.2; P = 0.17), gestational ages were 29.9 (±1.7) weeks and 29.5 (±2.0) weeks, respectively (P = 0.35). Infant clinical characteristics were not significantly different between groups.

We retrospectively collected the daily intake of macro- and micronutrients for all children in both groups during the first 7 weeks of life. During the first postnatal week, the intake of all macronutrients and the total energy intake were significantly higher in the Nutrium group (Table 9.2). During weeks 2 to 7, the daily intake of amino acids, carbohydrates, and total amount of calories were significantly higher in the Nutrium group, while the fat intake was not significantly different between groups. There was also an increased intake of fluid in the Nutrium group during the first week of life (Figure 9.3), which was due to the lack of highly concentrated parenteral nutrition solutions at the study hospital during this period.

Intakes of several minerals (potassium, calcium, phosphorus, magnesium, zinc, selenium, and copper) and vitamins were significantly closer to recommendations in the Nutrium group (data not shown).

We compared growth parameters at the time of birth, and at day 28 of life, at a post-menstrual age of 36 weeks and at the time of discharge from hospital (Figure 9.4), using a Swedish growth reference.[6] At birth, no significant differences were observed between the groups in patient characteristics or anthropometric measures (weight, length, and HC). From birth to 28 days, the mean weight SDS decreased in both groups but less so in the Nutrium group. At 28 days of life, the mean weight in the Nutrium group was 0.8 SDS higher than in the control group (p = 0.04) and this difference increased at the time of discharge to 0.9 SDS (p = 0.004).

There were even more pronounced differences in length, where the mean SDS dropped in control infants from –1.8 at birth to –3.0 SDS at 28 days of life and did not recover into normal values at the time of discharge (–2.7 SDS). The mean length SDS

TABLE 9.2

Macronutrient Intakes during the First Week of Life (mean ±SD)

Nutrient	Control	Nutrium (Tm)	P-Value
Fluid (mls/kg/d)	120 ±40	146 ±37	p < 0.001
Energy (kcal/kg/d)	70.4 ±30.4	88.7 ±29.1	p < 0.001
Amino Acids (g/kg/d)	1.66 ±1.00	2.95 ±1.03	p < 0.001
Carbohydrates (g/kg/d)	9.2 ±2.8	10.7 ±2.6	p < 0.001
Fat (g/kg/d)	2.84 ±1.96	3.60 ±1.79	p < 0.001

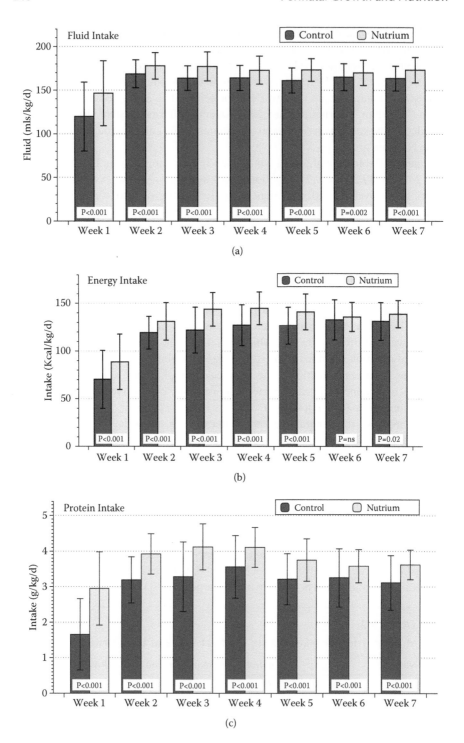

FIGURE 9.3 The intake of fluid, energy, and macronutrients in the control and Nutrium groups.

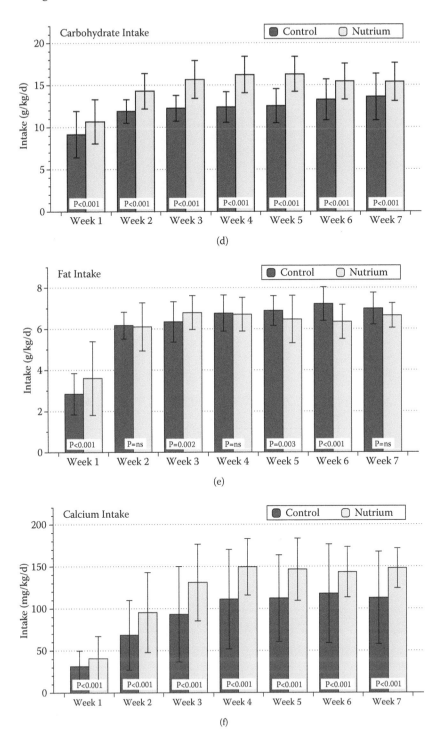

FIGURE 9.3 The intake of fluid, energy, and macronutrients in the control and Nutrium groups.

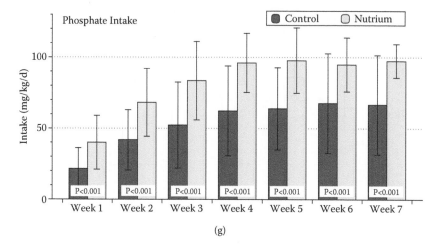

(g)

FIGURE 9.3 (CONTINUED) The intake of fluid, energy, and macronutrients in the control and Nutrium groups.

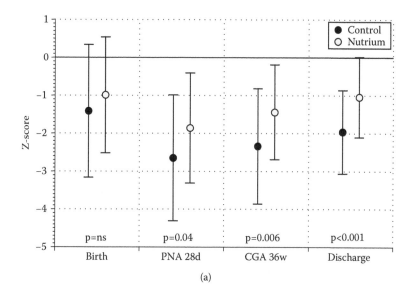

(a)

FIGURE 9.4 Body weight, length, and head circumference in control and Nutrium groups at the time of birth, at 28 days postnatal age, at 36 weeks corrected gestational age (post-menstrual age), and at discharge from the hospital. *(continued)*

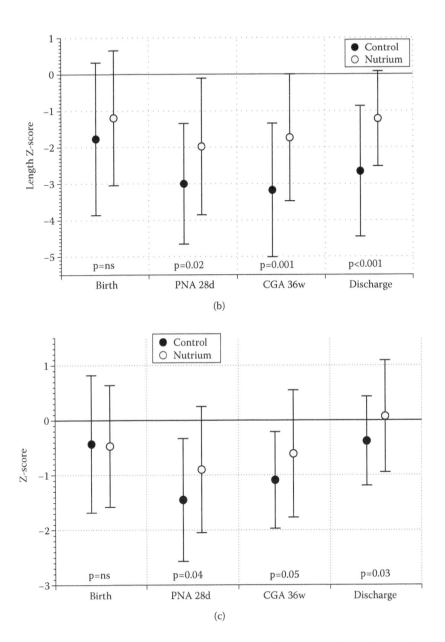

(b)

(c)

FIGURE 9.4 (CONTINUED) Body weight, length, and head circumference in control and Nutrium groups at the time of birth, at 28 days postnatal age, at 36 weeks corrected gestational age (post-menstrual age), and at discharge from the hospital.

in the Nutrium infants decreased from –1.2 SDS at birth to a minimum of –2.0 SDS at 28 days of life before recovering to –1.2 SDS at the time of discharge.

In control infants, the mean HC SDS decreased from –0.4 SDS to –1.4 SDS between birth and 28 days of age, before recovering to –0.4 SDS at discharge. In contrast, in the Nutrium group, mean SDS for HC showed a minimal drop of 0.4 SDS at day 28 of life and ultimately increased from birth (–0.5 SDS) to discharge (+0.1 SDS) (Figure 9.4).

CONCLUSION

Computer-aided prescription of enteral and parenteral nutrition reduces errors and, in NICUs where nutrition is not already optimized, use of such a system has been shown to result in improved intakes of macro- and micronutrients and improved growth (weight, length, and HC) in preterm infants. This is most likely due to improved compliance to recommended nutritional intakes.

Modern systems for computer-aided nutrition with a graphical and interactive user interface, such as the Nutrium system, are easy to use, save time, and our experience is that they increase interest and awareness of nutritional issues and improve knowledge about neonatal nutrition among neonatologists, dieticians, and neonatal nurses. These systems are also useful for plotting growth and nutrient intakes over time in individual patients or groups of patients and the data can easily be used for quality improvement and research purposes.

REFERENCES

1. Tsang RC, Uauy R, Koletzko B, Zlotkin S. *Nutritional Needs of the Preterm Infant. Scientific Basis and Practical Guidelines.* 2nd ed: Williams & Wilkins, 2005.
2. Agostoni C, Buonocore G, Carnielli VP, De Curtis M, Darmaun D, Decsi T, et al. Enteral nutrient supply for preterm infants: commentary from the European Society of Paediatric Gastroenterology, Hepatology and Nutrition Committee on Nutrition. *J Pediatr Gastroenterol Nutr* 2010;50(1):85–91.
3. Embleton NE, Pang N, Cooke RJ. Postnatal malnutrition and growth retardation: an inevitable consequence of current recommendations in preterm infants? *Pediatrics* 2001;107(2):270–3.
4. Fellman V, Hellstrom-Westas L, Norman M, Westgren M, Kallen K, Lagercrantz H, et al. One-year survival of extremely preterm infants after active perinatal care in Sweden. *JAMA* 2009;301(21):2225–33.
5. Stoltz Sjöström E, Ohlund I, Ahlsson F, Engström E, Fellman V,Hellström A, Köllön K, Norman M, Olhager E, Serenius F, Domellöf M. Nutrient intakes independently affect growth in extremely preterm infants: results from a population-based study. *Acta Paediatr.* 2013;102(11):1067–74.
6. Niklasson A, Albertsson-Wikland K. Continuous growth reference from 24th week of gestation to 24 months by gender. *BMC Pediatr* 2008;8:8.
7. Costakos DT. Of lobsters, electronic medical records, and neonatal total parenteral nutrition. *Pediatrics* 2006;117:e328–32.
8. Yeung MY, Smyth JP, Maheshwari R, Shah S. Evaluation of standardized versus individualized total parenteral nutrition regime for neonates less than 33 weeks gestation. *J Paediatr Child Health* 2003;39(8):613–7.

9. Senterre T, Rigo J. Reduction in postnatal cumulative nutritional deficit and improvement of growth in extremely preterm infants. *Acta Paediatr* 2012;101(2):e64–70.

10. Ball PA, Candy DC, Puntis JW, McNeish AS. Portable bedside microcomputer system for management of parenteral nutrition in all age groups. *Archives of Disease in Childhood* 1985;60(5):435–9.

11. Ball PA, De Silva DG, Candy DC, McNeish AS. The microcomputer: an aid to paediatric parenteral nutrition. *Intl J Clin Monit Comput* 1985;1(4):233–9.

12. Feldman MJ, Kizka DP. The use of a hand-held programmable calculator in performing neonatal parenteral nutrition solution calculations. *Drug Intel Clin Pharm* 1981;15(1):54–5.

13. Harper RG, Carrera E, Weiss S, Luongo M. A complete computerized program for nutritional management in the neonatal intensive care nursery. *Am J Perinatol* 1985;2(2):161–2.

14. Giacoia GP, Chopra R. The use of a computer in parenteral alimentation of low birth weight infants. *JPEN.* 1981;5(4):328–31.

15. Yamamoto LG, Gainsley GJ, Witek JE. Pediatric parenteral nutrition management using a comprehensive user-friendly computer program designed for personal computers. *JPEN.* 1986;10(5):535–9.

16. Dice JE, Burckart GJ, Woo JT, Helms RA. Standardized versus pharmacist-monitored individualized parenteral nutrition in low-birth-weight infants. *Am J. Hospital Pharm* 1981;38(10):1487–9.

17. Skouroliakou M, Konstantinou D, Papasarantopoulos P, Matthaiou C. Computer assisted total parenteral nutrition for pre-term and sick term neonates. *PWS* 2005;27(4):305–10.

18. Puangco MA, Nguyen HL, Sheridan MJ. Computerized PN ordering optimizes timely nutrition therapy in a neonatal intensive care unit. *J Am Dietetic Assoc* 1997;97(3):258–61.

19. Skouroliakou M, Koutri K, Stathopoulou M, Vourvouhaki E, Giannopoulou I, Gounaris A. Comparison of two types of TPN prescription methods in preterm neonates. *Pharm World Sci* 2009;31(2):202–8.

20. Eleni-dit-Trolli S, Kermorvant-Duchemin E, Huon C, Mokthari M, Husseini K, Brunet ML, et al. Early individualised parenteral nutrition for preterm infants. *Arch Dis Child Fetal Neonatal Ed* 2009;94(2):F152–3.

21. Ehrenkranz RA, Younes N, Lemons JA, Fanaroff AA, Donovan EF, Wright LL, et al. Longitudinal growth of hospitalized very low birth weight infants. *Pediatrics* 1999;104(2 Pt 1):280–9.

22. Mackay MW, Cash J, Farr F, Holley M, Jones K, Boehme S. Improving pediatric outcomes through intravenous and oral medication standardization. *J Pediatr Pharmacol Ther* 2009;14(4):226–35.

10 Customize or Generalize? Or the Imperfect Art of Fortifying Human Milk

Ekhard E. Ziegler

INTRODUCTION

It is generally agreed that human milk is the preferred feeding for preterm infants because of its many protective and other beneficial effects. It is also widely appreciated that the nutrients provided by human milk do not meet the high needs of preterm infants.[1,2] Nutrient supplementation (fortification) of human milk is therefore necessary. Fortification raises the concentration of specific nutrients to levels where infant needs are met whenever energy needs are satisfied. Fortification also increases the caloric density of milk.

The fundamental problem with the provision of adequate nutrient intakes for preterm infants is that the nutrient content of expressed milk is variable and hence not known to the caretaker. Although the content of all nutrients varies, variation of the protein content is what matters the most and poses the most problems in clinical practice. This is so because the needs for protein must be met at all times and because at the same time excessive intakes of protein may pose hazards to the infant and need to be avoided. At the time fortifiers were designed, safety was the overriding concern. The low protein content of most of today's fortifiers reflects the then dominant concern about the hazards of excessive protein intakes. Protein levels were therefore chosen that ensured that total protein intakes would never be excessively high, even when milk protein content happened to be high.

In broad terms, approaches to the fortification of human milk fall into two groups that differ with regard to the degree with which they rely on feedback from the infant. Generalizing methods use standard amounts of fortifiers and do not use feedback from the infant, whereas customizing approaches regularly utilize feedback from the infant or the mother with the aim of achieving a close match between protein intakes and needs. All fortification schemes provide satisfactory intakes of most specific nutrients.

255

1. Generalizing methods use standard (fixed) amounts of fortifier (powder or liquid) that are added to expressed milk. Modifications of this basic method are sometimes used with the aim of providing higher intakes of protein.
2. Customizing methods have been developed with the aim of achieving better matches between needs for and intakes of protein than the basic generalizing approaches provide. One of the customizing approaches, adjustable fortification,[3] uses the metabolic response of the infant to guide the addition of additional protein in the form of fortifier and modular protein. Another customizing approach, targeted fortification,[4] utilizes analysis of expressed milk to guide fortification to predetermined nutrient levels.

The two methods overlap somewhat in practice. Practitioners of generalized fortification will sometimes respond to feedback from the infant, such as poor growth, with an increase in protein content by adding modular protein or more than standard amounts of powder fortifier (superfortification).

FEEDING THE PREMATURE INFANT

NUTRIENT REQUIREMENTS

Our knowledge of nutrient requirements of preterm infants is fraught with uncertainties and limitations. Estimates of average requirements are derived from fetal body composition by the factorial method. These estimates inform us about nutrient intakes that are necessary if the preterm infant is to grow like the fetus. Fetal body composition has been derived from chemical analysis of a limited number of fetuses.[5] No information is available regarding variation of nutrient needs and we are left with estimates of average nutrient needs[6] without knowledge of the range of nutrient requirements within the population of very low birth weight (VLBW) infants. Because there is considerable evidence that inadequate intakes of protein lead to impaired neurodevelopment, protein requirements would ideally be defined as intakes that preserve normal neurodevelopment. Unfortunately, requirements cannot (yet) be defined in these terms and we are left with estimates of average needs that are largely based on fetal growth. Current best estimates of requirements for protein and energy are summarized in Table 10.1. It should be pointed out that needs for protein decrease with increasing size of the infant, whereas needs for energy increase. Empirical methods have yielded somewhat lower estimates of protein needs[7] than the factorial method. Also, alternative methods of estimating energy needs[8] have produced somewhat lower estimates than the factorial method. Values in Table 10.1 reflect in part these lower estimates. Needs for many other nutrients are indicated in Table 10.2.

NUTRIENT COMPOSITION OF HUMAN MILK

This is a short summary of facts about human milk composition that are relevant to the delivery of effective nutritional support to the preterm infant.

TABLE 10.1

Requirements of Protein and Energy Derived by the Factorial Method

	Body Weight (g)			
	500–1000	1000–1500	1500–2200	2200–3000
Fetal Weight Gain				
(g/d)	14.3	21.7	30.4	34.8
(g/kg/d)	19.0	17.4	16.4	13.4
Protein Needs (g/kg/d)				
Inevitable loss	1.0	1.0	1.0	1.0
Growth (accretion)	2.5	2.4	2.2	2.0
Required Protein Intake (g/kg/d)				
Parenteral[a]	3.5	3.4	3.2	3.0
Enteral[b]	4.0	3.9	3.7	3.4
Energy Needs (kcal/kg/d)				
Energy expenditure	61	66	70	73
Growth (accretion)	31	34	37	40
Required Energy Intake (kcal/kg/d)				
Parenteral[a]	92	100	107	113
Enteral[b]	106	115	123	130
Protein/Energy (g/100 kcal)				
Enteral and parenteral	3.8	3.4	3.0	2.6

[a] Sum of inevitable losses and needs for growth.

[b] Accounting for incomplete enteral absorption.

1. Amounts of all specific nutrients provided by human milk are inadequate to meet the needs of premature infants.
2. Although milk of mothers of premature infants has higher content of protein and certain minerals than milk of term mothers,[9] nutrients are still insufficient to meet VLBW infants' needs.
3. The protein content of milk decreases markedly with the duration of lactation. Whereas 7 days postpartum the mean protein concentration is 1.7 g/dl, it decreases rapidly and reaches a steady level of 1.2 g/dl ml after about 4 weeks.[10] Zinc also decreases during the early weeks of lactation. Shortfalls of these two nutrients therefore become more likely with time from birth.
4. Expressed mother's milk is highly variable in protein and energy content. More importantly, protein and energy content are not known to the caretaker (unless milk is analyzed). Bedside methods for analyzing milk are available; however, the proper use of these methods is not yet known.

TABLE 10.2

Typical Composition of Human Milk (HM) without and with Fortification, and Nutrient Requirements of Infants Weighing Less Than 1000 g

	HM (per dl)[a]	Fortified HM (per dl)[b]	Fortified HM (per 100 kcal)	Requirement (per 100 kcal)[c]
Energy (kcal)	68	80	•	•
Protein (g)	1.2	2.2	2.75	3.8
Calcium (mg)	25	125	156	170
Phosphate (mg)	15	75	94	116
Magnesium (mg)	3.3	5.3	6.6	6.4
Sodium (mmol)	1.2	1.9	2.4	3.0
Potassium (mmol)	1.3	2.1	2.6	2.2
Chloride (mmol)	1.7	2.3	2.9	2.6
Iron (mg)	0.1	1.5	1.9	1.85
Zinc (mg)	0.37	1.22	1.5	1.4
Copper (mcg)	38	82	102	111

[a] Typical composition at about 4 weeks of lactation.
[b] Powder fortifier with iron.
[c] Infant weighing <1000 g.

5. Donor milk is more constant in composition than mother's milk due to the fact that milk from multiple donors is pooled. With a typical protein content of 0.9 g/dl, fat at 4.0 g/dl, and caloric density at about 66 kcal/dl,[21] its protein content is appreciably lower than that of the average mother's milk.

RECENT CHANGES IN ATTITUDES RELEVANT TO NUTRITION

Attitudes toward the provision of nutrition to VLBW infants have undergone changes in recent years, which in the aggregate have had a noticeable impact on the delivery of nutritional support and have led to improved nutrient intakes.

1. Greater efforts to avoid growth failure and to meet nutrient needs are being made. Awareness of the widespread occurrence of postnatal growth failure and of its association with impaired neurodevelopment has increased since the publication of the report by Ehrenkranz et al. in 2006.[11] Once the primary cause of impaired growth was identified to be inadequate nutrient intakes,[12] the need for greater nutrient intakes was recognized. Higher nutrient intakes were achieved in part through greater willingness to accept risks thought to be attendant with higher levels of nutrient delivery.

2. Fear of protein has waned. The key obstacle to adequate protein intakes has for many years been the concern that "high" protein intakes must be avoided because they are dangerous. The details of the original study[13] are described next. As the protein intakes used in that study were no longer

known, what constituted a "high" protein intake could not be defined in quantitative terms. Thus, any protein intake that was higher than any other was deemed "high" and was considered dangerous. Given the variability of the protein content of human milk, the fear of protein dictated that fortifiers be sufficiently low in protein so that "high" protein intakes could not occur. This fear of protein seems to have subsided in recent years. For example, superfortification that some units have adopted in recent years is possible only with a low level of fear of protein.

3. Medical contraindications to nutrient provision, until the recent past, have curtailed delivery of nutritional support. For example, it used to be standard practice to withhold feedings during treatment for sepsis, whether proven or suspected. The lifting of this and similar proscriptions against feedings has had a positive impact on nutrient delivery.

APPROACHES TO FORTIFYING HUMAN MILK

STRATEGIES FOR HUMAN MILK FORTIFICATION

There is a certain hierarchy among nutrient requirements. For most nutrients, small deficits, especially if temporary, are of little consequence. In the case of protein and energy, on the other hand, if intakes are not adequate, growth cannot proceed at its normal rate and the infant is at risk of impaired neurodevelopment. A similar distinction applies to surfeit intakes. For most nutrients, modest surfeits are of little consequence, especially if they are temporary. However, in the case of protein, intakes exceeding requirements are considered hazardous, and in the case of energy, they are considered undesirable. These hierarchical distinctions have implications for strategies to meet nutritional needs. For most nutrients, the strategy can be to provide intakes that exceed by a modest margin the requirements, which are not known precisely in the first place. Not for protein. Excessively high intakes of protein are known to be hazardous for premature infants. This knowledge is based on the study of Goldman et al.[13] in which premature infants were fed formulas that provided either 3.0 to 3.6 g/kg/day or 6.0 to 7.2 g/kg/day of protein. Upon follow-up at 5 to 7 years of age, those with birth weight <1300 g who had received the high-protein formula showed a significantly increased incidence of low IQ scores. Similar data are unfortunately not available for intermediate levels of protein intake. The question as to where in this twofold range protein intakes become hazardous cannot be answered based on controlled trials. However, experience over recent years in the aggregate suggests that intakes greater than 3.6 g/kg/day, perhaps up to 4.5 g/kg/day, are very well tolerated and are safe in the short run.

As mentioned previously, in the past concerns about unduly high protein intakes have been strong and are responsible for the traditionally low protein content of fortifiers. The latter was the reason why customizing approaches to fortification have come into being. In recent years, awareness of the deleterious consequences of inadequate protein intakes has greatly increased. At the same time, confidence about the safety of moderately high protein intakes has also increased. This paradigm shift has led to a situation where it is now possible to aim for protein intakes that are adequate most of the time while being mildly excessive sometimes.

TIMING

Fortification of human milk is usually initiated when milk intake reaches 100 ml/kg/day, although earlier introduction would seem to be advantageous. In the study,[22] introduction at a feeding volume of 40 ml/kg/day was as well tolerated as introduction at 100 ml/kg/d. Parenteral nutrition is usually discontinued around the same time. Sometimes fortification is started at half strength and later advanced to full strength. The introduction of fortifier is often, but not always, accompanied by an increase in the size of gastric residuals or by the reappearance of gastric residuals.[14] Although this is often referred to as "intolerance," it simply is a manifestation of slower gastric emptying due to modest increases in osmolality of feeds brought about by the addition of fortifier.

FORTIFIERS

All fortifiers provide a source of energy (from carbohydrate and/or fat) that is designed to raise energy density from 67 to 80 kcal/dl. Protein is usually derived from bovine milk except for one liquid fortifier that derives protein from human milk. All fortifiers provide electrolytes, macrominerals, microminerals, and vitamins in amounts intended to augment the nutrient content of human milk to where it provides at least adequate amounts of all nutrients. As Table 10.2 shows, intakes of nutrients from fortified milk are in some cases a little shy of requirements, whereas in the case of most nutrients, intakes exceed requirements somewhat. There is considerable variation in nutrients provided by fortifiers, which is explained by the fact that the needs for many nutrients are not well understood. Some fortifiers provide selenium and iodine while others do not. Some fortifiers provide DHA and ARA.

The amount of protein provided by fortifiers varies greatly. Powder fortifiers add between 1.0 and 1.1 g per 100 ml of milk. Liquid fortifiers based on bovine protein increase protein concentration by 1.0 g/dl to 1.8 g/dl. The human milk based liquid fortifier (Prolacta Bioscience) increases protein concentration by between 0.92 g/dl and 2.3 g/dl depending on the ratio of fortifier to human milk.

GENERALIZING APPROACHES

The most widely used approach is the basic generalizing approach. It consists of the addition of a fortifier in standard amount regardless of the size or condition of the infant. This approach delivers most nutrients in amounts that meet or exceed the needs of the infant. The exception is protein. Powder fortifiers increase protein concentration by 1.0 to 1.1 g/dl, which is, as Table 10.2 shows, too little if milk protein content is 1.2 g/dl, which it typically is from 4 weeks on. Fortification by this and similar fortifiers leads to increased growth.[15] When actual intakes of protein achieved by the generalizing method have been determined, they were found to be considerably less than required intakes.[16, 17]

To achieve more adequate protein intakes, modifications of the basic approach are being used. One modification is the addition of modular protein in addition to standard multinutrient fortifier. Depending on the amount of protein added, this modification could achieve satisfactory intakes of protein. The protein powder requires exact weighing, which may be a reason why this method is not used widely. Another modification consists of the addition of greater than standard amounts of fortifier (superfortification). For example, six packets of powder fortifier may be used instead of the standard four packets. This achieves the desired greater protein intake, but at the expense of providing unnecessary high intakes of all other nutrients, including calcium and phosphorus. To safeguard against hypercalcemia, some units perform weekly determinations of serum calcium and phosphate in infants receiving superfortification. Finally, a third modification consists of the use of superfortification plus additional protein. This modification yields the highest protein addition and is sometimes used to fortify donor milk with its low protein content of 0.9 g/dl.

Some liquid fortifiers provide greater amounts of protein than powder fortifiers and other liquid fortifiers. One liquid fortifier adds (increases protein concentration by) 1.8 g/dl, an amount that is sufficient to raise protein intakes to satisfactory levels in almost all situations.[18] With this fortifier, when the protein content of milk is relatively high, the amount of protein delivered to the infant may exceed the required level of 3.8 g/100 kcal by some margin. Experience thus far indicates that such modest excesses of protein are inconsequential.[18] It is to be remembered that, due to the variability of milk protein content, high protein intakes are likely to occur only intermittently.

The advantage of generalizing approaches is their relative simplicity, including the absence of a need to measure fortifier powder. Because of that simplicity, generalizing approaches are assumed less prone to errors than other approaches.

Customizing Approaches

Customizing approaches fall into two categories: Approaches utilizing the metabolic response of the infant, and approaches based on analysis of milk with specific (targeted) addition of nutrients. An example of the former approach is the method described by Arslanoglu et al.[3] In this method, the amount of fortifier is increased as a first step, followed by additions of graded amounts of protein. Repeated determinations of blood urea nitrogen (BUN) are used to guide the stepwise increase of protein. This approach was shown to increase weight gain and head circumference gain and to increase BUN to a modest degree.[3] Protein intakes achieved with this method were later shown to approach requirement levels.[16] The use of BUN as feedback has the advantage that it provides assurance that protein intakes are not too high. It is not known how many NICUs are using the Arslanoglu approach, but the number is thought to be small. The biggest obstacle almost surely is that the additional fortifier and protein have to be measured precisely, a process that is cumbersome and susceptible to errors. The need for repeated BUN determinations may be another deterrent.

An example of the targeted fortification approach is that of Polberger et al.[4] In this approach, samples of milk are analyzed periodically, and protein and energy are added to expressed milk, in addition to fortifier, in amounts calculated to achieve adequate intakes. Improved growth is achieved by this method as protein intakes are brought to within approximately 10% of the target level of 3.5 g/kg/day.[4] Experience with more frequent milk analysis is limited. A recent report using analysis of 12-hour pools suggests that the method is feasible and practicable.[19] To date, there is no consensus regarding how frequently milk should be analyzed, nor whether pools or individual samples should be analyzed and fortified. Anecdotal reports indicate that bedside milk analyzers similar to the one used by Rochow et al.[19] are being used in some neonatal units. A concern about bedside analysis is that analyzers are calibrated to total nitrogen and therefore overestimate the amount of protein by approximately 17%.

Existing customizing approaches use either milk composition or the short-term metabolic response of the infant as feedback. Customizing approaches using infant growth as feedback have not been proposed. The reason is probably that growth has a long response time (5 to 7 days). However, even with such a response time a customizing approach would seem to be useful.

CONCLUSION

To customize or to generalize? All approaches achieve more or less satisfactory intakes of energy and of most other nutrients. They differ, however, with regard to how closely they meet protein needs.

Customizing approaches were developed with the aim of securing higher protein intakes than are achieved with the basic generalizing approach using powder fortifiers with the customary low protein content. The two existing customizing approaches achieve higher protein intakes and better growth. The customizing approaches have in common that they are relatively complicated and labor intensive. This is probably the reason why customizing methods have found limited acceptance

Generalizing approaches are used widely because of their simplicity. When using low-protein powder fortifiers, the only fortifiers available until recently, intakes of protein with this approach are inadequate most of the time. Modifications of the basic form can achieve adequate protein intakes, but do so at the expense of other disadvantages. Liquid fortifiers based on human milk can deliver satisfactory protein intakes. Liquid fortifiers based on bovine milk have recently become available. The one fortifier that raises protein content by 1.8 g/dl is likely to meet protein needs in almost all circumstances, if potentially exceeding them occasionally. This removes the major objection to the generalizing approach as used with low-protein powder fortifiers. It seems that use of the high-protein liquid fortifier obviates the need for customizing methods.

REFERENCES

1. Schanler RJ. Mother's own milk, donor human milk, and preterm formulas in the feeding of extremely premature infants. *Journal of Pediatric Gastroenterology and Nutrition.* 2007; **45 Suppl 3**: S175–7.
2. Schanler RJ. Evaluation of the evidence to support current recommendations to meet the needs of premature infants: the role of human milk. *American Journal of Clinical Nutrition.* 2007; **85**(625S–8S).

3. Arslanoglu S, Moro GE, Ziegler EE. Adjustable fortification of human milk fed to preterm infants: does it make a difference? *Journal of Perinatology.* 2006; **26**(10): 614–21.
4. Polberger S, Raiha NC, Juvonen P, Moro GE, Minoli I, Warm A. Individualized protein fortification of human milk for preterm infants: comparison of ultrafiltrated human milk protein and a bovine whey fortifier. *Journal of Pediatric Gastroenterology and Nutrition.* 1999; **29**(3): 332–8.
5. Ziegler EE, O'Donnell AM, Nelson SE, Fomon SJ. Body composition of the reference fetus. *Growth.* 1976; **40**(4): 329–41.
6. Ziegler EE. Meeting the nutritional needs of the low-birth-weight infant. *Annals of Nutrition & Metabolism.* 2011; **58 Suppl 1**: 8–18.
7. Kashyap S, Heird WC. Protein requirements of low birthweight, very low birthweight, and small for gestational age infants. In: Räihä NCR, Ed. *Protein Metabolism during Infancy.* New York: Raven Press; 1994. pp. 133–46.
8. Micheli J-L, Schutz Y. Protein. In: Lucas A, Uauy R, Zlotkin S, Eds. *Nutritional Needs of the Preterm Infant.* Baltimore: Williams & Wilkins; 1993.
9. Atkinson SA, Anderson GH, Bryan MH. Human milk: comparison of the nitrogen composition in milk from mothers of premature and full-term infants. *American Journal of Clinical Nutrition.* 1980; **33**(4): 811–5.
10. Lemons JA, Moye L, Hall D, Simmons M. Differences in the composition of preterm and term human milk during early lactation. *Pediatric Research.* 1982; **16**(2): 113–7.
11. Ehrenkranz RA, Dusick AM, Vohr BR, Wright LL, Wrage LA, Poole WK. Growth in the neonatal intensive care unit influences neurodevelopmental and growth outcomes of extremely low birth weight infants. *Pediatrics.* 2006; **117**(4): 1253–61.
12. Embleton NE, Pang N, Cooke RJ. Postnatal malnutrition and growth retardation: an inevitable consequence of current recommendations in preterm infants? *Pediatrics.* 2001; **107**(2): 270–3.
13. Goldman HI, Goldman J, Kaufman I, Liebman OB. Late effects of early dietary protein intake on low-birth-weight infants. *Journal of Pediatrics.* 1974; **85**(6): 764–9.
14. Moody GJ, Schanler RJ, Lau C, Shulman RJ. Feeding tolerance in premature infants fed fortified human milk. *Journal of Pediatric Gastroenterology and Nutrition.* 2000; **30**(4): 408–12.
15. Kuschel CA, Harding JE. Multicomponent fortified human milk for promoting growth in preterm infants. *Cochrane Database Syst Rev.* 2004; (1): CD000343.
16. Arslanoglu S, Moro GE, Ziegler EE. Preterm infants fed fortified human milk receive less protein than they need. *Journal of Perinatology.* 2009; **29**(7): 489–92.
17. Carlson SJ, Ziegler EE. Nutrient intakes and growth of very low birth weight infants. *Journal of Perinatology.* 1998; **18**(4): 252–8.
18. Moya F, Sisk PM, Walsh KR, Berseth CL. A new liquid human milk fortifier and linear growth in preterm infants. *Pediatrics.* 2012; **130**(4): e928–35.
19. N, Fusch G, Choi A, et al. Target Fortification of Breast Milk with Fat, Protein, and Carbohydrates for Preterm Infants. *J Pediatr* 2013; 163(4): 1001-7.
20. Rochow N, Fusch G, Choi A, Chessell L, Elliott L, McDonald K, et al. Target fortification of breast milk with fat, protein, and carbohydrates for preterm infants. *Journal of Pediatrics.* 2013.
21. Cooper AR, Barnett D, Gentles E, Cairns L, Simpson JH. Macronutrient content of donor human breast milk. *Arch Dis Child Fetal Neonatal Ed.* 2013;98(6):F539-41
22. Sullivan S, Schanler RJ, Kim JH, Patel AL, Trawöger R, Kiechl-Kohlendorfer U, Chan GM, Blanco CL, Abrams S, Cotten CM, Laroia N, Ehrenkranz RA, Dudell G, Cristofalo EA, Meier P, Lee ML, Rechtman DJ, Lucas A. An exclusively human milk-based diet is associated with a lower rate of necrotizing enterocolitis than a diet of human milk and bovine milk-based products. *J Pediatr.* 2010;156(4):562-7.e1

11 Customized Fortification of Human Milk

Sharon Groh-Wargo and Jae H. Kim

INTRODUCTION

Human milk (HM) is the preferred feeding for all infants, including low birth weight infants. Studies have established a wide range of advantages over formula including better feeding tolerance, faster progression to full enteral feedings, reduced rates of necrotizing enterocolitis (NEC) and late-onset sepsis, and improved neurodevelopmental outcomes.[1–7] The protection offered by HM is dose-dependent such that the more HM that is received, the greater the benefits.[5] Despite its many advantages, HM does not meet all nutrient needs of the rapidly growing preterm infant. Specifically, protein intake from HM is substantially below the protein requirement of preterm infants.[8] Commercial human milk fortifiers (HMF) or preterm formulas are routinely added to increase the nutrient density of HM.[9, 10] Without a known nutrient profile of the expressed HM fed to a baby, the composition of the fortified product is only an estimate. Current clinical practice assumes uniform composition when calculating nutrient intake of infants in the neonatal intensive care unit (NICU) who are fed expressed HM. This chapter will review known factors that explain the variability of HM composition, available evidence on "lactoengineering," equipment that can analyze HM, and strategies to operationalize an individualized approach to fortification. Our goal is to encourage the feeding of HM to all infants while meeting the increased nutritional requirements of the high-risk newborn.

VARIABILITY OF HUMAN MILK

The nutrient composition of HM varies depending on many factors including, but not limited to, length of gestation,[11–15] stage of lactation,[16–21] and time of day,[16, 19, 22, 23] as well as within a feeding[12, 19, 24] between mothers[16, 18, 23, 25] with various maternal factors and dietary intakes[19, 26–28] and whether the milk has been pooled, warmed, pasteurized, or frozen[29–32] (see Table 11.1). There are no good determinants of this variability with well nourished mothers.[33] Study results also demonstrate that milk synthesis differs in each mammary lobe even in the same breast. The degree of fullness in each mammary lobe seems to play the most important role in the fat content. The protein content in the milk from each mammary lobe is determined by other factors, presumably by the feedback inhibitor of lactation, accumulated in the corresponding mammary lobe.[34] Furthermore, in the first month of lactation, there is a loss of approximately 25% in total protein with a more gradual decline thereafter even out to six months of lactation.[12] Additionally, the composition of HM that is actually ingested by the baby can be affected by the handling, the method of feeding or pumping, and storage.[35–37]

TABLE 11.1
Factors that Influence the Composition of Human Milk

Factors	Impact on Composition
Length of gestation	Preterm milk has higher protein and sodium content compared to term milk[12–14, 20]
	Protein content higher in milk produced by mothers of extremely preterm than more moderately preterm infants[15]
Stage of lactation	Four stages: colostrum (first few days), transitional (first several weeks), mature (<7 months), and late (>7 months)
	Protein, sodium, carotenoid, IgA, and lactoferrin concentrations decrease with time[11, 12, 16, 18, 19]
	Volume of milk produced and fat concentration increase with time[19]
	Lactose content is relatively stable over time[12]
	Decrease in vitamins and mineral content in extended lactation (>7 months) compared to mature milk; decreasing milk volume during weaning associated with increased protein and sodium concentration[17, 21]
Time of day	Time elapsed since the last meal affects nutrient content[19]
	Protein content highly variable[16, 22]
	Fat content variable but tends to be lower in morning compared to later in the day[16, 23]
Within a feeding	Fat and energy content higher in hind- vs. foremilk[12, 19, 24]
Maternal factors (BMI, diet, health)	Between-mother variability is significant[16, 18, 23, 25, 78]
	Maternal BMI positively correlated with fat or protein content[18, 23]
	Severe malnutrition may decrease milk volume and fat content[19]
	Quality of dietary fatty acid intake affects content of fatty acids[26, 79]
	Intake of carotenoids directly correlated with carotenoid concentration[27, 28]
	Mastitis may decrease IgA, lactoferrin, and complement C-3; severe mastitis may destroy lactating tissue impairing mammary gland function, and current and future lactation[19]
Processing	Warming increases osmolality[30]
	Pasteurization or freezing decreases fat and protein concentration[31]
	Inadequate thawing or mixing after thawing can result in fat loss[32]
	24-hour pooling of expressed breast milk reduces caloric and nutrient variability without increasing bacterial counts[29]
Storage	Glass and hard food-grade plastic containers minimize loss of fat and immunologic factors compared to other containers[35, 36]
Feeding method	Loss of fat occurs due to separation and adherence to the sides of feeding tubes[71, 80, 81]
	Slow (1–2 hours) or continuous feeding results in fat loss compared to gravity or intermittent feeding[74, 81]
Pumping method	Hospital-grade pump helps establish optimal milk supply and complete emptying of the breast[37]

Protein

HM contains significant amounts of non-protein nitrogen (NPN). NPN components are the constituents remaining when proteins are removed by precipitation with tricholoracetic acid. NPN consists of urea, uric acid, creatinine, ammonia, peptides, nucleotides and nucleosides, and free amino acids, and accounts for approximately 24% of the total nitrogen in HM.[19] Although NPN components are largely unavailable for protein synthesis, approximately 27% is bioavailable. Total protein includes all nitrogen including NPN. The term "true protein" generally refers to total nitrogen minus NPN.[38] If total nitrogen values for HM are reported, bioavailable nitrogen can be calculated by summing 76% of total nitrogen (total − NPN) and adding 27% of the NPN (the bioavailable fraction on NPN). Nitrogen values can be converted to protein by multiplying the sum of nitrogen by 6.25 to determine bioavailable protein.[39] The whey:casein ratio of HM is variable with the proportion of whey to casein decreasing over the course of lactation.[38] Whey proteins are soluble in the liquid portion (whey) remaining in solution when milk is acidified to precipitate the caseins.[19] HM also contains a wide variety of protein-based protective factors including glycoproteins and immunoglobulins.[19] Figure 11.1 illustrates the various protein fractions in bovine and HM.

Carbohydrate

The carbohydrate content of HM comes primarily from the disaccharide lactose and from oligosaccharides. Lactose is second only to water as a major constituent of HM.

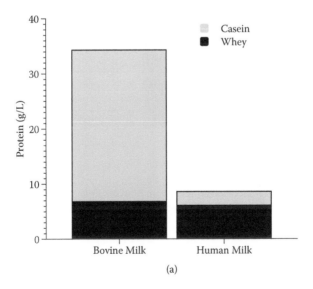

(a)

FIGURE 11.1 Differences between human and bovine milk in terms of casein and whey protein amount (a), casein protein content (b), and whey protein content (c). (Data from Reference 88.) *(continued)*

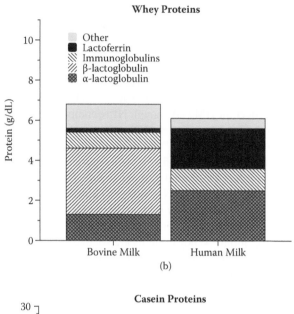

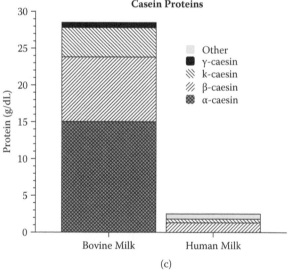

FIGURE 11.1 Differences between human and bovine milk in terms of casein and whey protein amount (A), casein protein content (B), and whey protein content (C). (Data from Reference 88.)

Lactose is one of the most stable of the macronutrients in HM. In addition to lactose, HM contains a wide variety of oligosaccharides. Oligosaccharides are complex, nondigestible carbohydrates that, in addition to glycoproteins, inhibit binding of pathogens to their receptors, promote a specific intestinal flora, and reduce infection in HM-fed babies.[19,40,41]

FAT

Fat contributes approximately 50% of the energy in HM. The quantity of fat is highly variable, as discussed previously, and the quality of the fat (i.e., the array of specific fatty acids) is greatly influenced by the quality of the fat in the diet of the mother.[40] Of particular interest are the long chain polyunsaturated fatty acids (LCPUFA) including the omega-3 fatty acid docosahexaenoic acid (DHA). HM responds to changes in the maternal diet and LCPUFA dietary supplementation increases DHA concentration in milk.[42] Although both the macronutrient and micronutrient content of HM can be affected by the mother's diet, in general, the diet of the mother affects the micronutrient content, specifically the vitamin content, more than the macronutrient content. An important exception is the fatty acid composition. The quality of dietary fat affects the types of fatty acids that predominate in mother's milk.[43] Overall, fat is the macronutrient that varies the most in HM.

DONOR HUMAN MILK

Donor human milk (DHM) is frequently fed to preterm and hospitalized newborns. The composition of DHM is known to differ from mother's own milk.[43] This is likely due to the relatively late stage of lactation that most donor mothers are in when they donate to a milk bank as well as the processing and storage to which DHM is exposed. The lower protein content of DHM and lack of lipase activity should be appreciated when feeding preterm infants with the thought of increasing protein and energy fortification when growth is suboptimal. DHM from mothers in the United States is known to have low concentrations of DHA.[44]

Table 11.2 summarizes milk composition values for key nutrients in several types of HM. Complete nutrient profiles of colostrum and mature milk from mothers of full-term infants are available.[45, 46]

HUMAN MILK ANALYSIS TECHNOLOGY

Current fortification methods of HM are blinded to the nutrient content and carry a very high error margin due to the inherent variability seen in nutrient quantity in HM. Lactoengineering is best possible when components of HM are directly measurable. Therefore, determining which technology offers the most accurate and precise measurement of HM components is essential for the success of the advancement of HM fortification.

The capacity to measure biochemical components of liquids in a rapid and reliable manner has been available to the dairy industry for many years. Applications for clinical use have been emerging with recent data suggesting validity of several of these methods. However, there are large challenges in the implementation of these new technologies into the NICU and acquisition of convincing clinical efficacy that targeted fortification with measurements changes clinical outcomes.

What in HM is most clinically important to measure? While there are also hundreds of compounds found in HM that have bioactivity beyond the basic macronutrient composition, the most pertinent nutritional concern with HM delivery has

TABLE 11.2

Composition of Human Milk per dl—Various Types and Selected Nutrients

	Colostrum[1]	Mature[1]	Late[2]	Preterm[3]	Donor
Energy (kcal)	58	70	71[8]	77[3]	65[8]
Protein (g)	2.3	0.9	1.2	2.1[3]	1.2[8]
Carbohydrate (g)	5.3	7.3	7.4	7.5[3]	7.8[8]
Fat (g)	2.9	4.2	4.1	4.5[3]	3.2[8]
Minerals					
Calcium (mg)	23	28	22	27[3]	26[9]
Phosphorus (mg)	14	15	—	6.5[3]	—
Sodium (mg)	48	18	9.4	24[3]	26[9]
Potassium (mg)	74	58	40	51[3]	50[9]
Iron (mcg)	45	40	21	98[4]	—
Zinc (mcg)	540	120	38	320[5]	—
Copper (mcg)	46	25	16	46[6]	—
Vitamins					
Vitamin A (mcg)	89	67	—	16[6]	—
B Carotene (mcg)	112	23	—	23[7]	—
Vitamin E (mcg)	1280	315	—	716[6]	—

[1] Reference 37

[2] Reference 17. §Calculated at 4 kcal/g carbohydrate and protein and 9 kcal/g fat

[3] Reference 15 (mean of three groups of preterm infants)

[4] Reference 82 (mean of first four weeks postpartum)

[5] Reference 20 (four weeks post-partum)

[6] Reference 83 (mean of first four weeks postpartum)

[7] Reference 84 (day of life 37)

[8] Reference 43

[9] Reference 85

been with macronutrient content, particularly protein and energy. The potential to measure other components found in HM such as micronutrients, bioactive factors, oligosaccharides, and contaminants offer additional benefits in HM profiling. For this section of this chapter, we will focus primarily on technologies enabling macronutrient point-of-care measurements for HM.

MACRONUTRIENTS

The measurement of fat, protein, and carbohydrates in HM is possible with several existing technologies. These include reference chemistry, creamatocrit, acoustic spectroscopy, and infrared spectroscopy. Real-time measurement of the nutritional content of HM by these technologies offers the potential for incorporating an individualized form of HM fortification. Measurements of total protein and true protein are also possible with some of these devices.

IDEAL FEATURES OF A MILK ANALYZER IN THE CLINICAL ENVIRONMENT

The ideal milk nutrient analyzer is capable of measuring the components in an accurate and precise manner (Table 11.3). The machine should have a small footprint, be easy to use, have high capacity for multiple measurements, be relatively inexpensive, require low maintenance, and use a small milk volume. Due to the great difficulties in milk production that challenge lactating mothers of preterm infants, it is important to be able to analyze with the smallest volume of milk possible. To be effective in the NICU, the device also needs to be incorporated into the clinical workflow and decision making of the nutritional management of the preterm infant. Several options are available that met some or all of these requirements to various degrees.

CHEMICAL ANALYSIS

There are several different reference chemistry (RC) methods that can be used for macronutrient measurements in HM. The primary choice for determining protein (or nitrogen) content is the Kjeldahl method.[89] This method first breaks down the protein by oxidation with sulfuric acid upon which the reduced nitrogen is converted chemically into ammonia and then back titrated to determine the amount of nitrogen present by detecting the amount of ammonia. Despite its history of more than a century, the Kjeldahl remains an accurate chemical standard for protein determination.

For overall fat content, the Mojonnier[90] method is considered one of the best standard chemistry methods. In this method, lipids are extracted using ethers and then following ether evaporation, the remaining solids are weighed.

For carbohydrate measurements, high-pressure liquid chromatography (HPLC) is the preferred technique because of its high degree of accuracy. Isolation of the carbohydrate fraction begins with elimination/precipitation of the proteins and extraction of the lipid fraction. With the remaining fluid, the sugars are run through a column, then separated over time and peaks of each sugar measured on the resulting graph.[91]

Collectively these methods can be used to reference other technologies to measure their accuracy in measuring macronutrient concentrations in HM.

TABLE 11.3

Features of an Ideal Human Milk Analyzer

Accurate and precise readings

Small volume of milk used

Fast measurement in point-of-care

Full macronutrient profile

Small equipment footprint

Ease of use

Durability for high traffic use

Computational capacity for targeted fortification algorithm

INFRARED SPECTROSCOPY

Infrared (IR) spectroscopy is widely used in determining organic constituents in a variety of foods and is one of the most common methods used in the dairy industry. The advantages are its ability to measure rapidly in a non-destructive and precise manner. Spectral analysis can occur in the near infrared (NIR, 800 to 2500 nm) or mid infrared (MIR, 2400 to 6000 nm) range. It measures the spectral absorption of C-H, N-H, and other organic bonds found in milk. Spectral analysis generally involves a partial least squares (PLS) regression to predict fat, protein, lactose, and urea after preprocessing IR data and selecting the most informative wave number variables.

The two major spectral ranges, NIR and MIR, have been examined for HM macronutrient profiling. The correlations between these two IR techniques and reference chemistry for making measurements of macronutrients in HM are excellent and well within the tolerance of clinical practice.[33, 47–50] These devices introduce a marked improvement in accuracy especially because HM samples can vary by even twofold in protein and energy and at least fivefold in fat.

A couple of approaches to spectral analyses are currently available for HM. More sophisticated, costlier machines collect the full spectrum across a range of wavelengths while simpler, cheaper devices collect spectral values with a small number of filters at preset informative wavelengths. In dairy milk, the full-spectrum analysis was found to be more accurate than filter analysis.[51] Unfortunately, there are no similar comparisons with HM, but the potential is there for less accuracy with a filtered device vs. a full-spectrum device. These differences may not be sufficient to overcome the large cost differential in the devices.[47, 48] The preparation of milk samples for spectroscopy requires warming of the samples to 40°C to help solubilize the fat content more than at refrigerated or room temperature. Homogenization of the milk is also important for better distribution of fat globules and improved accuracy. The costs of these machines are relatively high, in the range of $30,000 to $60,000, and therefore may be a prohibitive factor for routine use in the NICU. If milk analysis requires additional personnel to maintain the machine and measure milk on a regular basis, further expenses would be incurred.

CREAMATOCRIT

The technique of a creamatocrit (CMT) was first described in 1978.[52] The basic concept depends on the natural separation of HM fat globules from the aqueous fraction of the milk. While this happens naturally over time, taking a sample and spinning the milk down in a capillary tube can quickly separate the two fractions, a top portion of fat and a lower portion of aqueous, generating a fractional fat determination. Calibration calculations were derived based on RC methods including bomb calorimetry for fat and energy content. While initial studies have demonstrated a good correlation between creamatocrit and reference calorie measurements, others more recently have found that creamatocrit measurements can overestimate the amount of fat and total energy when compared to MIR and RC.[53–56] This method is simple to perform and has good inter-operator reliability.[57] The biggest limitation of

CMT measurements against other methods includes the inability to measure protein content, which is known to be variable.

ACOUSTIC SPECTROSCOPY

The detection of milk components using acoustic spectroscopy has been used in the dairy industry. The underlying premise for this technique involves the differences in acoustic attenuation and transmission with different milk densities and composition. The separation of fat globules from the aqueous components of milk is the most favorable distinguishable factor, but other key components such as protein or carbohydrates are less accurately detectable with this method.[58, 59] Like CMT, however, the inability to accurately measure protein poses a significant problem with this technology. Therefore, there are current limitations in the utility of this technique but especially that there are no HM studies based on this technique.

REGULATION/RULES

The use of any analytic equipment that provided information for the purposes of clinical decision making is regulated by the Food and Drug Administration (FDA). This also applies to equipment that analyzes food. HM analyzers are not currently approved for use as standard of care in the NICU in the United States. Therefore, the primary use of advanced targeted HM fortification is currently only under research protocol such as through investigational device exemption (IDE) application. Commercial owners of these technologies will need to file for appropriate 510K approval by the FDA. Table 11.4 compares several qualities in milk analysis equipment.

LACTOENGINEERING

The term *lactoengineering* has been coined to describe ways to individualize HM feeding and fortification. The fat content of HM can be manipulated to maximize the

TABLE 11.4
Comparison of Human Milk Analysis Methods

Method	Analysis Time	Footprint	Milk Volume	Costs	Limitations
NIR or MIR spectroscopy	Less than 15 minutes	Small	1–10 mL	High	Needs homogenization, needs manpower
Creamatocrit	Less than 15 minutes	Small	1 mL	Low	Lacks protein content, needs manpower
Acoustic spectroscopy	Less than 15 minutes	Small	10 mL	Low	Lacks protein content, needs manpower
Reference chemistry	1 day	Large	50 mL	High	High cost, manpower, expertise

use of HM. For example, the creation of fat-free HM is promoted as a way to bring the benefits of HM to infants with chylothorax.[60] A technique that produces milk with 0 grams of fat has been described.[61] The skim milk is fortified with additional fat, calories, and essential fatty acids to provide adequate nutrition while retaining the immune and nutritional benefits of HM without exacerbating the chylous effusions in the baby. High-fat hindmilk can be used to improve weight gain in VLBW infants fed HM.[62] Care is exercised to ensure adequate protein and an acceptable protein and mineral density when hindmilk is used for additional calories. More recently and because HM composition varies so much, interest in an individualized approach to HM feeding is increasing. Two approaches of interest are "adjustable fortification" (AF) and "targeted fortification" (TF).[63] There is no consensus in the literature if one approach is superior to the other.

ADJUSTABLE FORTIFICATION (AF)

AF adds more protein in a stepwise fashion using the baby's blood urea nitrogen (BUN) value as a monitor. If the BUN falls below a specific value, more protein is added and if the BUN rises, protein is removed. Table 11.5 summarizes the AF approach used by Arslanoglu and colleagues,[64] but briefly, when using an AF regimen, infants are started on standard fortification (Level 0) and adjustments are made in the amount of HMF or additional protein that is added based on twice-weekly BUN values. A BUN between 9 and 14 mg/dl is generally considered normal. Every time the BUN is below 9 ml/dl, fortification is increased one level. If the BUN is greater than 14 mg/dl, a decrease in fortification by one level is made. AF has been shown to be effective in achieving higher protein intakes and supporting improved growth.[64]

TARGETED FORTIFICATION (TF)

TF uses HM analysis to individualize nutritional management and milk is fortified based on the results of the HM analysis. Limited evidence supports the efficacy of TF. Polberger et al. randomly assigned 32 healthy preterm infants less than 1800 g at birth to two different protein-based fortifiers.[65] The protein content of the HM was analyzed

TABLE 11.5
Adjustable Fortification Schedule

Fortification Level	Amount of Protein Added to HM (g/100 ml)
3	2.1
2	1.7
1	1.3
0	1
−1	0.8
−2	0.5

Source: Adapted from Reference 64.

using the Kjeldahl method and fortification was targeted to provide 3.5 g/kg per day to study infants. Growth and tolerance was similar between groups.

Results from a study comparing preterm infants fed HM fortified in the traditional way vs. preterm infants fed HM that was analyzed daily and then individually fortified with medium chain triglycerides (MCTs) or HMF suggests that TF reduces the variability of nutrient intake, more closely provides recommended nutrient intakes, and may result in growth closer to the growth of preterm infants fed nutrient-dense preterm formula.[66] TF may include macronutrient milk analysis as well as measurement of osmolality. In a study of 20 matched infants (TF vs. routinely fortified), 12-hour batches of HM from the TF study infants were analyzed each day for macronutrient content with near-infrared spectroscopy and osmolality with a freezing point osmometer.[50] A specific prescription of fortification based on the milk analysis was written twice each day and included adjustment of all three macronutrients using the following targets: 4.4 g fat, 3 g protein, and 8.8 g carbohydrate (per 100 ml). The acceptable target range for osmolality was 400 to 480 mOsmol/kg. All 650 samples of milk collected and analyzed during the study required at least one macronutrient adjustment to meet targets. The average osmolality of fortified milk was 436 mOsmol/kg. TF increased the intake of macronutrients, met nutrient recommendations, and reduced the inter-day intake variability. Infants on TF had weight gain that significantly correlated with milk intake (P = 0.004).

AF and TF can be used with both own mother's milk feedings and when DHM is fed although additional well-controlled and randomized trials with sufficient sample sizes are needed before either method of lactoengineering can be used with confidence. Further, and as mentioned previously, milk analysis equipment needs regulatory approval before routine use in clinical care. Table 11.6 compares advantages and disadvantages of AF and TF.

CLINICAL IMPLEMENTATION AND OPERATIONAL CONSIDERATIONS

Quality of HM

The increasing use of HM has resulted in greater responsibility and accountability on the part of the NICU and their institution to manage the quality and traffic of HM

TABLE 11.6
Comparison of Adjustable Fortification and Targeted Fortification

	Adjustable Fortification	Targeted Fortification
Advantages	Directly monitors baby's metabolic response	Considers variability of HM composition
	Avoids excessive protein intake	Avoids excessive protein intake
	Practical for routine use with no need for special equipment	Improves and regulates energy or protein intake
Disadvantages	BUN may reflect renal immaturity more than protein intake especially during the first weeks of life in VLBW infants[86, 87]	Requires special equipment and trained staff

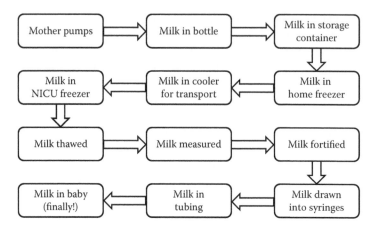

FIGURE 11.2   Milk traffic chain.

from the beginning of milk production to the delivery to vulnerable preterm infants (Figure 11.2). At each step there are potential risks for loss of quality of HM including loss of nutrient and biologic value. Due to the complex and organic nature of HM, the risk of deteriorating quality of HM is evident from the moment HM is expressed. These risks include damage by oxidation, photo-degradation, and bacterial contamination. In addition, excessive handling and transfer increases the risk of nutrient loss with each material surface with which the milk is in contact. Further risks can occur with repeated handling, freezing, and heating. Freezing destroys most immune cells such as neutrophils or macrophages, but does not damage bacteria significantly.

Milk Handling

The increasing use of HM along with varying and more complex fortification strategies has presented new problems of quality control. HM comes into the hospital in a multitude of ways and much of this is poorly controlled (Figure 11.2). Most mothers of preterm infants are required to pump because their infants cannot feed orally or breastfeed. Mothers pump at home or in the hospital, and bring in milk either fresh or frozen, with little quality control in regard to rules of cleaning, storage, or transport.

Milk Preparation and Fortification

Currently most NICUs in the United States have the preparation of HM carried out by the nurse at the bedside in the NICU. In some cases, a dedicated clean space is available but in others having quality controlled spaces that enable consistent and safe handling of milk is also helpful. The American Dietetic Association (now The Academy of Nutrition and Dietetics) publishes guidelines that support having a clean room for formula or milk preparation.[67]

Collection

Frequent pumping into individual containers generates a significant amount of work for mothers. Ideally, HM collection containers should be standardized to minimize contamination risks, improve nutrient content, and decrease maternal workload. The pumped milk needs to be labeled and dated, equipment needs to be cleaned, and mothers pump 6 to 8 times each day. Typically these pump sessions are collected in individualized milk collections. Pooling 24 hours worth of milk into a single container offers significant advantages in ease of use for mothers and less variability in nutrient content from feed to feed, with no disadvantage in higher bacterial counts.[29] The challenge with daily pooling is obtaining larger food grade bottles to store the milk and refrigerator space to store the bottles.

Transport

Transporting of HM from home should be standardized by maintaining cooled or frozen milk in an insulated container packed with ice or freezer packs to minimize warming of the transported milk.

Storage

Stored HM is generally kept in hospitals in a frozen state at −20°C. Recent data would support, however, the use of refrigerated (+4°C) HM for at least 96 hours.[68] This would eliminate any untoward effects that might occur with freezing.[69] Keeping HM in a refrigerated state for less than four days slightly decreased pH, reduced WBC, and reduced protein and gram-positive bacteria counts. Increases were seen in free fatty acids from active lipolysis. No changes in osmolality, secretory IgA, fat, gram-negative bacteria, and lactoferrin were noted. Thus, cold HM can retain an optimal nutrient profile and a safe content for 96 hours after expression.

Labeling

The concern for milk error, particularly wrong milk administration to a baby, has encouraged the milk labeling and tracking industry to grow over the past few years. The increasing standardization of electronic medical records (EMR) is enabling the integration of these labeling systems to provide improved workflow in tracking the movement of HM through the NICU across most of the milk chain. Ultimately, these improvements will permit the documentation and communication of sophisticated fortification strategies throughout the medical system.

Freezing

Optimal freezer organization includes individual covered bins, proper freezer alarms, and ready access of freezers to clinical care. All mammalian cells are lost with freezing due the lack of a cell wall and the expansion of water with freezing. This is partially effective for reducing the CMV containing cell burden in the milk but loss of immune cells such as neutrophils and macrophages does drop HM immune protective capacity. Prolonged freezing has minimal effects on milk bacterial quality, but can affect bioactive properties.[70, 71]

Warming HM

Bringing frozen or refrigerated milk to feeding temperature (either room temperature or body temperature) is not properly standardized in NICUs across the United States. Several commercial options are now available that offer controlled thawing or warming of HM. These are preferable as unmonitored heating may reduce bioactive factors in HM. Microwaving, in particular, should be avoided due to "hotspots" that can be generated and degradation of milk bioactivity.[70]

Role of a Milk Lab

With increasing complexity in HM feeding options and greater individualization of nutrient delivery, centralizing HM processing and fortification processes may be of benefit. A dedicated space with all available storage and supplies may increase the workflow productivity of a large unit while reducing the chance for milk contamination. Some NICUs employ milk technicians who are responsible for collecting the daily milk order, using standard recipes to mix daily feedings, warming milk through consistent practice, drawing up each feeding into syringes for enteral tube feeding or large bottles with oral feeding. Other benefits of a milk technician include reduction in nursing workload, consistent preparation practices, reduced number of staff to train, and overall better quality control of HM (www.spinprogram.ucsd. edu). Newer tasks may also include routine milk analysis to allow for optimization of the nutritional quality of the final milk product. Nurses spend less time away from the bedside and more time in patient care when milk is stored and prepared in a milk lab.[72] Resources for setting up a milk lab are available. The University of Michigan has a "Milk Room Practicum." More information is available at http:// www.med.umich.edu/pfans/services/confinfo.htm. A certificate program for technicians working in a milk lab is available through Columbus State Community College in Columbus, Ohio. This program has been shown to reduce preparation errors.[73]

Personnel

Adequate personnel are required to manage the full control of HM collection, processing, and delivery to infants. This includes the neonatal dietitian, milk technician, and lactation support. In particular, lactation support is a fundamental service for ensuring an adequate and safe HM production. Enhancing HM to alter the nutritional quality of the milk required, dedicated personnel and lactation services (neonatal dietitian, lactation consultants, and nurses with lactation education) are clear participants in these types of activities. This may include separation of fat-rich hindmilk from fore milk or spinning down milk to separate HM fat from the aqueous portion as some do for infants with chylothorax. However, more advanced lactoengineering such as custom fortification based on milk analyses are better to be handled by dedicated milk technicians.

Feeding of HM

The use of HM through enteral feeding systems has been shown to be a source of significant loss of nutrients.[71, 74] This is particularly relevant with syringe-loaded feeding systems where due to the separation and rise of the fat globules, a level or inverted position of the syringe is less favorable than an upright position (spout up). Because milk fat adheres to containers, it is important to reduce transfers from containers, minimize continuous syringe pump feedings, and keep syringes facing upward during feedings.

Donor Human Milk

The role for DHM is primarily a benefit as a bridge until mother's milk is available. The evidence for prevention of necrotizing enterocolitis is less compelling than for mother's own milk. A Cochrane review in addition to systematic reviews has been inconclusive in defining a clear benefit of exclusive HDM and NEC reduction.[75, 76] There are few pure studies that have randomized infants strictly to use of DHM. This would require the unethical randomization of infants to receive DHM even when mother's milk is present. There are two large DHM trials underway in North America that will be able to evaluate the effects of DHM on NEC, but again are not pure DHM trials (www.clinicaltrials.gov). Despite the benefit of having DHM bridge the gap when mother's milk is not available or short in supply, only 42% of the NICUs in the United States actually use DHM.[77] The majority therefore use infant formula as a substitute or a full replacement.

DESCRIPTION OF THE SPIN PROGRAM

In 2007, in response to the above-mentioned challenges in the practice of HM nutrition and a strong desire to standardize care in this area, UC San Diego Medical Center (UCSDMC) established the SPIN (Supporting Premature Infant Nutrition) program, a multifaceted, multidisciplinary program to improve neonatal nutrition practices and increase HM intake in preterm infants across the United States (http://spinprogram.ucsd.edu). It was prefaced in 2006 with becoming the first academic Baby Friendly Hospital Initiative (BFHI) in California. BFHI USA has demonstrated that rates of in-hospital breastfeeding initiation in healthy term newborns dramatically go up with the implementation of program strategies. Given the success of the BFHI for healthy term infants, these same benefits of HM delivery could be passed on to more vulnerable preterm infants in the NICU.

The major structural innovation of the SPIN program is the collaboration of the nutrition and lactation stakeholders in the hospital. This brings key stakeholders to develop common goals and objectives for the best interest in growing healthier preterm infants. The overarching mission statement for the SPIN program is to create a center of excellence in neonatal nutrition focused on the provision, analysis, and research of

---

TABLE 11.7

SPIN Program Top Ten Practices

1	Have a NICU nutrition/HM policy.
2	Educate all mother/baby staff in SPIN 10-steps.
3	Educate NICU families about optimal premature infant nutrition.
4	Prevent extra uterine growth restriction.
5	Standardize enteral feeding procedures.
6	Target 100% HM nutrition.
7	Maximize mothers' milk production.
8	Optimize milk quality and safety.
9	Encourage skin-to-skin care and breastfeeding.
10	Plan a nutritional discharge from NICU.

HM to improve nutritional and long-term health outcomes of premature babies. Other important facets of the program include following the SPIN Ten Steps (Table 11.7) and setting up outpatient follow-up (premature infant nutrition community [PINC] clinic), community outreach to other cities through lecture series, and HM nutrition research. Key aspects of our program that were foundational in this comprehensive program were to form a multidisciplinary group, administrative support, involvement of all stakeholders, performance of a self-assessment, setting specific goals and timelines, regular team meetings, providing staff updates, and collection of key outcome data. The SPIN program has stimulated behavior and attitude change by all health care professionals, and set a new standard for HM as the preferred feeding for preterm infants.

SUMMARY

The benefits of HM for the preterm infant support the increased use of HM in the NICU. The appreciation of the high variability in nutritional content of HM has increased the demand for individualized fortification strategies to drive optimal growth and development. New technologies have emerged to improve our capacity to have real-time measurements of different nutritional components of HM but insufficient data are available and in some cases, regulatory approval has not been established to bring this to the clinical arena. There is not enough clinical data to recommend clear guidelines for the individualized fortification of preterm infants, but the promise of lactoengineering is upon us and there is great optimism that advanced customized fortification will be available to improve the outcomes of our most vulnerable infants.

REFERENCES

1. Schanler RJ. The use of human milk for premature infants. *Pediatr Clin North Am.* 2001; **48**(1): 207–19.
2. Sisk PM, Lovelady CA, Gruber KJ, Dillard RG, O'Shea TM. Human milk consumption and full enteral feeding among infants who weigh </= 1250 grams. *Pediatrics.* 2008; **121**(6): e1528–33.
3. Ehrenkranz RA, Dusick AM, Vohr BR, Wright LL, Wrage LA, Poole WK. Growth in the neonatal intensive care unit influences neurodevelopmental and growth outcomes of extremely low birth weight infants. *Pediatrics.* 2006; **117**(4): 1253–61.
4. Schanler RJ. Evaluation of the evidence to support current recommendations to meet the needs of premature infants: the role of human milk. *Am J Clin Nutr.* 2007; **85**(2): 625S–8S.
5. Meinzen-Derr J, Poindexter B, Wrage L, Morrow AL, Stoll B, Donovan EF. Role of human milk in extremely low birth weight infants' risk of necrotizing enterocolitis or death. *J Perinatol.* 2009; **29**(1): 57–62.
6. Sisk PM, Lovelady CA, Dillard RG, Gruber KJ, O'Shea TM. Early human milk feeding is associated with a lower risk of necrotizing enterocolitis in very low birth weight infants. *J Perinatol.* 2007; **27**(7): 428–33.
7. Vohr BR, Poindexter BB, Dusick AM, McKinley LT, Wright LL, Langer JC, et al. Beneficial effects of breast milk in the neonatal intensive care unit on the developmental outcome of extremely low birth weight infants at 18 months of age. *Pediatrics.* 2006; **118**(1): e115–23.

8. Poindexter B, Denne SC. Protein needs of the preterm infant. *Neoreviews.* 2003; **4**: e52–9.

9. Groh-Wargo S, Sapsford A. Enteral nutrition support of the preterm infant in the neonatal intensive care unit. *Nutr Clin Pract.* 2009; **24**(3): 363–76.

10. Ziegler EE. Meeting the nutritional needs of the low-birth-weight infant. *Ann Nutr Metab.* 2011; **58 Suppl 1**: 8–18.

11. Butte NF, Goldblum RM, Fehl LM, Loftin K, Smith EO, Garza C, et al. Daily ingestion of immunologic components in human milk during the first four months of life. *Acta Paediatr Scand.* 1984; **73**(3): 296–301.

12. Saarela T, Kokkonen J, Koivisto M. Macronutrient and energy contents of human milk fractions during the first six months of lactation. *Acta Paediatr.* 2005; **94**(9): 1176–81.

13. Gross SJ, David RJ, Bauman L, Tomarelli RM. Nutritional composition of milk produced by mothers delivering preterm. *J Pediatr.* 1980; **96**(4): 641–4.

14. Lemons JA, Moye L, Hall D, Simmons M. Differences in the composition of preterm and term human milk during early lactation. *Pediatr Res.* 1982; **16**(2): 113–7.

15. Bauer J, Gerss J. Longitudinal analysis of macronutrients and minerals in human milk produced by mothers of preterm infants. *Clin Nutr.* 2011; **30**(2): 215–20.

16. Weber A, Loui A, Jochum F, Buhrer C, Obladen M. Breast milk from mothers of very low birthweight infants: variability in fat and protein content. *Acta Paediatr.* 2001; **90**(7): 772–5.

17. Dewey KG, Finley DA, Lonnerdal B. Breast milk volume and composition during late lactation (7–20 months). *J Pediatr Gastroenterol Nutr.* 1984; **3**(5): 713–20.

18. Michaelsen KF, Skafte L, Badsberg JH, Jorgensen M. Variation in macronutrients in human bank milk: influencing factors and implications for human milk banking. *J Pediatr Gastroenterol Nutr.* 1990; **11**(2): 229–39.

19. Kunz C, Rodriguez-Palmero M, Koletzko B, Jensen R. Nutritional and biochemical properties of human milk, Part I: General aspects, proteins, and carbohydrates. *Clin Perinatol.* 1999; **26**(2): 307–33.

20. Butte NF, Garza C, Johnson CA, Smith EO, Nichols BL. Longitudinal changes in milk composition of mothers delivering preterm and term infants. *Early Hum Dev.* 1984; **9**(2): 153–62.

21. Karra MV, Udipi SA, Kirksey A, Roepke JL. Changes in specific nutrients in breast milk during extended lactation. *Am J Clin Nutr.* 1986; **43**(4): 495–503.

22. Lammi-Keefe CJ, Ferris AM, Jensen RG. Changes in human milk at 0600, 1000, 1400, 1800, and 2200 h. *J Pediatr Gastroenterol Nutr.* 1990; **11**(1): 83–8.

23. Ruel MT, Dewey KG, Martinez C, Flores R, Brown KH. Validation of single daytime samples of human milk to estimate the 24-h concentration of lipids in urban Guatemalan mothers. *Am J Clin Nutr.* 1997; **65**(2): 439–44.

24. Daly SE, Di Rosso A, Owens RA, Hartmann PE. Degree of breast emptying explains changes in the fat content, but not fatty acid composition, of human milk. *Exp Physiol.* 1993; **78**(6): 741–55.

25. Hibberd CM, Brooke OG, Carter ND, Haug M, Harzer G. Variation in the composition of breast milk during the first 5 weeks of lactation: implications for the feeding of preterm infants. *Arch Dis Child.* 1982; **57**(9): 658–62.

26. Brenna JT, Varamini B, Jensen RG, Diersen-Schade DA, Boettcher JA, Arterburn LM. Docosahexaenoic and arachidonic acid concentrations in human breast milk worldwide. *Am J Clin Nutr.* 2007; **85**(6): 1457–64.

27. Canfield LM, Clandinin MT, Davies DP, Fernandez MC, Jackson J, Hawkes J, et al. Multinational study of major breast milk carotenoids of healthy mothers. *Eur J Nutr.* 2003; **42**(3): 133–41.

28. Schweigert FJ, Bathe K, Chen F, Buscher U, Dudenhausen JW. Effect of the stage of lactation in humans on carotenoid levels in milk, blood plasma and plasma lipoprotein fractions. *Eur J Nutr.* 2004; **43**(1): 39–44.

29. Stellwagen LM, Vaucher YE, Chan CS, Montminy TD, Kim JH. Pooling expressed breastmilk to provide a consistent feeding composition for premature infants. *Breastfeed Med.* 2013; **8**: 205–9.

30. Fenton TR, Belik J. Routine handling of milk fed to preterm infants can significantly increase osmolality. *J Pediatr Gastroenterol Nutr.* 2002; **35**(3): 298–302.

31. Vieira AA, Soares FV, Pimenta HP, Abranches AD, Moreira ME. Analysis of the influence of pasteurization, freezing/thawing, and offer processes on human milk's macronutrient concentrations. *Early Hum Dev.* 2011; **87**(8): 577–80.

32. Jones F. *Handling Milk. Best Practice for Expressing, Storing and Handling Human Milk in Hospitals, Homes, and Child Care Settings.* Fort Worth, TX: Human Milk Banking Association of North America; 2011.

33. Sauer CW, Kim JH. Human milk macronutrient analysis using point-of-care near-infrared spectrophotometry. *J Perinatol.* 2011; **31**(5): 339–43.

34. Mizuno K, Nishida Y, Taki M, Murase M, Mukai Y, Itabashi K, et al. Is increased fat content of hindmilk due to the size or the number of milk fat globules? *Int Breastfeed J.* 2009; **4**: 7.

35. Bankhead R, Boullata J, Brantley S, Corkins M, Guenter P, Krenitsky J, et al. Enteral nutrition practice recommendations. *JPEN J Parenter Enteral Nutr.* 2009; **33**(2): 122–67.

36. Lessen R, Sapsford A. Expressing human milk. In: Robbins ST, Meyers R, Eds. *Infant Feeding: Guidelines for Preparation of Human Milk an Formula in Health Care Facilities.* Chicago, IL: American Dietetic Association; 2011, 40–70.

37. Jones F. *Education of Mothers. Best Practice for Expressing, Storing and Handling Human Milk in Hospitals, Homes, and Child Care Settings.* Fort Worth, TX: Human Milk Banking Association of North America; 2011.

38. Lonnerdal B. Nutritional and physiologic significance of human milk proteins. *Am J Clin Nutr.* 2003; **77**(6): 1537S–43S.

39. Fomon SJ. Requirements and recommended dietary intakes of protein during infancy. *Pediatr Res.* 1991; **30**(5): 391–5.

40. Picciano MF. Nutrient composition of human milk. *Pediatr Clin North Am.* 2001; **48**(1): 53–67.

41. Boehm G, Stahl B. Oligosaccharides from milk. *J Nutr.* 2007; **137**(3 Suppl 2): 847S–9S.

42. Lapillonne A, Groh-Wargo S, Gonzalez CH, Uauy R. Lipid needs of preterm infants: updated recommendations. *J Pediatr.* 2013; **162**(3 Suppl): S37–47.

43. Wojcik KY, Rechtman DJ, Lee ML, Montoya A, Medo ET. Macronutrient analysis of a nationwide sample of donor breast milk. *J Am Diet Assoc.* 2009; **109**(1): 137–40.

44. Valentine CJ, Morrow G, Fernandez S, Gulati P, Bartholomew D, Long D, et al. Docosahexaenoic acid and amino acid contents in pasteurized donor milk are low for preterm infants. *J Pediatr.* 2010; **157**(6): 906–10.

45. Lawrence RA, Lawrence RM. *Breastfeeding: A Guide for Medical Professionals.* Maryland Heights, MO: Mosby; 2011.

46. Picciano MF. Representative values for constituents of human milk. *Pediatr Clin North Am.* 2001; **48**(1): 263–4.

47. Silvestre D, Fraga M, Gormaz M, Torres E, Vento M. Comparison of mid-infrared transmission spectroscopy with biochemical methods for the determination of macronutrients in human milk. *Matern Child Nutr.* 2012.

48. Casadio YS, Williams TM, Lai CT, Olsson SE, Hepworth AR, Hartmann PE. Evaluation of a mid-infrared analyzer for the determination of the macronutrient composition of human milk. *J Hum Lact.* 2010; **26**(4): 376–83.

49. Corvaglia L, Battistini B, Paoletti V, Aceti A, Capretti MG, Faldella G. Near-infrared reflectance analysis to evaluate the nitrogen and fat content of human milk in neonatal intensive care units. *Arch Dis Child Fetal Neonatal Ed.* 2008; **93**(5): F372–5.
50. Rochow N, Fusch G, Choi A, Chessell L, Elliott L, McDonald K, et al. Target fortification of breast milk with fat, protein, and carbohydrates for preterm infants. *J Pediatr.* 2013; **163**(4): 1001–7.
51. Lefier D, Grappin R, Pochet S. Determination of fat, protein, and lactose in raw milk by Fourier transform infrared spectroscopy and by analysis with a conventional filter-based milk analyzer. *J AOAC Int.* 1996; **79**(3): 711–7.
52. Lucas A, Gibbs JA, Lyster RL, Baum JD. Creamatocrit: simple clinical technique for estimating fat concentration and energy value of human milk. *Br Med J.* 1978; **1**(6119): 1018–20.
53. O'Neill EF, Radmacher PG, Sparks B, Adamkin DH. Creamatocrit analysis of human milk overestimates fat and energy content when compared to a human milk analyzer using mid-infrared spectroscopy. *J Pediatr Gastroenterol Nutr.* 2013; **56**(5): 569–72.
54. Meier PP, Engstrom JL, Zuleger JL, Motykowski JE, Vasan U, Meier WA, et al. Accuracy of a user-friendly centrifuge for measuring creamatocrits on mothers' milk in the clinical setting. *Breastfeed Med.* 2006; **1**(2): 79–87.
55. Wang CD, Chu PS, Mellen BG, Shenai JP. Creamatocrit and the nutrient composition of human milk. *J Perinatol.* 1999; **19**(5): 343–6.
56. Mizuno K, Nishida Y, Salurai M. Accuracy of creamatocrit technique and its efficacy in preterm infants' management. *J Japan Pediatric Soc.* 2006; **110**: 1242–6.
57. Meier PP, Engstrom JL, Murtaugh MA, Vasan U, Meier WA, Schanler RJ. Mothers' milk feedings in the neonatal intensive care unit: accuracy of the creamatocrit technique. *J Perinatol.* 2002; **22**(8): 646–9.
58. Dukhin AS, Goetz PJ, Travers B. Use of ultrasound for characterizing dairy products. *J Dairy Sci.* 2005; **88**(4): 1320–34.
59. Lehmann L, Buckin V. Determination of the heat stability profiles of concentrated milk and milk ingredients using high resolution ultrasonic spectroscopy. *J Dairy Sci.* 2005; **88**(9): 3121–9.
60. Lessen R. Use of skim breast milk for an infant with chylothorax. *ICAN.* 2009; **1**(303–10).
61. Chan GM, Lechtenberg E. The use of fat-free human milk in infants with chylous pleural effusion. *J Perinatol.* 2007; **27**(7): 434–6.
62. Valentine CJ, Hurst NM, Schanler RJ. Hindmilk improves weight gain in low-birth-weight infants fed human milk. *J Pediatr Gastroenterol Nutr.* 1994; **18**(4): 474–7.
63. Arslanoglu S, Moro GE, Ziegler EE, The Wapm Working Group On N. Optimization of human milk fortification for preterm infants: new concepts and recommendations. *J Perinat Med.* 2010; **38**(3): 233–8.
64. Arslanoglu S, Moro GE, Ziegler EE. Adjustable fortification of human milk fed to preterm infants: does it make a difference? *J Perinatol.* 2006; **26**(10): 614–21.
65. Polberger S, Raiha NC, Juvonen P, Moro GE, Minoli I, Warm A. Individualized protein fortification of human milk for preterm infants: comparison of ultrafiltrated human milk protein and a bovine whey fortifier. *J Pediatr Gastroenterol Nutr.* 1999; **29**(3): 332–8.
66. de Halleux V, Rigo J. Variability in human milk composition: benefit of individualized fortification in very-low-birth-weight infants. *Am J Clin Nutr.* 2013; **98**(2): 529S–35S.
67. Robbins ST, Meyers R, Eds. *Expressing Human Milk.* Chicago, IL: American Dietetic Association; 2011.
68. Slutzah M, Codipilly CN, Potak D, Clark RM, Schanler RJ. Refrigerator storage of expressed human milk in the neonatal intensive care unit. *J Pediatr.* 2010; **156**(1): 26–8.
69. Silprasert A, Dejsarai W, Keawvichit R, Amatayakul K. Effect of storage on the creamatocrit and total energy content of human milk. *Hum Nutr Clin Nutr.* 1987; **41**(1): 31–6.

70. Quan R, Yang C, Rubinstein S, Lewiston NJ, Sunshine P, Stevenson DK, et al. Effects of microwave radiation on anti-infective factors in human milk. *Pediatrics.* 1992; **89**(4 Pt 1): 667–9.

71. Tacken KJ, Vogelsang A, van Lingen RA, Slootstra J, Dikkeschei BD, van Zoeren-Grobben D. Loss of triglycerides and carotenoids in human milk after processing. *Arch Dis Child Fetal Neonatal Ed.* 2009; **94**(6): F447–50.

72. Gabrielski L, Lessen R. Centralized model of human milk preparation and storage in a state-of-the-art human milk lab. *ICAN.* 2011; **3**: 225–32.

73. Dumm M, Peel L, Jones A, Hunter C, Kendall-Harris M. Technician training reduced formula preparation errors. *ICAN.* 2010; **2**: 258–60.

74. Rogers SP, Hicks PD, Hamzo M, Veit LE, Abrams SA. Continuous feedings of fortified human milk lead to nutrient losses of fat, calcium and phosphorous. *Nutrients.* 2010; **2**(3): 230–40.

75. Quigley MA, Henderson G, Anthony MY, McGuire W. Formula milk versus donor breast milk for feeding preterm or low birth weight infants. *Cochrane Database Syst Rev.* 2007; (4): CD002971.

76. Boyd CA, Quigley MA, Brocklehurst P. Donor breast milk versus infant formula for preterm infants: systematic review and meta-analysis. *Arch Dis Child Fetal Neonatal Ed.* 2007; **92**(3): F169–75.

77. Parker MG, Barrero-Castillero A, Corwin BK, Kavanagh PL, Belfort MB, Wang CJ. Pasteurized human donor milk use among US level 3 neonatal intensive care units. *J Hum Lact.* 2013; **29**(3): 381–9.

78. Smithers LG, Markrides M, Gibson RA. Human milk fatty acids from lactating mothers of preterm infants: a study revealing wide intra- and inter-individual variation. *Prostaglandins Leukot Essent Fatty Acids.* 2010; **83**(1): 9–13.

79. Chulei R, Xiafang I, Hongseng M, Xiulan M, Guizheng I, Gianhong D, et al. Milk composition in women from five different regions of China, the great diversity of milk fatty acids. *J Nutr.* 1995; **125**: 2993–8.

80. Martinez FE, Desai ID, Davidson AG, Nakai S, Radcliffe A. Ultrasonic homogenization of expressed human milk to prevent fat loss during tube feeding. *J Pediatr Gastroenterol Nutr.* 1987; **6**(4): 593–7.

81. Narayanan I, Singh B, Harvey D. Fat loss during feeding of human milk. *Arch Dis Child.* 1984; **59**(5): 475–7.

82. Mendelson RA, Anderson GH, Bryan MH. Zinc, copper and iron content of milk from mothers of preterm and full-term infants. *Early Hum Dev.* 1982; **6**(2): 145–51.

83. Moran JR, Vaughan R, Stroop S, Coy S, Johnston H, Greene HL. Concentrations and total daily output of micronutrients in breast milk of mothers delivering preterm: a longitudinal study. *J Pediatr Gastroenterol Nutr.* 1983; **2**(4): 629–34.

84. Chappell JE, Francis T, Clandinin MT. Vitamin A and E content of human milk at early stages of lactation. *Early Hum Dev.* 1985; **11**(2): 157–67.

85. Schanler RJ, Oh W. Composition of breast milk obtained from mothers of premature infants as compared to breast milk obtained from donors. *J Pediatr.* 1980; **96**(4): 679–81.

86. Ridout E, Melara D, Rottinghaus S, Thureen PJ. Blood urea nitrogen concentration as a marker of amino-acid intolerance in neonates with birthweight less than 1250 g. *J Perinatol.* 2005; **25**(2): 130–3.

87. Roggero P, Gianni ML, Morlacchi L, Piemontese P, Liotto N, Taroni F, et al. Blood urea nitrogen concentrations in low-birth-weight preterm infants during parenteral and enteral nutrition. *J Pediatr Gastroenterol Nutr.* 2010; **51**(2): 213–5.

88. Heine WE, Klein PD, Reeds PJ. The importance of alpha-lactalbumin in infant nutrition. *J Nutr.* 1991; **121**(3): 277–83.

89. Lonnerdal B, Woodhouse LR, Glazier C. Compartmentalization and quantitation of protein in human milk. *J Nutr.* 1987;117(8):1385-95.

90. Kleyn DH, Trout JR, Weber M. Determination of fat in raw milk: comparison of Mojonnier (ether extraction) and Gerber method. *J Assoc Off Anal Chem* 1988;71(4):851–3.
91. West LG, Llorente MA. High performance liquid chromatographic determination of lactose in milk. *J Assoc Off Anal Chem.* 1981;64(4):805–7.

12 Mathematical Description of Postnatal Growth
Z-Scores and Statistical Control Process Analysis

Ian J. Griffin

A BRIEF HISTORY OF GROWTH CHARTS

The assessment and interpretation of growth is an essential part of care of the newborn infant, and its importance has been appreciated for most of the history of neonatology. Pierre Budin devotes a large part of his textbook from 1900, *Le Nourrisson: Alimentation et hygiene. Enfants debiles et enfants nes a terme,*[1] to the description and assessment of the growth of the newborn infant. Building on the earlier work of Quetelet[2] and Bowditch,[3] he uses growth charts that will be immediately familiar to a modern reader. Against a grid composed of horizontal divisions marked in age, and a vertical axis of weight, he plots the weight of the individual infant and the "average" growth of "normal" infants[1] (Figure 12.1). From the start of Lecture VI we read:

> I have represented graphically the progress of the average infant's weight during the first year... If a point be placed each week on this chart, in the space corresponding to the weight and age of the infant, the joining of the points will show the curve of its growth, and by comparison, whether it is inferior, equal, or superior to the normal. These charts are of great service both in hospital and in private practice.[1] (p. 86)

One thing may strike us as unusual about Budin's charts; his reference curve consists of a single smoothed line based on the average weight of an infant during the first year of life. No estimate of the variability around this average is presented, nor are differences between the genders mentioned.

In 1948, Dancis[4] published his "growth grid" based on 100 low birth weight infants; the first true "peer" reference dataset.* For the first time, the reference data

---

* Although the title of Dancis's paper refers to "premature infants," it uses the historical definition of prematurity of a birth weight < 2.5 kg, a population that would now be called low birth weight.

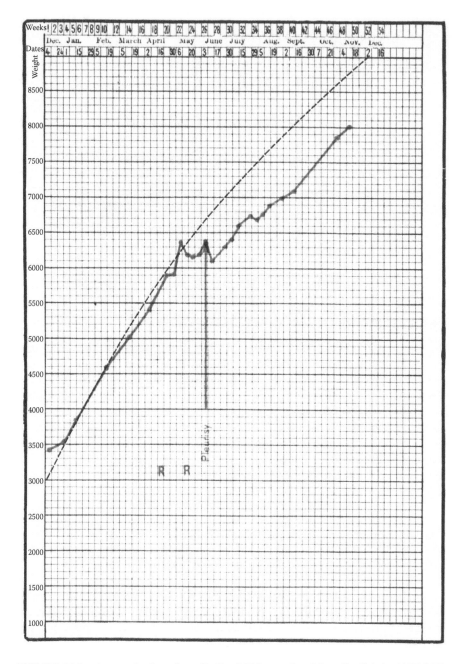

FIGURE 12.1 A growth chart from Budin (1900, translated into English in 1907).[1] The growth of a female infant is plotted (solid line) and compared to the expected growth of newborns (broken line). The infant grew well until approximately 20 weeks of age when "the infant was brought to me . . . as the mother was attacked with acute pleurisy [and] her doctor had forbidden nursing." The infant was started on sterilized milk but grew poorly until the fluid intake was increased from 600 g/d to 675 g/d.

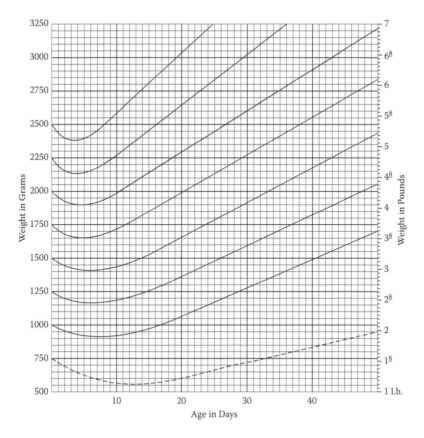

FIGURE 12.2   The "growth grid" of Dancis.[4] Expected weight gain for LBW infants born at 750 g, 100 g, 1250 g, 1500 g, 1750 g, 2000 g, 2250 g, and 2500 g are shown. (Figure © Elsevier Ltd, Kidlington, UK. With permission.)

is represented by a series of similar but diverging curves. However, these curves do not represent percentiles; instead, they represent the expected (i.e., average) growth rates at different initial weights.

A significant advance in presentation of growth standards is seen in Lubchenco's intrauterine growth curves.[5] Using data from live born infants between 24 and 42 weeks gestation, she produced curves showing both the mean weight and the 10th, 25th, 75th, and 90th percentiles of the population. Now the growth chart provides data not only on the mean weight at different ages, but also on the expected variability around that mean. These charts and those related to them[5–7] have established the *de facto* format of most growth charts, including the most recent growth charts for preterm infants[8–10] (e.g., Figure 12.2).

VISUAL INTERPRETATION OF GROWTH CHARTS

Most current growth curves are presented as a family of upward sloping lines (as in Figure 12.3), and by the time of hospital discharge most preterm infants lie below the

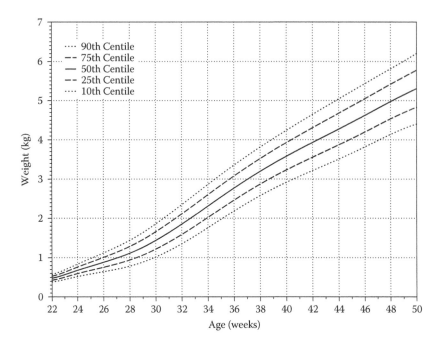

FIGURE 12.3 Weight data from Fenton 2003 charts for preterm infants calculated from Reference 8. Weight data is shown as mean, and 10th, 25th, 75th, and 90th percentiles.

lowest reference line.[11] Identification of catch-up growth depends on perceiving that the growth curve of the infant is approaching the percentile line above. This type of graph, where the quantity of interest is the difference between two curves, is called a curve-difference graph, and it is much more difficult to interpret visually than a plot of the difference itself.[12,13] For example, in Figure 12.4a, four 1-week long line segments are shown, each beginning 300 g below the 10th percentile. The question is, which (if any) are showing catch-up growth? Although it can be difficult to tell by visual inspection, line B is increasing at the same rate as the 10th percentile, lines A and C are increasing 10% more than the 10th percentile, and line D is increasing 20% more than the 10th percentile. The difficulty of visually assessing data presented in this format can lead to misperceptions that could lead to failure to detect growth that is diverging from surrounding percentile lines (growth faltering) or converging with them (catch-up growth, or excessive growth). However, if the curve-difference chart (Figure 12.4a) is replaced with a plot of the absolute difference between the line segment and the 10th percentile (Figure 12.4b), it is much easier to see that in three of the cases (A, C, and D) the distance from the 10th percentile is decreasing, that is, catch-up growth is occurring.

The difficulty correctly interpreting the data in Figure 12.4 not surprising, as visual perception of angles and slopes is frequently inaccurate.[13,14] However, it is better for horizontally and vertically orientated lines than for those placed at other angles.[13,15,16] Indeed, such misperception of angles is the basis of the well-known Poggendorff illusion (Figure 12.5). Two parallel lines, A and B, enter the lower

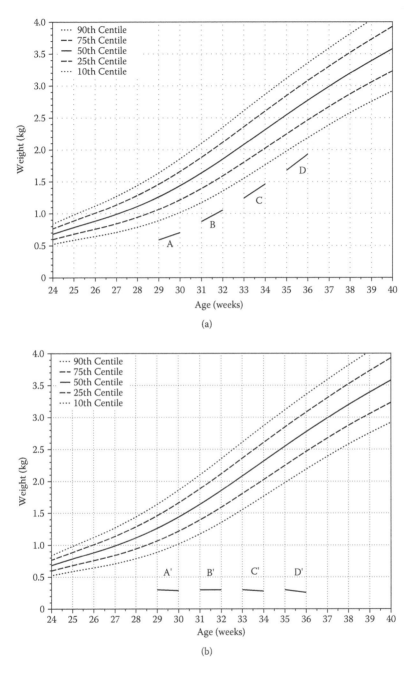

FIGURE 12.4 (a) Four 1-week-long line segments representing short-term growth presented against the backdrop of the Fenton (2003) percentile from 24 to 40 weeks. Which, if any, segment is catching up to the 3rd percentile line? (b) The same data is shown, but as a difference between the 10th percentile and the line segment. Horizontal and vertical axis scales remain the same as for (a).

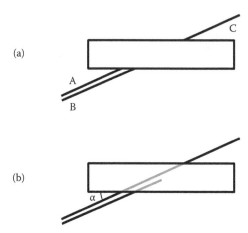

FIGURE 12.5 (a) and (b) The Poggendorff illusion. Due to a tendency to overestimate acute angles, line C is often misperceived to be continuation of line B (upper panel), whereas it is actually a continuation of line B (see lower panel).

border of a masked box, and one emerges from the upper border (Figure 12.5a). A common misperception is that line C is a continuation of line B. However, C is a continuation of B (Figure 12.5b). This illusion results from a tendency for humans to overestimate the angle α. In the preterm infant, the rate of catch-up growth could be perceived to be greater than it really was as the angle between the infant's growth curve and the nearest percentile would be overestimated.

Alternatively, the distance between percentile lines and individual points may be interpreted by estimating the vertical distance (length) between the 10th percentile and the start and the end of the line. However, length is only slightly better perceived than are angle and slope in scientific charts.[13] Furthermore, the percentile lines on growth charts diverge with increasing age (see Figure 12.3). These diverging lines could lead to misperception of length. For example, in the cigarette illusion (or forced perceptive illusion, Figure 12.6) two cylinders (cigarettes) of equal length are shown against a grid of lines. The grid produces the illusion of perspective and this leads to the right-hand cigarette being misperceived as being longer than the left-hand one. The same effect can be produced with more subtle visual cues. In the Ponzo illusion (Figure 12.7), the upper horizontal line is usually perceived to be longer than the lower horizontal line, even though they are actually the same length. In growth charts, such a misperception may lead to a relative underestimation of the distance from a percentile line when percentile lines are further apart. In theory, this could lead to over-estimation of the degree of catch-up growth, or a false perception of catch-up growth that is not, in fact, present.

Visual interpretation of data on growth charts is therefore likely to be difficult to interpret and analyze visually. Small (but clinically important) changes in growth may be missed or perceived to be present when they are not.

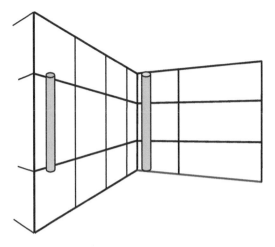

FIGURE 12.6 The cigarette illusion. Two identical cigarette-shaped objects are shown against a grid on straight lines. Due to an attempt to interpret the image in three dimensions, a false perspective is imposed on the image causing the left-hand cigarette to appear smaller than the right-hand one.

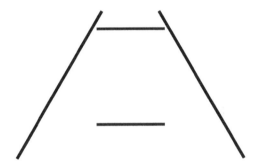

FIGURE 12.7 The Ponzo illusion. The upper horizontal line appears to be longer than the lower one, even though they are really the same length.

OPTIMIZED PRESENTATION OF ANTHROPOMETRIC DATA

Most current neonatal growth charts are difficult to interpret due to the following

1. They are curve-difference charts. The data for both the individual and the comparison population is constantly changing with age, and assessment of growth relies on correctly interpreting the differences between two curves.
2. Growth is signified by an upward sloping line, and the assessment of adequacy of growth depends on comparing that oblique line to one or more other oblique lines. However, these comparison lines are non-parallel, but gradually diverge as age increases. This can lead to misperceptions, as humans are relatively poorly able to assess accurately slope and angle, especially for oblique lines.[13–16]

CHARACTERISTIC OF A BETTER GROWTH CHART

Given these limitation, a better growth chart would

1. Present data as the absolute difference between the individual and the comparison population.
2. Present normal growth as a horizontal or vertical line, rather than as an oblique line.
3. Avoid the presence of obliquely orientated lines that may skew perception.[15]

All of these requirements are met by the use of Z-score growth charts.

Z-Scores

The Z-score, or standard deviation score (SDS), represents the relative position of an individual data point relative to a distribution. It is calculated from population mean and standard deviation (SD) using the following equation:

$$Z\text{-score} = \frac{(\text{Observed value} - \text{Population mean})}{\text{Population standard deviation}}.$$

In our instance, where we want to compare the data for an individual to that of a comparison population, the equivalent equation is:

$$Z\text{-score} = \frac{(\text{Individual's value} - \text{Comparison population mean})}{\text{Comparison population standard deviation}}.$$

Z-scores are, by definition, normally distributed with a mean of 0 and a standard deviation of 1. A Z-score of 0 is therefore equivalent to the population mean, a Z-score of +1 is 1 standard deviation greater than the mean, and a Z-score of –2 is 2 standard deviations below the mean. Z-scores can be converted to percentiles using the distribution of the standard normal distribution.

Historically, it has been difficult to calculate Z-scores as some growth data, especially weight, is highly skewed and a single SD cannot represent the data at any age.[17] However, in recent years, improved statistical methods such as Cole's LMS method have helped to resolve this problem. This method represents the distribution of data against time using three variables:[17,18]

M = the age-specific mean
L = the age-specific Box-Cox power needed to normalize the distribution
S = the age-specific SD of the Box-Cox transformed data

The age-specific values for L, M, and S can be used to convert an individual value (x) into a Z-score using the equation

$$\text{Z-score} = \frac{(x / M)^{L} - 1}{L.S}$$

and the value (x) at any particular Z-score can be calculated from the equation

$$x = M.(1 + L.S.Z)^{(1/L)}.$$

The LMS method or an alternative (Healy's moving box[19,20]) is used by about half of recent neonatal growth standards,[21] including three of the largest populations.[8–10, 22] Summary tables of LMS values for weight, length, and head circumference have been published for those three large neonatal references[9, 10, 22] and are also available for term infants as the WHO Growth Standards[23] and the 2000 U.S. growth charts produced by the CDC.[24]

DEVELOPMENT OF Z-SCORE CHARTS

The published summary tables of L, M, and S values for neonatal charts are published as weekly values, rather than as the underlying equations.[9, 10, 22] These data are not well suited to the construction of a continuous model of neonatal growth, unless intermediate values are interpolated.

For example, the published L, M, and S values for the 2003 Fenton growth charts are available as summary values for every week between 22 weeks and 50 weeks,[22] but intermediate values can be calculated by modeling. The values for L do not change with age, and are 1.0 for weight and for length, and 1.5 for head circumference.[22] The M and S values for weight, length, and head circumference were fitted by age using a modified multiple fractional polynomial method[25, 26] where the quantity of interest (M or S) is regressed against age raised to the power of +2, +1, +0.5, 0, −0.5, −1, and −2 (or age squared, age, the square root of age, Ln(age), and to the reciprocals of age squared, age and square root of age).[25] The power terms were added and removed sequentially, until no subjectively meaningful change in fit was seen.[25]

The regression coefficients for the six fits are shown in Table 12.1, and fit the reported M and S variables closely. The adjusted r^2 values for the models are good, but are a little poorer for the S term (especially for head circumference S) than for the M terms. The summary values for the main percentiles also closely fit the modeled data (data not shown).

INTERPRETATION OF Z-SCORE CHARTS

Growth, shown on a Z-score chart, is easy to interpret. The position on the vertical (y) axis shows the infant's relative position compared to the comparison population. An individual with a y-value of +1 is one standard deviation above the comparison population mean. A normal rate of growth (i.e., the same as the comparison population) is denoted by a horizontal line. Slower than expected growth (including growth faltering) is shown by a line sloping downward, while an upward sloping line is indicative of faster growth than the reference population (including catch-up growth).

TABLE 12.1

Coefficients from Multiple Fractional Polynomial Regression for the M and S Values for Weight, Length, and Head Circumference

	Weight M	Weight S	Length M
Age^2	−15.67125577	+2.8817066950	+11.88127569
Age	+21488.42066	−3884.763051	−16205.06800
$Age^{0.5}$	−799683.4466	+143240.9514	+601977.4516
Ln(Age)	+3254232.336	−577420.0712	−2446787.66
$1/Age^{0.5}$	+26659484.15	−4684872.851	−20034032.14
$1/Age$	−23880211.67	+4155235.628	+1794500.419
$1/Age^2$	+19344601.34	−3298147.860	−14553061.47
Intercept	−11411607.48	+2013797.599	8576027.995
Model adjusted r^2	>0.9999	0.9998	>0.9999

	Length S	Head Circumference M	Head Circumference S
Age^2	+0.21648380	−3.016271302	+0.149353382
Age	−292.0762707	+3253.736651	−171.7921212
$Age^{0.5}$	+10773.57986	−106983.3047	+5808.043555
Ln(Age)	−43432.5636	+383881.4743	−2.13338761
$1/Age^{0.5}$	−352315.5970	+2769549.619	−156571.5381
$1/Age$	+312343.9500	−2185747.182	+124520.3508
$1/Age^2$	−247519.878	+1388657.7558	−76718.14401
Intercept	+151468.1984	−1248887.295	+70288.64532
Model adjusted r^2	0.9955	>0.9999	0.9990

Source: From Reference 22.

For example, the growth of a hypothetical infant who is born weighing 1 kg at 27 weeks of gestation, and who then gains weight at a rate of 1.2% of bodyweight each day is shown in Figure 12.8. The infant's weight (Figure 12.8a) is near the 50th percentile at birth, but subsequent growth is slower than the *in utero* rate and by 36 weeks the baby lies below the 10th percentile. Between 36 and 44 weeks, some catch-up in weight is seen. The same data is show on a Z-score growth chart (Figure 12.8b). The infant's weight Z-score at birth is approximately 0. Between birth and 37 weeks, the Z-score declines, showing that the infant is growing more slowly than the reference population. This decline does not mean that the infant's weight is decreasing, only that the infant is growing slower than the reference population. After about 36 weeks, weight gain is faster than the comparison population; that is, there is catch-up growth. The onset of catch-up growth is much more easy to appreciate in the Z-score chart (lower panel) where the growth curve begins to increase, than it is from the weight chart (upper panel) where it occurs when the slope of the line begins to increase, rather than decrease.

Also shown in Figure 12.8b is the weight Z-score calculated from the published summary data for L, M, and S. Calculations using the published weekly values lead to an artificial saw-tooth pattern in weight Z-score (Figure 12.8b, broken line).

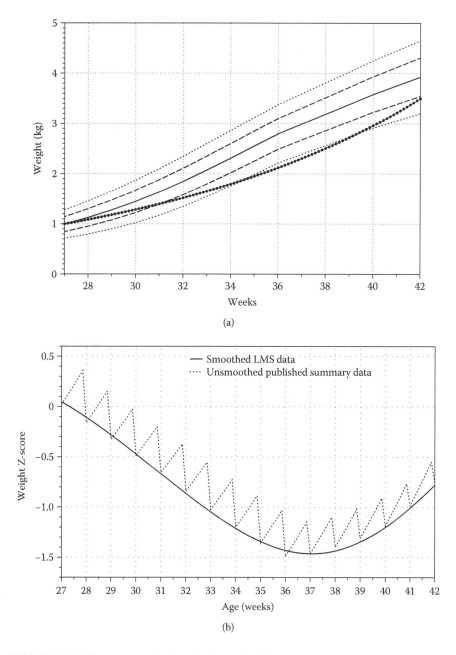

(a)

(b)

FIGURE 12.8 Z-score growth chart for a hypothetical 1 kg, 27 weeks gestation infant who gains 1.2% of body weight every day. (a) Data is shown for absolute weight, and for the Z-score calculated from weekly published summary[22] (broken line) (b) and for fitted data (solid line).

However, using modeled values of M and S leads to much smoother change in weight Z-score (solid line).

Also shown (Figures 12.9a and 12.9b) are approximate mean data for three cohorts of infants from the NICHD network—those born at 24 or 25 weeks gestation, those at 26 or 27 weeks gestation, and those at 28 or 29 weeks gestation.[11] The

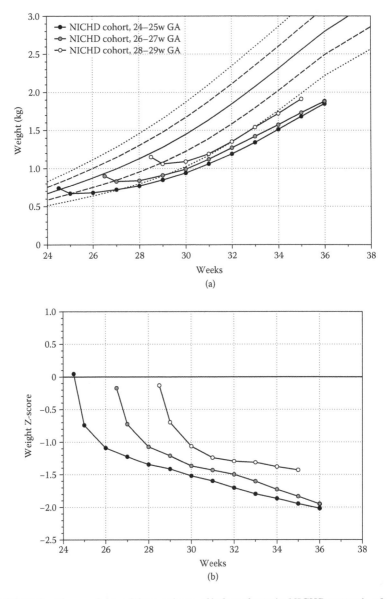

FIGURE 12.9 Mean weights of three cohorts of infants from the NICHD network, of gestational age 24 to 25 weeks, 26 to 27 weeks, and 28 to 29 weeks.[11] Approximate data extracted from the figures in Reference 11 are compared to the Fenton comparison cohort as both weight-for-age charts (a) and as weight Z-scores for age (b).

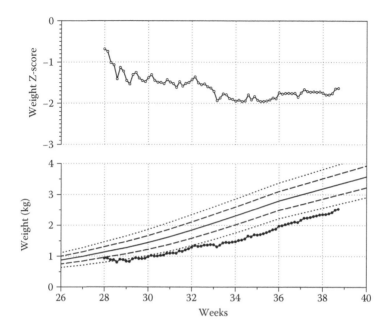

FIGURE 12.10 Growth charts for a 28 weeks gestation infant with a relatively straightforward course who was discharged at 39 weeks. The upper panel shows the growth expressed as weight Z-scores, and the lower panel shows the weight in kilograms.

mean weight for all three cohorts begins near the 50th percentile (Figure 12.9a) or close to a Z-score of 0 (Figure 12.9b), but all three groups decline relative to the comparison population to lie below the 10th percentile or below a Z-score of –1.29. Even after 34 to 35 weeks corrected gestational age, all three cohorts are growing more slowly than the comparison population, and this is clearer from downward sloping lines on the Z-score growth chart than it is for the raw weight data. Finally, growth data is shown for a preterm infant with relatively unremarkable neonatal courses, both as weight charts and as weight Z-score charts (Figure 12.10).

STATISTICAL ANALYSIS OF Z-SCORE CHARTS

The conversion of growth data to Z-scores also allows for simple statistical comparisons between the data for an individual and for the comparison population, as the normal range for Z-scores should be, by definition, ±1.96.

We have used two simple analyses to identify outliers and trends in the Z-score data.

Identification of Outliers

To identify outliers, we have borrowed from statistical control process analysis. This is a method used to assist in manufacturing quality control that is increasingly being applied to epidemiology and health care.[27] One tool of statistical control process is the control chart (Figure 12.11), which plots sequential measures of a parameter against time. Upper and lower control limits (typically ±3 SD from the mean) are

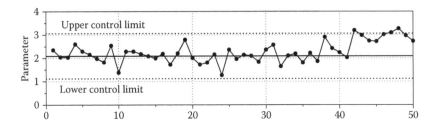

FIGURE 12.11 A control chart. The output of an industrial process is measured sequentially, and the result is plotted on the y-axis against its number in the sequence. Upper and lower control limits (mean ±SD) are shown. Toward the end of the sequence of measurement an unknown change occurs, and the parameter increases to lie above the upper control limit.

drawn, and if the observed parameters exceed these limits it may be a sign of a change in the process governing the outcome.[27]

We have modified this approach to identify individual measurements that diverge from the mean and standard deviation over a 5-day or 10-day period.

For example, for each day "n" the anthropometric measure is converted to a Z-score (Z_n). The mean Z-score (X) and standard deviation for the 5-day period including that day "n" and the preceding (n–4) are calculated in the usual manner:

$$X_{(n,n-4)} = (Z_n + Z_{n-1} + Z_{n-2} + Z_{n-3} + Z_{n-4})/5$$

and

$$SD_{[n,n-4]} = \sqrt{\Sigma((X_{[n,n-4]} - Z_n)^2 + (X_{[n,n-4]} - Z_{n-1})^2 + (X_{[n,n-4]} - Z_{n-2})^2}$$
$$+ (X_{[n,n-4]} - Z_{n-3})^2 + (X_{[n,n-4]} - Z_{n-4})^2)/4.$$

The outlier score over 5-days is calculated from

$$(Z_n - X_{[n,n-4]})/SD_{[n,n-4]}.$$

This describes how far that day's value is from the 5-day mean value, expressed in multiples of the 5-day rolling SD. This can be shown graphically with an outlier plot, where the outlier score for each day is shown (Figure 12.12a).

A similar method is used to estimate the outlier score over 10 days.

Identification of Trends

For new weight measurement, the 5-day slope of the regression line of Z-score against age is calculated and the significance value of the line compared to zero is calculated using standard statistical methods. Once again the slope is plotted against time to show whether the 5-day or 10-day slope is significantly greater than or less than zero, and to show how significant the difference is ($p < 0.05$ or $p < 0.01$) (Figure 12.12b).

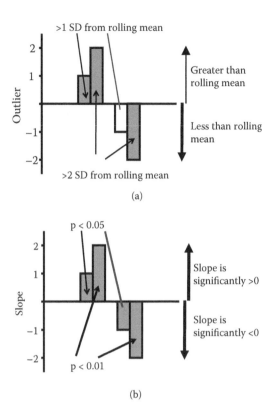

(a)

(b)

FIGURE 12.12 Format of outlier plots and slope plots. (a) Outlier plots show when that day's Z-score is >1 or >2 SD from the rolling mean, and whether the outlier is greater or less than the rolling mean. (b) Trend plots show if the recent trend is significantly greater than or less than 0, and whether the p-value is <0.05 or <0.01.

INTERPRETATION OF TREND AND OUTLIER PLOTS

The Z-score growth chart for an individual growing along his or her percentile line would be an approximately horizontal line with random fluctuations around it. The 5-day and 10-day rolling means would be similar to one another, as would the 5-day and 10-day SD. Approximately 16% of points would be expected to have an outlier score of +1 or more, and a further 16% would have an outlier score of −1 or less; 2.3% would be >+2 and 2.3% <−2.

However, the growth of preterm infants is not so uniform. Initially, it is usually slower than the comparison population, and the Z-score growth line trends downward (Figures 12.9 and 12.10). Sometimes, catch-up growth will be observed, most often when infants are changed to *ad libitum* feeds before discharge, and the Z-score growth line will slope upward during these periods. A Z-score growth chart with outlier and trend data for a 27 weeks gestation infant is shown in Figure 12.13. Between 28 and 31 weeks there is growth faltering and the weight Z-score begins to fall. In this case, this is first seen as a negative outlier score and later by significant negative scores on the trend analysis.

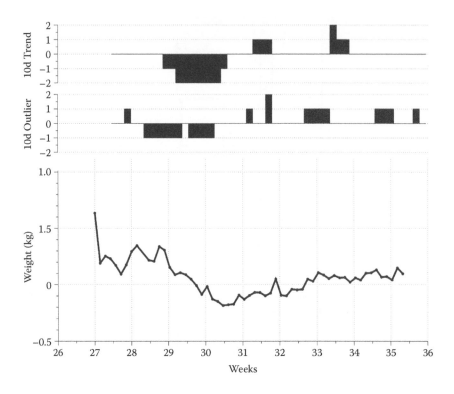

FIGURE 12.13 Z-score chart for weight for a 27 weeks gestation preterm infant. Also shown are the 10-day slope (trend) chart, and the 10-day outlier chart (see Figure 12.12 for details of outlier and trend charts).

Whether the prevailing trend is upward or downward, the mean Z-score calculated over 5 days will be closer to the current value than the value calculated over 10 days. Even though the SD calculated at 5 days is also smaller than that calculated over 10 days, the net result is that the outlier score (the difference from rolling mean divided by the standard deviation) is larger when calculations are carried out over 10 days than over 5 days. However, the 5-day outlier score identifies outliers sooner than does the 10-day score. This is a double-edged sword; if growth rate does change, then the 5-day outlier score will identify it sooner than the 10-day score. However, errors in measurement or in data entry are more likely to be identified as outliers when calculated over 5 days rather than 10 days.

The Z-score trend is less affected whether they are calculated over 5 days or 10 days. Even if a single day's measurement is unexpectedly high or low, this may be identified more easily on the 10-day trend than the 5-day trend, especially if the previous trend was relatively flat.

It has been our subjective clinical experience that the use of the 10-day trend is most helpful for identifying new growth faltering or the onset of catch-up growth. For example, a Z-score growth chart is shown for a 24 weeks gestation infant with 10-day trend and outlier plots (Figure 12.14) and with 5-day trend and outlier plots

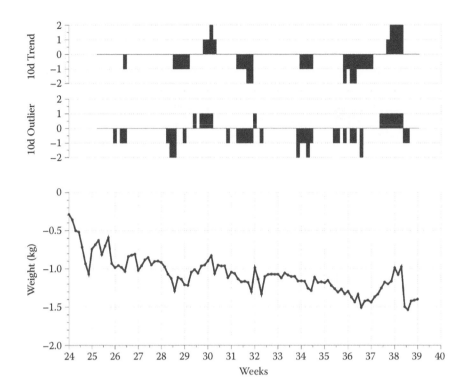

FIGURE 12.14   Z-score chart for weight for a 24 weeks gestation preterm infant. Also shown are the 10-day slope (trend) chart, and the 10-day outlier chart (see Figure 12.12 for details of outlier and trend charts).

(Figure 12.15). The use of the 10-day trend can be supplemented by the 5-day or 10-day outlier analysis. As 5-day outlier scores >1 or <−1 are not infrequent, we would typically await two such scores within a 3-day period before responding.

COMPUTERIZED CALCULATION OF Z-SCORES, OUTLIERS, AND TRENDS

The mathematics underlying the conversion of weight, length, and head circumference data to Z-scores, and the estimation of outlier scores and trends is simple in theory, but somewhat cumbersome in practice. However, the mathematics can easily be built into a spreadsheet. An example using the 2003 Fenton dataset[8, 22] is available online (http://www.iangriffin.net or http://members.shaw.ca/growthchart/). Patient demographic data (including gestational age and date of birth) and anthropometric measures (weight, length, and head circumference) are entered on one page of the workbook (Figure 12.16). Weight, length, and head circumference Z-scores are calculated automatically. In addition, 5-day and 10-day outlier scores are displaced numerically showing how many SDs that day's weight Z-score is from the 5-day or 10-day rolling mean Z-score (−2, −1, +1, +2, etc.). The 5-day and 10-day weight Z-score slope is calculated and a value displayed if the slope is significant. Positive

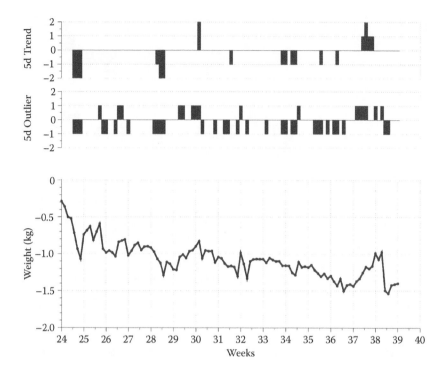

FIGURE 12.15 Z-score chart for weight for the infant shown in Figure 12.14. Also shown are the 5-day slope (trend) chart and the 5-day outlier chart (see Figure 12.12 for details of outlier and trend charts).

slopes are shown as positive numbers that denote how significant the slope diverges from zero ($1 = p < 0.05$, $2 = p < 0.01$, $3 = p < 0.001$). Negative slopes are shown in a similar manner with slopes of -1, -2, and -3 representing slopes of $p < 0.05$, $p < 0.01$, or $p < 0.001$, respectively. Finally, Z-score growth charts for weight (Figure 12.17) and for weight, length, and head circumference (not shown) are generated and plotted automatically.

Similar workbooks using other reference standards, including the Olson data of 2010 for preterm infants,[9] or the WHO 2006 dataset for term infants[23,28] can be produced in the same way and several are available online (http://www.iangriffin.net).

LIMITATIONS OF Z-SCORE CHARTS

Although our experience is that Z-score growth charts, and to a lesser extent outlier and trend plots, improve the assessment of growth in preterm infants, problems remain. These approaches do nothing to improve the quality of the raw anthropometric data. Measurement error in neonatal growth assessments can be surprisingly high,[29–31] even for weight under optimum condition.[32]

Computerized generation of growth charts, however, does remove systemic errors in plotting gestational age[33] as well as the random plotting errors that are relatively

NAME:	Baby Boy SMALL
ID	
DoB (mm/dd/yy)	12/12/12
Birth-weight	0.46 kg
Gestation	23 w
	1 d
Gender	M

Date	PNA (d)	PMA (d)	PMA (w)	Wt (kg)	L (cm)	HC (cm)	Wt Z	LZ	HC Z	5d outlier	10d outlier	5d trend	10d trend
12/12/12	0	162	23 1/7	0.46	28.5	20.5	(1.26)	(0.88)	(0.37)	•	•	•	•
12/13/12	1	163	23 2/7	0.46			(1.36)	•	•	•	•	•	•
12/14/12	2	164	23 3/7				•	•	•	•	•	•	•
12/15/12	3	165	23 4/7	0.445			(1.69)	•	•	•	•	•	•
12/16/12	4	166	23 5/7	0.445			(1.77)	•	•	•	•	•	•
12/17/12	5	167	23 6/7	0.49		20.4	(1.46)	•	(0.97)	•	•	•	•
12/18/12	6	168	24	0.51		20.5	(1.38)	•	(1.00)	•	•	•	•
12/19/12	7	169	24 1/7	0.53			(1.30)	•	•	1	•	1	•
12/20/12	8	170	24 2/7	0.54			(1.29)	•	•	0	•	1	•
12/21/12	9	171	24 3/7	0.54	29		(1.36)	(1.50)	•	0	•	-	•
12/22/12	10	172	24 4/7	0.51		20.5	(1.64)	•	(1.40)	(1)	•	-	•
12/23/12	11	173	24 5/7	0.52		20.2	(1.62)	•	(1.69)	(1)	•	(1)	•
12/24/12	12	174	24 6/7	0.49			(1.87)	•	•	(1)	(1)	(2)	-
12/25/12	13	175	25	0.52			(1.71)	•	•	0	0	-	-
12/26/12	14	176	25 1/7	0.52		20.5	(1.75)	•	(1.78)	0	(1)	-	(1)
12/27/12	15	177	25 2/7	0.54			(1.67)	•	•	0	0	-	(1)
2/1/13	51	213	30 3/7	1.01	36.2	25.6	(1.49)	(1.96)	(1.80)	(1)	0	-	-
2/2/13	52	214	30 4/7	1.025		25.8	(1.51)	•	(1.75)	(1)	(1)	(1)	-
2/3/13	53	215	30 5/7	1.06		25.8	(1.47)	•	(1.83)	0	0	-	-
2/4/13	54	216	30 6/7	1.085			(1.47)	•	•	0	0	-	-
2/5/13	55	217	31	1.105		26.3	(1.47)	•	(1.67)	0	0	-	(1)
2/6/13	56	218	31 1/7	1.135			(1.46)	•	•	0	0	-	-
2/7/13	57	219	31 2/7	1.16	36.5	26.5	(1.45)	(2.29)	(1.70)	1	0	-	-
2/8/13	58	220	31 3/7	1.185	36.8		(1.45)	(2.24)	•	0	0	-	-
2/9/13	59	221	31 4/7	1.215			(1.44)	•	•	1	0	1	-
2/10/13	60	222	31 5/7	1.24			(1.44)	•	•	0	1	1	2
2/11/13	61	223	31 6/7	1.265			(1.44)	•	•	0	0	-	1

Instructions | Z-scores | Wt Chart | Wt, L & HC Chart | +

FIGURE 12.16 Data entry page of Z-score calculation spreadsheet. Patient demographics are entered in cells C2:C9, and weight, length, and head circumference data are entered in the appropriate cells in columns J, K, and L. Weight, length, and head circumference Z-scores are calculated automatically and displaced in the corresponding cells in columns M, N, and O. Outlier scores for the previous 5 days and 10 days are displaced in the corresponding cells in columns P and Q, and the 5-day and 10-day trends in columns R and S.

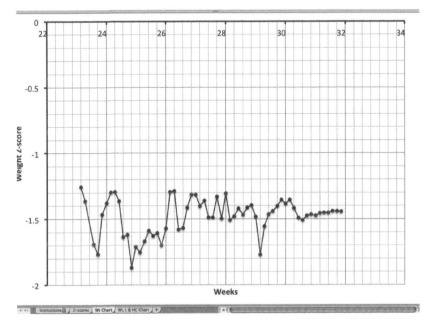

FIGURE 12.17 Weight Z-score plot generated from data-entry sheet (see Figure 12.16).

common in the use of neonatal growth charts.[32, 34] Some of these errors, however, will be replaced by transcription errors, as data is entered incorrectly into the computer spreadsheets.

Although the LMS method allows easy calculation of Z-scores, the Standard Errors for calculated Z-scores or percentiles are worse for lower Z-scores if L is positive.[18] This results in growth retarded infants being less accurately placed within the distribution than larger infants.[18] This error increases as L increases and as S increases.[18]

Finally, the growth charts suffer from regression to the mean.[35] This is the tendency for values at the tails of the normal distribution to move toward the distribution mean when repeated, rather than to move to more extreme values.[35] The practical result of this is that an increase in Z-score of +1 is much more likely to occur in a subject whose initial Z-score is −3 than for one whose initial Z-score is −2 or −1.[35] This effect could be accounted for by using conditional growth charts,[35] but this would require a major change in how growth standards are interpreted in clinical practice.

SUMMARY AND CONCLUSIONS

The presentation of growth data on growth charts has not changed substantially for over 100 years. The current methods of displaying such data are difficult to interpret visually and make comparisons between the growth rate of an individual and the comparison population prone to visual misperceptions. Rather than present the data in such a *curve-difference* format, we suggest presenting the data as a Z-score growth chart, which allows improved interpretation of the data and is less prone to misperception.

Computer-generated plotting of Z-score data makes this process straightforward and allows for statistical analysis of the growth data to identify early signs of growth acceleration or deceleration.

REFERENCES

1. Budin P. *The Nursling: The Feeding and Hygiene of Premature and Full-Term Infants.* London, England: The Caxton Publishing Company; 1907.
2. Quetelet MA. *Anthropométrie au mesure des différentes facultés de l'homme.* Brussels, Belgium; 1870.
3. Bowditch HP. *Eighth Annual Report of the State Board of Health of Massachusetts.* Boston, Massachusetts; 1875.
4. Dancis J, O'Connell JR, Holt LE, Jr. A grid for recording the weight of premature infants. *J Pediatr* 1948;33:570–2.
5. Lubchenco LO, Hansman C, Dressler M, Boyd E. Intrauterine growth as estimated from liveborn birth-weight data at 24 to 42 weeks of gestation. *Pediatrics* 1963;32:793–800.
6. Lubchenco LO, Hansman C, Boyd E. Intrauterine growth in length and head circumference as estimated from live births at gestational ages from 26 to 42 weeks. *Pediatrics* 1966;37:403–8.
7. Babson SG. Growth of low-birth-weight infants. *J Pediatr* 1970;77:11–8.
8. Fenton TR. A new growth chart for preterm babies: Babson and Benda's chart updated with recent data and a new format. *BMC Pediatr* 2003;3:13.
9. Olsen IE, Groveman SA, Lawson ML, Clark RH, Zemel BS. New intrauterine growth curves based on United States data. *Pediatrics* 2010;125:e214–24.

10. Bertino E, Spada E, Occhi L, et al. Neonatal anthropometric charts: The Italian Neonatal Study compared with other European studies. *J Pediatr Gastroenterol Nutr* 2010;51:353–61.

11. Ehrenkranz RA, Younes N, Lemons JA, et al. Longitudinal growth of hospitalized very low birth weight infants. *Pediatrics* 1999;104:280–9.

12. Cleveland WS, McGill R. Graphical perception: Theory, experimentation and application to the development of graphical methods. *J Am Stat Assoc* 1984;79:531–4.

13. Cleveland WS, McGill R. Graphical perception and graphical methods for analyzing scientific data. *Science* 1985;229:828–33.

14. Bouma H, Anderson JJ. Perceived orientation of isolated line segments. *Vision Res* 1968;8:493–507.

15. Bouma H, Anderson JJ. Induced changes in the perceived orientation of line segments. *Vision Res* 1970;10:333–49.

16. Keene GC. The effect of response codes on the accuracy of making absolute judgments of lineal inclinations. *J Gen Psychol* 1963;69:37–50.

17. Argyle J. Approaches to detecting growth faltering in infancy and childhood. *Ann Hum Biol* 2003;30:499–519.

18. Cole TJ. The LMS method for constructing normalized growth standards. *Eur J Clin Nutr* 1990;44:45–60.

19. Healy MJ, Rasbash J, Yang M. Distribution-free estimation of age-related centiles. *Ann Hum Biol* 1988;15:17–22.

20. Pan HQ, Goldstein H, Yang Q. Non-parametric estimation of age-related centiles over wide age ranges. *Ann Hum Biol* 1990;17:475–81.

21. Bertino E, Giuliani F, Occhi L, et al. Benchmarking neonatal anthropometric charts published in the last decade. *Arch Dis Child Fetal Neo Ed* 2009;94:F233.

22. Fenton TR, Sauve RS. Using the LMS method to calculate z-scores for the Fenton preterm infant growth chart. *Eur J Clin Nutr* 2007;61:1380–5.

23. *WHO Child Growth Standards: Length/Height-for-Age, Weight-for-Age, Weight-for-Length, Weight-for-Height and Body Mass Index-for Age.* Methods and Development. Geneva, Switzerland: World Health Organization; 2006.

24. Kuczmarski RJ, Ogden CL, Guo SS, et al. 2000 CDC Growth charts for the United States: methods and development. Vital and health statistics Series 11, data from the national health survey 2002:1–190.

25. Royston P, Altman DG. Regression using fractional polynomials of continuous covariates: Parsimonious parametric modelling. *Appl Stat* 1994;43:429–67.

26. Griffin IJ, Cole TJ, Duncan KA, Hollman AS, Donaldson MD. Pelvic ultrasound measurements in normal girls. *Acta Paediatr* 1995;84:536–43.

27. Benneyan JC, Lloyd RC, Plsek PE. Statistical process control as a tool for research and healthcare improvement. *Quality and Safety in Health Care* 2003;12:458–64.

28. Borghi E, de Onis M, Garza C, et al. Construction of the World Health Organization child growth standards: selection of methods for attained growth curves. *Stat Med* 2006;25:247–65.

29. Griffin IJ, Pang NM, Perring J, Cooke RJ. Knee-heel length measurement in healthy preterm infants. *Archives of Disease in Childhood Fetal and Neonatal Edition* 1999;81:F50–5.

30. Lawn CJ, Chavasse RJ, Booth KA, Angeles M, Weir FJ. The neorule: a new instrument to measure linear growth in preterm infants. *Arch Dis Child Fetal Neo Ed* 2004;89:F360–3.

31. Johnson TS, Engstrom JL, Warda JA, Kabat M, Peters B. Reliability of length measurements in full-term neonates. *J Obstret Gynecol Neo Nurs* 1998;27:270–6.

32. Gibson AT, Carney S, Cavazzoni E, Wales JK. Neonatal and post-natal growth. *Horm Res* 2000;53:42–9.

33. Rochow N, Raja P, Straube S, Voigt M. Misclassification of newborns due to systematic error in plotting birth weight percentile values. *Pediatrics* 2012;130:e347–51.
34. Cooney K, Pathak U, Watson A. Infant growth charts. *Arch Dis Child* 1994;71:159–60.
35. Cole TJ. Growth monitoring with the British 1990 growth reference. *Arch Dis Child* 1997;76:47–9.

Section III Conclusions

We have seen how our best estimates of the nutritional requirements are relatively imprecise (Chapter 8). This is partly unavoidable due to the heterogeneity of the patient population. Given the rapid changes in growth rate during the third trimester it should come as no surprise that the nutrient requirements change rapidly as well. For example, the protein requirements of preterm infants decrease as they grow and mature, but their energy requirements increase (Table III.1).[1] Rapid changes are also seen for the requirements for trace minerals such as zinc. Fractional zinc requirements (per kg body weight) fall for 500 mcg/kg/d at weight 1 kg to 20 mcg/kg/d at weight 10 kg (Table III.2).[2]

So one can ask: Do we require different formulas for different gestational ages? Or for different weight preterm infants? If so, does the newborn 28 weeks gestation infant have the same requirements as a 4-week-old infant born at 24 weeks gestation? Do we include the requirements for "catch-up" growth in the design of our nutritional supplements?

Ideally, we would be able to customize nutrient intakes for each individual preterm infant (Chapter 10) to account for the inter-individual differences in nutrient requirements. These differences can be very large. For example, in one study (Cooke and Griffin, unpublished observations) 11 preterm infants (BW 1.06 ± 0.22 kg, GA 28.9 ± 2.9 w) had two 72-h metabolic balances carried out 7 days apart, allowing us to separate out the variability in the data due to measurement error from that due to between-subject differences. The first balance was carried out at a postnatal age of 29 ± 14 days, and the second, 7 days later. The effects of nutrient intake, birth weight, gestational age at birth, gender, postnatal age at the time of the balance, weight and the time of the balance, and between-subject random effects on nutrient retention (%) were assessed using a mixed effect linear model. Models were carried out sequentially as the effect of intake, birth demographics (birth weight and gestational age), balance details (postnatal age and weight at the time of the balance), and subject were sequentially added. The subject's dietary intakes were very similar, so the effect of intake on retention was relatively small (adjusted $r^2 < 0.20$ for all minerals). Addition of birth details (birth weight and gestational age) to the model did little to improve the model, nor did current weight or postnatal age increase the amount of variability in retention explained by model (with the exception of iron). However, including "subject" significantly increased the amount of variance in nutrient retention explained, with the largest effects seen for fat, nitrogen, iron, and zinc, and less so for calcium or magnesium (Table III.3). Of all of these factors, therefore, between-subject factors were the major source of variation in retention, and neither weight nor age at birth or at the time of the balance accounted for this effect.

Although metabolomics holds the promise of allowing us to customize the amount of nutrients we provide to an individual infant based on his or her individual needs, or based on the response to those intakes (Chapter 2), no such metabolomic methods are available at present. Twice-weekly assessments of BUN have been used

TABLE III.1
Enteral Protein and Energy Requirements for Preterm Infants at Different Weights

Weight (kg)	Enteral Energy Requirement (kcal/kg/d)	Enteral Protein Requirement (g/kg/d)	Protein/Energy Ratio (g/100 kcal)
0.5–0.7	105	4.0	3.8
0.7–0.9	108	4.0	3.7
0.9–1.2	119	4.0	3.4
1.2–1.5	127	3.9	3.1
1.5–1.8	128	3.6	2.8

Note: Data from Reference 1.

TABLE III.2
Requirements for Absorbed Zinc at Difference Weights in Preterm Infants and during the First Year of Life

Weight (kg)	Zinc Requirement (mcg/kg/d)
1.0	500
1.5–2.0	400
2.5–3.5	200–300
6	80
8	50
10	25

Note: Data from Reference 2.

TABLE III.3
The Contribution of Nutrient Intake (mg/kg), Birth Weight (BW), Gestational Age at Birth (GA), Weight at Time of Study (Wt), Postnatal Age at Time of Study (PNA), and "Subject" to the Adjusted r^2 (Variability) in Fat, Nitrogen, Calcium (Ca), Magnesium (Mg), Iron (Fe), and Zinc (Zn) Retention (% of intake) in Preterm Infants

Modeled Variables	Fat	Nitrogen	Ca	Mg	Fe	Zn
Intake	0.11	<0.10	0.17	0.14	<0.10	0.14
Intake + Birth details (BW, GA)	0.11	0.24	0.26	0.17	<0.10	<0.10
Intake + Birth details (Wt, GA, gender) + Balance details (Wt, PNA) +	0.20	0.17	0.57	0.20	<0.10	0.25
Intake + Birth details (Wt, GA, gender) + Balance details (Wt, PNA) + Subject	0.59	0.62	0.71	0.30	0.57	0.63

to adjust protein intake and this approach has been shown to improve growth in preterm infants (Chapter 10). However, this method has been successful in large part by providing practitioners reassurance that it was safe to increase protein intakes nearer to those recommended for preterm infants. For example, in the study by Arslanoglu et al.,[3] the maximum protein intake was 3.4 g/kg/d (SD 0.5) in the group whose fortification was adjusted based on BUN. This is not significantly different from the estimated requirement of 3.6 g/kg/d[2] (p = 0.13) in preterm infants generally. The control group, which received standard levels of fortification, received significant less protein (2.8 g/kg/d, SD 0.2)[2] than the 3.6 g/kg/d currently recommended (p < 0.0001) and probably less than they required. The improved group of the adjustable fortification group could probably have been achieved simply by giving all subjects a protein intake nearer 3.6 g/kg/d.

Despite the limitations of our understanding of nutritional requirements in preterm infants and our inability to individualize nutrition intakes, it is clear that if we carefully assess the intakes we are delivering (Chapter 9) and the growth of our patients (Chapters 9 and 12), and aggressively manage our nutritional regimens to optimize nutrient delivery and growth, we can greatly improve nutrient intakes and short-term growth as well. Advances in near-point-of-care analysis (Chapter 11) and advances in nutritional products available for preterm infants should only help us to more closely approximate the nutrient intakes that our patients require.

Clearly, preventing *ex utero* growth restriction and normalizing long-term growth of preterm infants is a worthwhile goal, and one we should strive to reach. We have plenty of room to improve.

Our fears are traitors, and make us lose the good we oft might win, by fearing to attempt.

Lucio, *Measure for Measure*

REFERENCES

1. Thureen, P. J. (2007). The neonatologist's dilemma: catch-up growth or beneficial undernutrition in very low birth weight infants-what are optimal growth rates? *J Pediatr Gastroenterol Nutr* 45 Suppl 3: S152–154.
2. Klein, C. J. (2002). Nutrient requirements for preterm infant formulas. *J Nutr* 132(6 Suppl 1): 1395S–1577S.
3. Arslanoglu, S., G. E. Moro and E. E. Ziegler (2006). Adjustable fortification of human milk fed to preterm infants: does it make a difference? *J Perinatol* 26(10): 614–621.

Index

β-Sympathomimetics effect on energy
    expenditure, 47
1-Hematocrit in calculation of serum protein
    mass, 23

A

Abdominal distention and sepsis, 49
Absorption and retention of nutrients, 236–239
Accumulation of feeding deficits, 51–54
Accuracy of assessment measurements, 28–29
ACE, *see* Angiotensin-converting enzyme (ACE)
Acoustic spectroscopy of breast milk, 273
Acronyms list (partial), 41, 185
Adequate intake (AI), definition, 229
Adipokine levels, 136
Adiponectin
    levels, 136
    polymorphism and LGA infants, 124
Adiposity
    into adulthood, 161
    catch-up growth and, 43
    catch-up growth timing and, 89
    confounding factors in evaluation, 159–160
    distribution of, 156–157
    fat distribution through childhood, 161–162
    fetal malnutrition as cause, 153
    growth rate effects, 165–167
    intervention effects, 168–169
    in preterm infants, 176–177
    as proxy measurement for metabolic
        syndrome prediction, 156–157
    trajectory of accumulation around time of
        birth, 160–161
Adiposity rebound, 132
Adjustable fortification (AF) of breast milk, 274
Adolescent mothers recommended weight gains,
    123
Adreno-receptors down-regulation, 155
Adult disease risk affected by conditions *in utero*,
    65
Adult-onset diseases association with early
    growth rate, 11
AF, *see* Adjustable fortification (AF) of breast
    milk
African-Americans
    adult metabolic risk and weight gain timing,
        165
    carry lower risk of LGA births, 124
    mothers' recommended weight gains, 123

AGA, *see* Appropriate for gestational age (AGA)
    infants
"Aggressive nutrition", 49–50
Agouti mice, 98–99
AI, *see* Adequate intake (AI)
Air-displacement plethysmography for fat mass
    estimation, 31
Albumin in serum; *see also* Transthyretin
    (pre-albumin)
    monitoring of, 23–24
    and protein intake, 24
ALSPAC, *see* Avon longitudinal study of parents
    and children (ALSPAC)
American Academy of Pediatrics endorsement of
    Denver charts, 5
American infants' measurements, 6
Amino acid form and lipogenesis, 154
Angiotensin-converting enzyme (ACE)
    heritability factors, 102
    I/D polymorphism effects, 106–107
    I/D polymorphisms, 102
Anorexia and sepsis, 49
Anthropometry considered in growth evaluation,
    54
Appropriate for gestational age (AGA) infants
    body size and neurodevelopmental outcomes,
        191–198
    catch-up growth and blood pressure, 129
    comparison with SGS infants, 84–86
    effects of faster and slower growth, 63
    effects of size at birth, 66
    EUGR in, 46–47
    growth and neurodevelopment in term
        infants, 204–209
    growth rate and adiposity, 164
    and insulin resistance, 128–129
    postnatal growth and neurodevelopment,
        198–200
    risk factors associated, 67–68
Asphyxiated babies urinary metabonomics, 33
Assessments as predictors of ultimate
    development, 28–29
Audit of clinical care function, 22
Australian infants' measurements, 6
Auxological factors in nutritional assessment, 20
Avon longitudinal study of parents and children
    (ALSPAC), 73, 78–82
    catch-up growth and central fat, 128
Axin fused mice, 99

313